Cultural Issues in Pediatric Mental Health

Guest Editors

SHASHANK V. JOSHI, MD
ANDRES J. PUMARIEGA, MD

CHILD AND ADOLESCENT PSYCHIATRIC CLINICS OF NORTH AMERICA

www.childpsych.theclinics.com

Consulting Editor
HARSH K. TRIVEDI, MD

October 2010 • Volume 19 • Number 4

SAUNDERS an imprint of ELSEVIER, Inc.

W.B. SAUNDERS COMPANY

A Division of Elsevier Inc.

Elsevier Inc. • 1600 John F. Kennedy Boulevard • Suite 1800 • Philadelphia, Pennsylvania 19103-2899

http://www.childpsych.theclinics.com

CHILD AND ADOLESCENT PSYCHIATRIC CLINICS OF NORTH AMERICA Volume 19, Number 4
October 2010 ISSN 1056–4993, ISBN-13: 978-1-4377-2433-2

Editor: Sarah E. Barth
Developmental Editor: Jessica Demetriou

Child and Adolescent Psychiatric Clinics of North America (ISSN 1056-4993) is published quarterly by Elsevier Inc., 360 Park Avenue South, New York, NY 10010-1710. Months of issue are January, April, July, and October. Business and Editorial Offices: 1600 John F. Kennedy Boulevard, Suite 1800, Philadelphia, PA 19103-2899. Periodicals postage paid at New York, NY and additional mailing offices. Subscription prices are $275.00 per year (US individuals), $425.00 per year (US institutions), $139.00 per year (US students), $318.00 per year (Canadian individuals), $513.00 per year (Canadian institutions), $176.00 per year (Canadian students), $378.00 per year (international individuals), $513.00 per year (international institutions), and $176.00 per year (international students). International air speed delivery is included in all Clinics subscription prices. All prices are subject to change without notice. **POSTMASTER:** Send address changes to Child and Adolescent Psychiatric Clinics of North America, Elsevier Health Sciences Division, Subscription Customer Service, 3251 Riverport Lane, Maryland Heights, MO 63043. **Customer Service: 1-800-654-2452 (U.S. and Canada); 314-447-8871 (outside U.S. and Canada). Fax: 314-447-8029. E-mail: JournalsCustomerService-usa@ elsevier.com (for print support) or journalsonlinesupport-usa@elsevier.com (for online support).**

Reprints. For copies of 100 or more articles in this publication, please contact the Commercial Reprints Department, Elsevier Inc., 360 Park Avenue South, New York, New York 10010-1710 Tel.: (212) 633-3812; Fax: (212) 462-1935, E-mail: reprints@elsevier.com.

Child and Adolescent Psychiatric Clinics of North America is covered in *MEDLINE/PubMed (Index Medicus), ISI, SSCI, Research Alert, Social Search, Current Contents,* and *EMBASE/Excerpta Medica.*

Printed in the United States of America.

Contributors

CONSULTING EDITOR

HARSH K. TRIVEDI, MD
Associate Professor of Psychiatry, Vanderbilt University School of Medicine;
and Executive Medical Director, and Chief-of-Staff, Vanderbilt Psychiatric Hospital,
Nashville, Tennessee

CONSULTING EDITOR EMERITUS

ANDRÉS MARTIN, MD, MPH

FOUNDING CONSULTING EDITOR

MELVIN LEWIS, MBBS, FRCPSYCH, DCH

GUEST EDITORS

SHASHANK V. JOSHI, MD
Assistant Professor of Psychiatry, Pediatrics, and Education, Director of Training in Child
and Adolescent Psychiatry, Lucile Packard Children's Hospital and Stanford University
School of Medicine, Stanford, California

ANDRES J. PUMARIEGA, MD
Professor of Psychiatry and Behavioral Sciences, Temple University School of Medicine,
Philadelphia; Chief, Section of Child and Adolescent Psychiatry, The Reading Hospital and
Medical Center, Reading, Pennsylvania

AUTHORS

CHERYL S. AL-MATEEN, MD, FAACAP, DFAPA
Associate Professor of Psychiatry and Pediatrics, Virginia Commonwealth University
School of Medicine, Richmond, Virginia

MARGARITA ALEGRIA, PhD
Professor of Psychology, Department of Psychiatry, Harvard Medical School, Boston;
Director, Center for Multicultural Mental Health Research, Cambridge Health Alliance,
Somerville, Massachusetts

RAPHAEL BERNIER, PhD
Associate Professor of Psychiatry and Behavioral Sciences, University of Washington,
Seattle, Washington

L. LEE CARLISLE, MD
Assistant Professor, Department of Psychiatry and Behavioral Sciences, University of Washington, Seattle, Washington

GABRIELLE CERDA, MD
Clinical Professor, Department of Psychiatry, University of California, San Diego, San Diego, California

BRIAN A. COLLINS, PhD
Assistant Professor, Hunter College, New York, New York

NISHA DOGRA, BM, DCH, MA, PhD, FRCPsych
Senior Lecturer in Child and Adolescent Psychiatry; Honorary Consultant, Greenwood Institute of Child Health, University of Leicester, Leicester, United Kingdom

APRIL E. FALLON, PhD
Professor, School of Psychology; Fielding Graduate University, Santa Barbara, California; Associate Professor, Department of Psychiatry, Drexel University College of Medicine, Philadelphia, Pennsylvania

R. RAO GOGINENI, MD
Associate Professor, Department of Psychiatry, Robert Wood Johnson Medical School, UMDNJ, Piscataway; Head, Division of Child and Adolescent Psychiatry, Cooper University Hospital, Camden, New Jersey

TOI BLAKLEY HARRIS, MD
Assistant Professor, Menninger Department of Psychiatry and Behavioral Sciences, Baylor College of Medicine, Houston, Texas

SHASHANK V. JOSHI, MD
Assistant Professor of Psychiatry, Pediatrics, and Education; Director of Training in Child and Adolescent Psychiatry, Lucile Packard Children's Hospital and Stanford University of School of Medicine, Stanford, California

NIRANJAN S. KARNIK, MD, PhD
Assistant Professor of Psychiatry and Behavioral Neuroscience, Department of Psychiatry, The University of Chicago, Pritzker School of Medicine, Chicago, Illinois

SHERYL KATAOKA, MD, MSHS
Associate Professor in Residence, University of California Los Angeles-Jane and Terry Semel Institute for Neuroscience and Human Behavior and David Geffen School of Medicine, Department of Psychiatry and Biobehavioral Sciences, Los Angeles, California

JAMES LAKE, MD
Adjunct Clinical Assistant Professor, Department of Psychiatry and Behavioral Sciences, Stanford University, Stanford, California; Visiting Clinical Assistant Professor, Department of Medicine, Arizona Center for Integrative Medicine, University of Arizona College of Medicine, Tucson, Arizona

WILLIAM B. LAWSON, MD, PhD
Professor and Chair, Department of Psychiatry and Behavioral Sciences, Howard University, Washington, District of Columbia

FRANCIS G. LU, MD
Director of Cultural Psychiatry and Associate Director, General Psychiatry Residency Training Program, Luke & Grace Kim Endowed Professor in Cultural Psychiatry, Department of Psychiatry and Behavioral Sciences, University of California-Davis, Sacramento, California

MANSOOR MALIK, MD
Assistant Professor, Department of Psychiatry and Behavioral Sciences, Howard University, Washington, District of Columbia

ALICE MAO, MD
Associate Medical Director, Depelchin Children's Center; Associate Professor of Psychiatry, Baylor College of Medicine, Houston, Texas

AYESHA I. MIAN, MD
Assistant Professor, Menninger Department of Psychiatry and Behavior Sciences, Baylor College of Medicine, Houston, Texas

DOUGLAS K. NOVINS, MD
Professor of Psychiatry, Centers for American Indian and Alaska Native Health Research and Departments of Psychiatry, and Community and Behavioral Health, University of Colorado Anschutz Medical Campus, Aurora, Colorado

ANNELLE B. PRIMM, MD, MPH
Associate Professor, Department of Psychiatry, Johns Hopkins School of Medicine, Baltimore, Maryland; Deputy Medical Director and Director, Minority and National Affairs, American Psychiatric Association, Arlington, Virginia

ANDRES J. PUMARIEGA, MD
Professor of Psychiatry and Behavioral Sciences, Temple University School of Medicine, Philadelphia; Chief, Section of Child and Adolescent Psychiatry, The Reading Hospital and Medical Center, Reading, Pennsylvania

NYAPATI R. RAO, MD, MS
Professor of Clinical Psychiatry, SUNY Downstate Medical Center, Brooklyn, New York; Chairman, Department of Psychiatry and Behavioral Sciences, Nassau University Medical Center, East Meadow, New York

EUGENIO M. ROTHE, MD
Professor of Psychiatry and Public Health, Herbert Wertheim College of Medicine, Florida International University, Miami, Florida

JOHN SARGENT, MD
Professor of Psychiatry, Tufts Medical Center, Boston, Massachusetts

CATHERINE DECARLO SANTIAGO, PhD
Postdoctoral Fellow, University of California Los Angeles-Jane and Terry Semel Institute for Neuroscience and Human Behavior and David Geffen School of Medicine, Department of Psychiatry and Biobehavioral Sciences, Los Angeles, California

SUZAN SONG, MD
Medical Director, Asian Americans for Community Involvement, San Jose, California

CLAUDIO O. TOPPELBERG, MD
Project Director, Child Language and Developmental Psychiatry Research Lab;
Research Scientist; Director of Psychiatry, Manville School, Judge Baker Children's
Center; Assistant in Psychiatry, Children's Hospital Boston; Assistant Professor
of Psychiatry, Harvard Medical School, Boston, Massachusetts

DAN TZUANG, MD
Child, Adolescent, and Adult Staff Psychiatrist, Student Health Center at UC-Irving,
Irvine, California

MELISSA VALLAS, MD
Fellow in Child and Adolescent Psychiatry, Lucile Packard Children's Hospital
at Stanford, Stanford, California

JENNIFER YEN, MD
Depelchin Children's Center, Baylor College of Medicine, Houston, Texas

Contents

> Although culture has long been recognized as having a significant impact on human development and its variations, many child and adolescent psychiatrists and mental health clinicians assume a universal nonvariance to normal development, with the risk of identifying variations as pathologic. This article reviews the conceptual basis for the role of culture in human development, particularly psychosocial and cognitive development, presents evidence and support from field observations of children in diverse cultures, and discusses the emerging evidence from the field of cultural neuroscience. Implications for these different perspectives on future research, childhood education, and even intercultural relations are presented.

> The rapidly changing demographic landscape of the United States, brought about by immigration, has resulted in an increasingly multiracial and multicultural population. These changes have become accentuated by the phenomenon of globalization, which occurs when there is an acceleration of movement of people, ideas, and products between nations, which also brings about an increase in the complexity of everyday problems. This article discusses the concept of identity formation and how the stresses of immigration and acculturation and the factors of resiliency and risk affect immigrant children, adolescents, and their families, so that clinicians treating these populations can be prepared to understand divergent, and often well-hidden, world views, which may cause intrafamilial conflicts and interfere with the child's developmental process.

> In this article the authors discuss first why it is crucial, from a clinical and public health perspective, to better understand the development as well as risk and protection processes for the mental health of immigrant children. The authors then shift focus to the main tenet of this article, namely, that

specific aspects of the dual language development of immigrant children are highly relevant to their mental health and adaptation. This argument is illustrated with empirical studies on Latino immigrant children, as they represent the majority of immigrant children in America and as a way of exemplifying the risks and circumstances that are potentially shared by other immigrant groups. Finally, the authors conceptually differentiate dual language development and its mental health impact from the dual-culture (bicultural) development and circumstance of immigrant children and their mental health impact.

This article briefly reviews the history of the inclusion of culture within child and adolescent psychiatry. This history is a reflection of broader trends within medical education and psychiatry, more generally. The authors then present an approach for incorporating culture within the clinical setting termed the cultural sensibility model. In addition to outlining the model and its philosophical basis, they present brief case examples and a sample curriculum in support of this model.

Child and adolescent psychiatrists are already serving an increasing population of culturally and ethnically diverse patients and families in their practices and in different agency settings. This article discusses adaptations to practice that enable child and adolescent psychiatrists to address the diverse clinical and cultural needs of this emerging population. Special attention is given to work in psychotherapy and in agency settings where diverse children and youth are found in large numbers.

Disparities remain in mental health status and care for racial and ethnic minority youth, despite national attention to disparity reduction. This article offers a comprehensive picture of the status of pediatric disparities, by addressing the major areas affecting minority youth mental health, including: prevention of problems, need for services, access to care, mental health treatment types, and treatment outcomes. The authors address relevant factors in the family, community and socioeconomic context, and describe various local and national programs that aim to tackle the obstacles and fill the gaps in high-quality care for racial/ethnic minority youth. The article concludes by offering recommendations for improvement that acknowledge the importance of understanding preferences and attitudes toward treatment, ensuring that screening and diagnosis is appropriate to minority youth, and ensuring that evidence-based programs are available at multiple levels to best service children and succeed in addressing their needs.

Ethnic minority children continue to have substantial unmet mental health needs, and evidence-based treatments (EBTs) have proved challenging to disseminate widely among ethnic minority communities. Indeed, policy makers have made an important distinction between EBTs, interventions that have proven efficacy in clinical trials, and evidence-based practice, which involves "the integration of the best available research with clinical expertise in the context of patient characteristics, culture, and preferences." The present research evidence suggests that several interventions have been found to be effective in ethnic minority populations without a need for major adaptations of the original interventions. However, this article highlights the need to deliver evidence-based practice, which is defined as the implementation of EBTs delivered with fidelity and with the integration of important cultural systems and community factors.

There are important ethnic variations in metabolism, response, and tolerability of psychotropic medications. There has been a dramatic expansion of use of psychotropic medications in children in recent years. This article reviews the literature on the role of race and ethnicity in psychopharmacology as it relates to children and adolescents, examines what is known thus far about complementary and alternative medicine approaches in pediatric psychopharmacology, and presents a method to engage patients and families of varying educational and cultural backgrounds in pharmacotherapeutic treatment.

Diversity and Our Practitioners

The changing face of the United States urges the field of child and adolescent psychiatry toward more culturally sensitive care. This article gives a comprehensive review of the history of cultural education, empirical findings that speak to its need, and the challenges that may be faced in the conception and implementation of a cultural competency curriculum. The American Academy of Child and Adolescent Pscyhiatry's model curriculum is presented to help child and adolescent residency programs design one that is specific to their resources and needs.

This article reviews, consolidates, and enhances current knowledge about the issues and problems child and adolescent psychiatry international medical graduates face. Their training, work force issues, and establishment and advancement of professional identity are presented. Acculturation and immigration dynamics include facing prejudice and discrimination, social mirroring, and difficulties with language. Treatment issues are discussed with a special focus on therapeutic alliance, resistance, transference, countertransference, and child rearing practices. Recommendations for training and future goals are considered.

Special Challenges for Diverse Children and Families

Autism spectrum disorders (ASDs) are now considered to be the most common of the developmental disorders, although the effect of cultural influences on the diagnosis and treatment of ASDs has received limited attention. The existing literature on this topic suggests that both macrolevel and microlevel cultural factors can affect the characterization, diagnosis, and treatment of ASDs. As a result, it is important for clinicians to consider cultural factors throughout the diagnostic, treatment planning, and intervention implementation processes. In this article, cultural influences on the prevalence of autism and the diagnostic and treatment processes are reviewed and synthesized through a consideration of the developmental context and through clinical practice suggestions.

It has been estimated that as many as two-thirds of American youth experience a potentially life-threatening event before 18 years of age and that half have experienced multiple potentially traumatic events. Race, ethnicity, and culture influence the frequency and nature of these traumas and also the ways in which children react to traumatic events. The authors discuss the varied influences of cultural background on these reactions to trauma, the varying presentations of diverse children experiencing troubling reactions, and the need to provide treatment to children and their families in a fashion that is culturally sensitive and acceptable to diverse families.

FORTHCOMING ISSUES

RECENT ISSUES

THE CLINICS ARE NOW AVAILABLE ONLINE!

Access your subscription at:
www.theclinics.com

Foreword
So, What's in a Name?

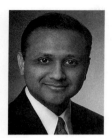

Harsh K. Trivedi, MD
Consulting Editor

At a recent faculty recruitment dinner, one of our pregnant faculty members was asked a simple question. Have you thought of a name for your baby? The answer we received, while direct and logical, led to a thought-provoking and insightful conversation about race, culture, gender roles, family ancestry, and self-identity. We heard about families of origin, countries of origin, the meaning of family names, and even the changing of those names upon entry to the United States. What was remarkable was the significant effort placed by these soon-to-be parents in making meaning of their rich and diverse multicultural backgrounds. The purpose of this exercise was to reach a new understanding such that each of their stories could be synthesized to create the new parchment unto which their child's experience of culture could be written.

In creating this issue of *Child and Adolescent Psychiatric Clinics of North America*, I thank our guest editors for embarking down a similar process in creating a new parchment for telling this story. Their purposeful inclusion of what unites the experiences of many cultures is both fresh and quite welcome. Having grown up in New York City, the arguable melting pot of the world, I am all too aware that the human experience is a common one despite which country we come from or language we speak. Though the lens may be different and the particular experiences may vary, there is a commonality that can be discovered by exploring each of these stories. Of note, rest assured that this exercise is not one that belittles or devalues any particular experience.

I thank Shashank Joshi and Andres Pumariega for guest editing this issue. They have indeed provided a meaningful 'context' from which to understand this topic as well as to incorporate a culturally informed perspective to clinical care. I am also

Child Adolesc Psychiatric Clin N Am 19 (2010) xiii–xiv
doi:10.1016/j.chc.2010.09.005   **childpsych.theclinics.com**

grateful to each of our contributors for sharing their knowledge and expertise. May our better understanding of culture allow us to better meet the needs of our patients, their families, and our communities.

Harsh K. Trivedi, MD
Vanderbilt Psychiatric Hospital
1601 23rd Avenue South, Suite 1157
Nashville, TN 37212, USA

E-mail address:
harsh.k.trivedi@vanderbilt.edu

Preface
America's New Kids

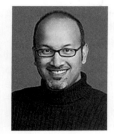 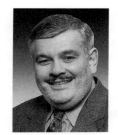

Shashank V. Joshi, MD   Andres J. Pumariega, MD
Guest Editors

As *Child and Adolescent Psychiatric Clinics* begins its 20th year, it seems appropriate that this edition be focused on making us more attuned to the changing needs of our increasingly diverse children, youth, and families. Borrowing a phrase from our colleague, Claudio Toppelberg, we refer to this new population of children (who by 2030 will be the majority in our nation) as "America's new kids." In the pages that follow, the authors use an array of related terms with *culture* or *cultural* as the first word. As readers of this edition are likely aware, the evolving demographics of the United States have necessitated that clinicians be, at the very least, more culturally informed—and at the very best, culturally curious, skilled, and competent. Yet, the published literature on evidence-based practice regarding cultural issues in pediatric mental health has struggled to keep pace with the multiethnic and multicultural growth of the past 30–40 years.

In compiling the list of articles and authors, we are struck by the cultural and academic diversity within our group of writers. Among the editors, one of us (SVJ) is reminded of how, during a clinical clerkship in medical school, I would get regular comments about "what a nice guy I was," and how patients and families "really felt I listened to their concerns." Yet, although that was a necessary condition for being a successful student or intern, it was not sufficient. For although *I* thought that I was providing the very best care, families didn't always agree. As, for example, when the patient's mother thought that I could have been more deferential to the elder visiting (despite his history of being physically and emotionally abusive to family members). A simple therapeutic engagement strategy such as subtly (but definitely) acknowledging this patriarchal figure first when I entered the patient's room may have been enough to get his buy-in, thus allowing the family to wholeheartedly embrace outpatient psychotherapy for this teenager with chronic reactive airways disease and a depressive disorder. So, my chief resident would remind me (in her thick Brooklyn accent), "It's not enough to be *nice*, SVJ. You gotta be *good*." The lesson I took away was this—I could be the most culturally aware student, or practice with a cultural curiosity that honors the patient's or family's narrative of whatever is afflicting their

Child Adolesc Psychiatric Clin N Am 19 (2010) xv–xvii
doi:10.1016/j.chc.2010.08.001

child. But ultimately, it is most important to be *culturally effective*. In this edition of the *Clinics,* we hope the reader, too, will be effectively drawn in by the unique perspectives and styles of the authors, as much as with the subject matter itself.

We have avoided organizing the articles in ethnically focused sections. This approach has its place in the medical anthropologic literature when highlighting issues which may be unique in a given ethnic/racial population. For this edition, however, we believe there is greater value in emphasizing more generalizable principles, knowledge, and skills for cultural effectiveness. Although some cultural groups may be highlighted more than others, they are meant to serve as examples of how to conduct culturally sensible practice, rather than to be focused on as a disadvantaged group per se. We and others[1,2] are striving to change the "misguided perspective that the close relationship between culture and illness occurs strictly in the lives of ethnocultural minorities (only)". Rather, we believe this relationship and these connections are human ones, and occur in persons of all races and ethnicities.

The first section of this edition focuses on development across cultures, and there are numerous new research findings highlighted from the fields of cultural neuroscience and cultural anthropology. A highly practical article on acculturation and child development follows by Eugenio Rothe, Dan Tzuang, and Andres Pumariega. Drs Toppleberg and Collins then frame the discussion on an understudied but crucial piece of development across cultures, that of language development.

Next, you'll read about conceptual approaches to achieving cultural nirvana: from being culturally aware (perhaps where we all need to start), to developing cultural attunement, to a more process-oriented approach that is eloquently described by Drs Karnik and Dogra. To conclude this section, Drs Pumariega, Rothe, Song, and Lu review the literature and present the key ingredients of culturally informed practice.

The section that follows focuses on evidence-based practice (EBP) as it relates to disparities in care and also examines interventions that are either known to work or need to be highlighted. Optimistically speaking, Drs Kataoka, Novins, and Santiago remind us that despite the relatively few treatment studies in child and adolescent psychiatry that have an ethnic minority focus, most EBPs can be adapted for work within minority communities by culturally attuned clinicians (the "tuned in" practitioner skillfully finds just the right frequency, a sort of metaphorical radio dial, to make the cultural connection). In their article on disparities, Drs Alegria, Vallas, and Pumariega emphasize the need for vigilance in our efforts to reach those in greatest need, offering some hypotheses about how disparities are developed and perpetuated, and proposing approaches to achieve equitable outcomes in underserved racial and ethnic populations. Drs Malik, Lake, Lawson, and Joshi focus on the intersection between diversity and biology in treatment. They highlight that a *good enough alliance* may bring even the most reluctant family back for the follow-up visit, so that all pharmacotherapeutic options, from allopathic to CAM treatments, can be fully explored. This must be done while staying aware of ethnic variations in pharmacokinetics that underlie the philosophy of 'starting (super) low and going (super) slow' for certain patients.

The next section reflects an increasingly important statistic, which is that we could have renamed this preface, *America's New Docs*. Currently, at least 50% of all psychiatric residents in the U.S. are either women or ethnic minorities.[3] In the next couple of articles, first Ayesha Mian, Cheryl Al-Mateen, and Gabrielle Cerda teach us more about the crucial role of training programs in raising the next generation of culturally effective child and adolescent psychiatrists. Then Drs Gogineni, Fallon and Rao highlight how international medical graduates (IMGs) have been and will continue to be important contributors in our field, while at the same time requiring support for the challenges they face in cultural adaptation, often in parallel with those of their patients.

Finally, some of the diverse patients and families we take care of will face unique challenges, especially those with developmental disabilities and those whom have suffered trauma or loss. In the last two articles of the edition, Drs Bernier and Mao, and then Drs Harris, Carlisle, Sargent, and Primm write about how cultural attunement and sensitivity become especially important in providing effective care to the most vulnerable among us.

Editing this issue has been an illuminating and rewarding experience. Yet, we readily admit to the challenging and sometimes stressful nature of this endeavor, as we are fully aware of the responsibility for framing and sharing this rarely collected knowledge and these perspectives with the rest of the field. Our hope is that this issue will be useful for practitioners serving America's new kids and for future scholars in inspiring and continuing the advancement of this work. We thank our dedicated, industrious authors for meeting tight deadlines and responding to our translation of this responsibility. We also wish to honor three pioneers who came before us and championed the culturally effective perspective in child and adolescent psychiatry: Jeanne Spurlock, John McDermott, and Harry Wright. Without their advocacy and scholarly inspiration, much of this work would either not have occurred or not seen the light of day. Above all, we honor the courage and perseverance of diverse children, youth, and families as they adapt to their environments and shape the future of our nation.

Shashank V. Joshi, MD
Division of Child and Adolescent Psychiatry
Lucile Packard Children's Hospital at Stanford
401 Quarry Road, MC 5719
Stanford, CA 94305, USA

Andres J. Pumariega, MD
Temple University School of Medicine
Philadelphia, PA 19106, USA
Section of Child & Adolescent Psychiatry
The Reading Hospital and Medical Center
Reading, PA 19611, USA

E-mail addresses:
svjoshi@stanford.edu (S.V. Joshi)
pumarieg@verizon.net (A.J. Pumariega)

REFERENCES

1. Choi H. Understanding adolescent depression in ethnocultural context. ANS Adv Nurs Sci 2002;25(2):71–85.
2. Al-Mateen C, Mian A, Cerda G, et al. American Academy of Child & Adolescent Psychiatry (AACAP) Model Curriculum in Cultural Competence, 2011, in press.
3. APA Resident Census 2008–2009. Washington, DC: American Psychiatric Association; 2009.

Culture and Development in Children and Youth

Andres J. Pumariega, MD[a,b,*], Shashank V. Joshi, MD[c]

KEYWORDS

- Culture • Development • Neuroscience • Cultural psychiatry
- Cultural neuroscience

At the time of this writing, the United States is undergoing unprecedented growth in its racial, ethnic, and cultural diversity.[1] And over the past 10 years, it has become a reality that most parents in the United States are living in cultural milieus other than those in which they were raised.[2,3] Thus, child and adolescent psychiatrists must approach all of their work under the presumption of multiculturalism, particularly if a broad definition of culture is chosen that is not limited to ethnic or racial makeup, but rather (as McDermott wrote in 1996) one that embraces the variable values, attitudes, beliefs, and behaviors shared by a people, and that is transmitted between generations. Multiculturalism is based on the assumption that no single "best" way exists to conceptualize human behavior or explain the realities and experiences of diverse cultural groups.[2] Rather, it is more useful, particularly for clinicians, to assume that everyone has a unique culture, and that cultural influences are woven into personality like a tapestry.[4]

From this perspective, three of the major tasks for clinicians include (1) developing a broad knowledge base about cross-cultural variations in child development and childrearing; (2) integrating this knowledge in a developmentally relevant way to make more informed clinical assessments and case formulations; and (3) developing a culturally sensitive attitude and therapeutic stance in all interactions with patients and families, including those of the same background as the clinician.[5] Thus, standard assumptions about developmental trajectories may need to be reexamined when considering culture—both across and within cultures. Many contextual factors (including socioeconomic milieu, unique family history and narrative, whether from a rural or urban setting, or temperamental variations) may contribute to the expression

[a] Department of Psychiatry and Behavioral Sciences, Temple University, Temple Episcopal Campus, 100 East Lehigh Avenue, Philadelphia, PA 19125, USA
[b] The Reading Hospital and Medical Center, 6th Avenue and Spruce Street, K Building, West Reading, PA 19612, USA
[c] Lucile Packard Children's Hospital at Stanford, 401 Quarry Road MC 5719, Stanford, CA 94305, USA
* Corresponding author. The Reading Hospital and Medical Center, 6th Avenue and Spruce Street, K Building, West Reading, PA 19612.
E-mail address: pumariegaa@readinghospital.org

Child Adolesc Psychiatric Clin N Am 19 (2010) 661–680
doi:10.1016/j.chc.2010.08.002
1056-4993/10/$ – see front matter © 2010 Elsevier Inc. All rights reserved.

childpsych.theclinics.com

of culture within a child or teen's emerging personality. When in the therapeutic engagement process, the culturally attuned clinician may benefit from adopting an ethnographic perspective. As Storck and Stoep[6] described in a seminal paper from an earlier volume of the *Child and Adolescent Psychiatry Clinics*, the ethnographic approach in psychiatry has evolved from its anthropologic roots into a process of inquiry wherein the clinician adopts a sort of participant–observer status in the patient or family's life. This perspective is enhanced by learning the language, meanings, and community affiliations of children and their families.

With eyes and ears open, psychiatrists may engage in ethnographic fieldwork while attending family meetings, consulting at the bedside in an intensive care unit, or walking the high-school halls to consult with a treatment team. Families often must engage in the same type of ethnographic work to understand their children and to understand hospitals and clinics. As ethnographers, clinicians and parents are wondering, "What is it like for my patient/child to navigate this setting?"[6(p138)]

HISTORICAL AND CONCEPTUAL BACKGROUND

Today there is wide recognition that cultural values and beliefs are transmitted primarily by the family to the developing child, and later reinforced by other social institutions (eg, school, church, other religious or community institutions). Historically, however, many developmental theories tended to emphasize the commonality and invariance of child development across societies and cultures. Freud[7] hypothesized stages of psychological development that were marked by invariability in its timing and sign-posts (such as feeding, toilet training, expression of sexual and competitive urges, and achievement of intimacy), which primarily expressed themselves within dyadic and nuclear family relationships and determined the individual's psychological outcome, and which he believed were fairly constant in their expression across different cultural settings. He also characterized emotions as primarily irrational and, along with other mental functions, invariant across cultures, with cultures primarily providing symbolic means to assist the individual in recognizing and attenuating their impact. James[8] posited the individual having a unique sense of self that was present from birth and evolved in its scope of consciousness as the individual developed psychologically and cognitively. He viewed emotions as more rational and manageable in the normal individual, and as important motivators for social change. However, he viewed certain cultural beliefs and expressions, such as religion, as symbolic of the conflicts between individually determined drives and their prohibitions.

Among others, five important developmental theorists who have placed individual development within the context of cultural and social influence include Vygotsky, Erikson, Montessori, Bandura, and Mead. The essence of L.S. Vygotsky's work was based on the assertion that all human mental functioning is socioculturally, historically, and institutionally based, and that various individual mental phenomena have their origins in social activity. He viewed development as a process of transformation of individual functioning, while various forms of social practice became internalized.

Four domains of development were important to Vygotsky's view of development: phylogenesis, sociocultural history, ontogenesis, and microgenesis. Phylogenetically, he viewed the use of tools provided by a culture and the social organization involved in labor as the qualitative changes that advanced humans beyond the developmental capacities of primates. Socioculturally, he believed that individual mental processes have their origin in social interaction, and that a child's cultural development proceeded on two parallel and interacting planes: interpersonal and intrapsychological, with internalization of the interpsychological process then reciprocally affecting interpersonal processes. He believed that ontogeny recapitulates phylogeny, but that its recapitulation occurred in the context of culture as the body of accumulated human knowledge and beliefs. He formulated the concept of the zone of proximal development, which was the distance between actual development, self-generated through problem-solving, and potential development, a higher level determined through problem-solving under capable adult or peer guidance. He viewed identity formation as shaped by (and shaping) action involving a complex interplay among the use of cultural tools, the sociocultural and institutional context of the action, and the purposes embedded in the action. Identity is then not a static, inflexible structure of the self, but rather a dynamic dimension or moment in action that may change from activity to activity, depending on how the activity, its purpose, form, cultural tools, and contexts are coordinated.[9,10]

Erik Erikson's[11] work on psychosocial development represented an additional breakthrough in the recognition of the significance of culture in psychosocial development, in terms of both differences and similarities. He believed in psychosocial stages of development that spanned the total lifecycle and which were both biologically and socioculturally determined. Each stage had common tasks, but had variations in how these were expressed and in the timing of their expression or evolution. His major focus was on adolescence, which was not a very well-understood stage nor found to be particularly significant at that time in history.

He regarded identity formation as the central psychosocial task of adolescence and identified key aspects of optimal identity: (1) experiencing a subjective sense of comfort with the self; (2) having a sense of direction in life and a continuity of the self from the past, to the present, and to the anticipated future; and (3) expressing an identity that is affirmed by a community of important others. Erikson borrowed his basic definition of identity from James: "a subjective sense of an invigorating sameness and continuity."[11(p19)] This sense of sameness is an inner sense of feeling active and alive, always in dynamic tension with no guarantee of permanent stability by either society (or ideology) or inner certainty.

Erikson's formulation of identity was the unity of two components: personal identity and cultural identity. This concept was in large part influenced by his observations and psychoanalytic interpretations of cultural practices, worldviews, and childrearing among Yurok and Sioux tribes. He was also influenced by Freud, whose only reference to identity was used to denote ethnicity and the impact of the subjugation of Jews in Western culture on his "clear consciousness of inner identity."[11(p20)] Erikson described how a key problem for individuals in identity formation was the degree to which their own cultural identity is nurtured by members of their own culture and how it is validated by others in the community, in many ways foreseeing the dilemmas faced by youth from diverse cultural backgrounds living in host cultures. In this vein, he argued that the central problem for Native Americans (American Indians) was that the powerful psychological salience of their history could not be integrated with a future taught by non-Indian educators of Native American children.

Erikson was one of the first theorists who saw the importance of adolescence as the key stage for identity consolidation and the importance of racial/ethnic identity, including recognition of the value of maturational rituals in traditional cultures. At the same time, he had a negative view of non-Western adolescent achievement of personal identity formation because of the more collectivist orientation of their cultures and their de-emphasis on individualization, a psychoanalytic concept that is bound to and biased by Western culture.[10]

Maria Montessori considered culture an essential element in her three first planes of development. She viewed the first 3 years of life (the first part of the first phase) as being outside morality, but as laying the groundwork for the internalization of positive religious and cultural values, empathic attitudes, and ethical behavioral patterns, with these being expanded on during ages 3 to 6 years (the second part of the first phase). Cognitively, creation of mind, the development of language, and the formation of consciousness and self-awareness are based on many basic cultural elements (as also proposed by Vygotsky) and are the precursors of identity.[12] During the second phase (ages 6–12 years), she viewed both social and cognitive development as oriented toward children learning how to live as members of their society and culture, with cultural lessons serving as an important part of learning exposure, and moral development being focused on children learning to serve self and others.[13]

The third phase (ages 12–18 years) features youth working on their social and occupational roles as not only serving the self but also society, morally working on larger ethical dilemmas and developing an orientation to serve humanity, and cognitively acquiring the skills to interact within a complex society consisting of diverse viewpoints, and also multiple technologies and sources of knowledge.[14]

Albert Bandura[15] placed his theory of social cognitive development within the context of culture and its influence on the developing child. Unlike B.F. Skinner, Bandura believed that humans are distinguished from lower animals by cognitive abilities that enable them to shape their environment and not purely be shaped by it, with self-efficacy being the core belief that drives humans as effective agents. The concept of human agency is the construct that symbolizes the human's abilities to influence personal functioning and circumstances. His theory distinguishes three modes of agency: personal agency (which is oriented to self-regulation), proxy agency (through which people achieve desired outcomes by influencing others to act on their behalf), and collective agency, through which people work in concert to shape their environment and future. He addressed one of the key issues in cultural value orientation (individualism vs collectivism) through this concept, seeing the successful blend of these modes of agency as varying cross-culturally but not being polar opposites.

Cross-cultural variations in values systems, beliefs, roles, and behaviors, as viewed by Bandura, are variations in patterns of agency accumulated over time and reinforced by the culture and society. Developmentally, in reviewing various studies of cross-national and -cultural education, he found that children in collectivist cultures also had significant levels of perceived self-efficacy, whereas those taught within authoritarian educational systems had a lower sense of efficacy in pursuing independent learning. He also subscribes to an agentic theory of morality, in which moral reasoning is linked to moral conduct through self-regulatory mechanisms in the face of external inducements. In this view, individuals develops their own constructs of right and wrong that serve as guides for conduct, and refrain from violating these standards out of self-condemnation. However, Bandura also proposed that the individual can disengage from their standards through the use of cognitive rationalizations, including disavowal of personal agency in adverse outcomes, and that children of weak self-regulatory efficacy who easily disengage from their moral standards exhibit high levels of antisocial behaviors, regardless of whether they reside in individualistic or collectivist cultures.[15]

Supporting the views of these theorists, anthropologic studies of different cultures have shown significant differences in both childrearing patterns and the process of developmental progression. Despite these findings, there was a general lack of application of knowledge from anthropology to understanding culturally based developmental variations. Margaret Mead[16,17] was a pioneer in this research, focusing mainly on male and female gender roles, child development, and temperament, and how these differed in varied cultural contexts. Her field work examining the adolescent transition of Samoan girls in the 1920s was fueled by curiosity about the problems that

American adolescents faced in their transition to adulthood. Mead concluded that adolescent rebellion and difficulties in adolescent transition are universal developmental givens but differ significantly between cultures. She concluded that Samoan teenagers transitioned smoothly into adulthood because of the values and maturational rituals of their culture. This theory led to much controversy in the United States and the West, because for the first time it placed "lesser-developed" cultures in equal or even advantageous positions in comparison. Mead's approach was termed *culture and personality*, and sought to explain the relationship between childrearing customs and human behaviors. She saw the individual as a product of cultural values and beliefs, which shaped the person in unique ways. These cultural characteristics are learned by the individual from infancy and are reinterpreted and reinforced as the individual proceeds through subsequent developmental stages. She proposed that differences in norms and behaviors among people across different cultures are imparted from childhood, with the interaction between individuals and culture being a dynamic and complex process that results in individuals learning how to function within their society.

The major change that has occurred in recent years since the writings of Vygotsky, Erikson, Montessori, and Mead has been a greater awareness and depth of knowledge of the importance of culture in influencing patterns of human development, behavior, and identity formation and adaptation, and the adverse impact and cultural dissonance or conflict on the mental health of children and youth. This shift has been particularly true in adolescent development, in which the study of the formation of racial/ethnic identity and acculturation has shed light on their impact on mental health. See the article by Rothe and colleagues elsewhere in this issue and Pumariega and Rothe[18] review how racial/ethnic identity influences the mental health outcomes of youth and how the acculturation process has significant implications for individual and family adaptation.

CULTURE: DEVELOPMENTAL CONSIDERATIONS

Consistent with the ideas of these theorists, cultural influences are now widely recognized as having a major impact on psychological, emotional, and even cognitive development. This impact and the diversity of developmental patterns across cultures has been recognized by cultural anthropologists as having ultimate adaptive value for humans, allowing them to overcome challenges in more diverse environments and circumstances more rapidly than natural biologic evolution would have allowed. Alvard[19] proposes that development is the mechanism through which humans, through observational learning of accumulated cultural knowledge, recapitulate the evolution of these adaptations.

From birth onward, cultures set out different expectations around parenting and childrearing, and different expectations of developmental progression for children at their different stages. For example, Pachter and Dworkin[20] found significant differences among parents from different American ethnic and immigrant groups (90 Puerto Rican, 59 African American, 69 European-American, and 37 West Indian–Caribbean) in responses for 9 of 25 developmental milestones. The differences were mainly seen among personal and social milestones, with Puerto Rican mothers expecting children to attain these milestones at a later age than other mothers, although no differences in responses were seen between Spanish- and English-speaking Puerto Rican mothers. European-American mothers expected children to take first steps and become toilet trained at a later age.

Hopkins and Westra[21] studied 124 mothers from three cultural groups living in the same British city, asking them to give the ages at which they expected their

1-month-old infants to achieve three motor milestones. Jamaican mothers expected their infants to sit and walk much earlier than their English and Indian counterparts, whereas Indian mothers gave later estimates for crawling than those of the other two groups. The actual ages at which the abilities were attained closely reflected the cultural differences in expectations among the Jamaican, Indian, and English mothers.

Another aspect of early childhood psychological development that is highly culture-bound is that of attachment, including its degree of emotional intensity and its projection to a single primary parent versus multiple caretakers, which have been thought to be the underpinning of object relations theory.[22] Outgrowths of Western concepts of attachment also include the development of transitional objects[23] and the process of psychological hatching, or separation–individuation, as critical to psychological health.[24] Significant evidence shows that all of these concepts in psychological development are variable across cultures and even somewhat culture-bound. For example, Bornstein and colleagues[25] examined and compared characteristics of maternal responsiveness to infant activity during home-based naturalistic observations of mother–infant dyads in New York City, Paris, and Tokyo. They found that differences in maternal responsiveness across these cultures occurred in response to infant looking (at the mother) rather than infant vocalization, and in mothers emphasizing interactions within the mother–infant dyad versus outside or beyond the dyad.

Choi,[26] based on multiple studies, found that American culture encourages autonomous and independent behaviors from infants, whereas in Korean culture mothers expect infants to be more passive and dependent. American mothering is individually fashioned and relies on the expertise of health care providers, whereas Korean culture is highly ritualistic, so mothering is molded more by societal rules and folklore than by individual or expert design. American mothers tend to rear their infants in a nuclear family setting, whereas Korean mothers rear their infants in an extended family or a highly social environment.

Choi and Hamilton[27] studied infant behavior, maternal attitudes toward childrearing, and maternal–infant interaction in 39 Korean and American mother–infant dyads at 2 to 3 days after delivery. They found significant differences in the Brazelton Neonatal Behavioral Assessment Scale, including more rapid habituation by Korean infants ($P \leq .01$) and better state regulation by American infants ($P \leq .01$). On the Cohler's maternal scale, Korean mothers were found to view their infants as more passive and dependent than American mothers did. They found no differences in maternal reciprocity on the Maternal-Infant Adaptation Scale or maternal sensitivity on the Maternal-Infant Play Interaction Scale.

Van Ijzendoorn and Kroonenberg[28] studied almost 2000 Strange Situation classifications obtained in eight different countries. Aggregation of samples per country and continent allowed for a firmer empirical basis for cross-cultural analysis. Substantial intracultural differences were found, with samples from one country often resembling those in other countries more than their own. The data also suggested a pattern of cross-cultural differences, in which A classifications (insecure-avoidant) emerged as relatively more prevalent in Western European countries, and C classifications (insecure-resistant) more prevalent in Israel and Japan.

Applegate[29] reviewed the literature on the presence and nature of transitional objects across cultures, and found a wide normative sociocultural variation in transitional object attachments, as opposed to British psychoanalyst and pediatrician D.W. Winnicott's assertion of the universality of transitional object formation.[23] Rothbaum and colleagues[30] reviewed cross-cultural research on separation–individuation and family dynamic theory and concluded that the dynamics described in both theories partly reflect Western ways of thinking and Western patterns of relatedness. They cite, for example, evidence from Japan that extremely close ties between mother and child are perceived as adaptive and more common, and that children experience fewer adverse effects from these relationships than do children in the West. They also found that Japan puts less emphasis on the importance of the exclusive spousal relationship and has less need for mothers and fathers to find time alone to rekindle romantic, intimate feelings and openly communicate differences to resolve conflict. They concluded that the pattern frequently cited by Western theorists as maladaptive (that consisting of an extremely close mother–child relationship, an unromantic conflictual marriage characterized by little communication, and a peripheral, distant father) may function very differently in other cultures.

During the preschool and latency periods, the teaching of primary social norms, beliefs, values, and imperatives parallels the child's continued work on emotional regulation, increased engagement in the world of peers and the educational system, and the acquisition of the beginnings of a more analytic cognitive style.[13] Strong evidence shows that cultural context again plays significant roles in all of these processes.

For example, Farver and colleagues[31] studied 48 Korean and 48 Anglo-American children in preschool settings to examine the role of culture in organizing children's activities and shaping their pretend-play behavior. Observers recorded the presence or absence of preselected social behaviors and levels of play complexity. Although parents completed a questionnaire about play in the home, teachers rated children's social competence and children were given the Peabody Picture Vocabulary Test-Revised (PPVT-R) and a sociometric interview. Korean parents also completed an acculturation questionnaire. The researchers found significant cultural differences in children's social interaction, play complexity, adult–child interaction and home versus preschool play, adult beliefs about play, scores on the PPVT-R, and children's social functioning with peers. The results suggest that children's social interaction and pretend play behavior are influenced by culture-specific socialization practices that serve adaptive functions.

Cole and colleagues[32] studied cultural influences on children's emotional reactions by examining beliefs about revealing emotion in 223 second-, fourth-, and fifth-grade children from three cultures: Brahman (Indian), Tamang (Nepali), and the United States. Interviewers asked descriptions of how children would feel, whether they would want others to know their feelings, why they would or would not, and what they would do in difficult interpersonal situations. They found three distinct cultural patterns. Tamang youth were more likely to appraise difficult situations in terms of shame than were Brahman and United States children, who endorsed anger. Brahman children, however, were more likely to not communicate negative emotion than were Tamang and United States children. The responses of United States children seemed to be more problem-focused and action-oriented than those of Brahman and Tamang children. Age influenced the degree to which children used emotion-focused coping, and also affected decisions about communicating anger in Tamang and United States children.

Lin and Fu[33] studied the mothers and fathers of 138 children enrolled in kindergarten, first grade, and second grade in Taiwan and the United States to investigate differences and similarities in childrearing practices among second-generation Chinese, immigrant Chinese, and Caucasian-American parents. They focused on parental control, encouragement of independence, expression of affection, and emphasis on achievement. Using multiple analyses of variants (MANOVA's) for group differences, they found that both second-generation and immigrant Chinese parents tended to rate higher on parental control, encouragement of independence, and emphasis on achievement than Caucasian-American parents.

In adolescence, learning and preparing for social/occupational roles and the development of a stable identity are key developmental tasks. The processes through which youth learn and internalize these roles and skills are increasingly complex, and may occasionally result in an ill-defined adolescent stage and transition process. Traditional cultures have clearer prescribed maturational rituals for youth that, even now, have been shown to be beneficial to their adaptation and mental health.[34] Ethnic/racial/cultural identity is one aspect of adolescent development that is highly influenced by not only the youth's culture of origin but also their multicultural milieu. Rothe and colleagues elsewhere in this issue review the roots of ethnic identity development in earlier child development. Phinney[35] reviewed conceptual models and research on ethnic identity in both adolescents and adults. She proposes that ethnic identity is dynamic and changing over time and context, but also recognizes that several of the definitions of ethnic identity include its achievement through an active process of decision-making and self-evaluation. Although recognizing that there have been racially and ethnically specific models of identity development and achievement, she found commonalities across these models and proposed a three-stage progression from an unexamined ethnic identity, through a period of ethnic exploration, to an achieved or committed ethnic identity. The initial stage is characterized for minorities by a preference for the dominant culture, although they may also not have been interested in ethnicity and had given it little thought (with a diffuse ethnic identity). Alternatively, they may have absorbed positive ethnic attitudes from parents or other adults, but not have thought through the issues for themselves. The second stage is often triggered by a significant experience of self-awareness of one's ethnicity, often a discrimination experience. It involves more intense immersion in one's own culture through activities such as reading, discussions, and attending or participating in ethnic-specific cultural events, and may also involve rejecting dominant group values. The end result of this process is often that the individual develops a deeper understanding and internalization of their ethnicity. This culmination requires coming to terms with two fundamental problems for ethnic minorities: (1) cultural differences between their own group and the dominant group and (2) the lower or disparaged status of their group in society.

If the dominant group in a society holds an ethnic group and its characteristics in low esteem, then ethnic group members are potentially faced with a negative social identity and ethnic self-hate. This experience can be the result of racism and xenophobia, both of which have been recognized as having adverse mental health consequences at an individual and public health level.[36,37] Individuals may seek to avoid identification with their ethnic group by "passing" as members of the dominant group, but this solution may have negative psychological consequences and is not available to individuals who are racially distinct. Alternative solutions are to develop a sense of ethnic pride, to reinterpret characteristics deemed inferior as strengths, and to stress distinctiveness aspects of one's ethnicity.[35] Added challenges exist for youth who develop at the interface between their ethnic group of origin and its traditional cultural values (with social mirroring of cultural values from their family in the home environment) and the host dominant culture (with mirroring from peers and mainstream social institutions).[18] Theorists have postulated that the development of a bicultural identity is the most adaptive resolution for ethnic identity, wherein individuals are rooted in their own culture but can selectively adopt traits of both traditional and host culture[18] (see the article by Rothe and colleagues elsewhere in this issue for further exploration of this topic). Studies have supported that the development of a strong ethnic identity by minority youth within a host culture[38] and by immigrant groups in various nations[39] that has bicultural elements, including ethnic and national identifications, is associated with positive adaptation.

CULTURE AND DEVELOPMENT: EMPIRIC FINDINGS

In addition to the extensive psychosocial developmental research cited, significant cross-cultural research is emerging in the areas of theory of mind, neural mapping, object representation, and emotional reactivity. *Theory of mind* is the mental representation of concepts and activities that enable humans to posit the mental states of others. One paradigm that has been used for cross-cultural research on theory of mind is the false belief paradigm (which tests whether a child can understand that another person holds a false belief once the circumstances around it have changed; for example, understanding that a child still believes that a toy is still hidden in his room even after his mother moved it).

Wellman and colleagues[40] conducted a meta-analysis of 178 separate studies examining false belief understanding, and found cross-cultural consistency in the developmental trajectory of the acquisition of false beliefs concepts. However, differences exist in timing, with some cultures being more mentalistic (ie, projecting others' mental states from their actions) in their content and expression. Vinden[41] in another cross-cultural study, found that most children from various cultures eventually develop an understanding of belief as it affects behavior. Children from all cultures studied were also able to make correct desire-based judgments about emotion. However, the children from Western cultures came to understand belief-based emotion shortly after they came to understand false belief, whereas almost all children from non-Western cultures had difficulty predicting an emotion based on a false belief about the world.

Based on this research, Lillard[42] proposes a culturally based theory of mind, in which universal attributes exist, but also cultural differences, such as behavioral attribution (or how people explain action), with many cultures invoking more situational and contextual perspectives. She proposes a model of theory of mind construction that incorporates culture, introspection, analogy, and ontogeny.

Markus and Kitayama[43] reported that cultural variations in self-representations (more individualistic in Westerners vs collectivist in Asian cultures) were found to affect emotional and cognitive processes. The new tools of neuroimaging are now facilitating research in cultural neuroscience to examine these differences.

Ambady and Bharucha[44] suggest a framework for this research with two objectives: cultural mapping (mapping brain function from pattern characteristics of cultures to their neural processing) and source analysis (attempts to determine the sources of observed commonalities and differences). Cultural mapping can show how the same environmental stimuli are processed differently by individuals from different cultures. Source analysis examines the source or causes of brain mappings, such as genetic heritage, impact of learning on the brain, or similarity in cultural environments.

Examples of culture mapping include differences in cognitive processes, such as different activation of numerical and nonnumerical tasks for native English speakers (perisylvian cortical areas associated with language processing) and Chinese speakers (visual premotor association area),[45] and the recruitment and activation of different brain regions for complex figure recognition (East Asian–Americans in object processing areas in the ventral visual cortex, whereas non-Asians in left occipital and fusiform areas, classically associated with figure–ground relations).[46] They also include differences in social functions, which have implications for individualistic or collectivist object representations. Caucasians tend to have more self-referential cognitive processing of adjectives mapped solely in the medial prefrontal cortex, classically associated with self-representation, whereas Chinese individuals also map onto this area when they are processing adjectives that refer to relatives, including their mothers.[47]

Chiao and colleagues[48] examined whether priming cultural values of individualism and collectivism in bicultural individuals affect neural activity in cortical midline structures underlying self-relevant processes using functional MRI (fMRI). Biculturals primed with individualistic values showed increased activation within medial prefrontal cortex (MPFC) and posterior cingulate cortex (PCC) during general self-judgments, whereas biculturals primed with collectivistic values showed increased response within MPFC and PCC during contextual self-judgments. Degree of cultural priming was positively correlated with degree of MPFC and PCC activity during culturally congruent self-judgments. These findings illustrate the dynamic influence of culture on neural representations underlying the self and, more broadly, suggest a neurobiological basis through which people acculturate, and that bicultural adaptation is cognitively based and neurally represented.

Source analysis investigations include studies on variations in cultural learning or environment, and include examining neural processing in bilinguals versus learners of a second language. For example, Pallier and colleagues[49] found that adult Koreans adopted as young children by French families (who do not recall their native language) and children who were French natives had similar patterns of activation to sentences spoken in French, Korean, or other foreign languages. However, Kovelman and colleagues[50] found that bilinguals had distinct patterns of neural activation compared with monolinguals, with both activating Broca's area, but bilinguals also activating the left inferior frontal cortex.

Some source studies have involved neural responses to fear recognition, with greater amygdalar activation[51] and greater bilateral posterior superior temporal sulci recruitment[52] when using pictures of same-culture members with both Japanese and Caucasian Americans. However, Moriguchi and colleagues[53] found activation to Japanese fear expressions in emotion-related areas of the brain in Caucasians who had lived in Japan for more than a year, suggesting that cultural exposure can affect neural processes for emotional expressions, and concurs with traditional tests for theory of mind that involve the inference of intentions and emotions from pictures of eyes.[54]

Kobayashi and colleagues[55] studied 12 American monolingual children and 12 Japanese bilingual children with second-order false-belief story and cartoon tasks using fMRI. Although some brain regions, such as the ventromedial prefrontal cortex and precuneus, were recruited by both cultural/linguistic groups, several brain areas, including the inferior frontal gyrus and temporoparietal junction, were used in a culture/language-dependent manner during the theory of mind tasks, suggesting that the neural correlates of theory of mind may vary according to cultural/linguistic background from early in life.

Even the underlying biologic evolutionary factors in these adverse cultural processes such as discrimination and xenophobia have been studied objectively, with some developmental consequences. Animal models using multiple separations can produce social discrimination and xenophobia, such as in baby chicks[56,57] and monkeys.[58,59] Research has shown that negative prejudice is damaging and disruptive to social interactions and social justice.[60,61] Prejudice has been shown to be common across cultures, time, languages, and national boundaries.[60] Some research has supported the hypothesis that prejudice is an affective state and therefore has a motivational force, usually to discharge tension or anxiety.[62]

Prejudice is associated with stereotypes, which are beliefs and categories that are readily available and established in children's minds in early childhood before they are taught to critically evaluate perceptions.[63] However, some recent research also suggests that children are prone to categorization bias, with same-race facial preference being shown by infants as early as 3 months.[64] This early developmental propensity makes children highly susceptible to implicit stereotypical prejudices and rejection of the "other," especially because most racism and discrimination is now subtle rather than overt.[65]

SPECIAL TOPICS/CURRENT CONTROVERSIES
Biculturalism

As Northrup and Bean[66] wrote in a seminal paper on bicultural identity formation, adolescence may be experienced as a stressful time for many youth in Western cultures, because it involves establishing a unique identity while also navigating peer group norms and societal expectations. Multiracial adolescents may face a more difficult challenge than their monoracial peers in that they must develop this new identity and decide how, or even if, they can reflect positive aspects of all heritages while simultaneously rejecting certain societal expectations and stereotypes.[67,68] A multiracial or multiethnic heritage can further complicate this process.

By adolescence, most multiracial children have been made aware of any racial/ethnic differences between classmates and themselves. Often they are reminded of these differences as they attend school and are asked isolating questions such as "what are you?" from classmates puzzled or threatened by their racially or ethnically mixed appearance. These alienating questions often contribute to the feeling that no one understands them, not even their monoracial parents.[69] Concerns about not "fitting in" are magnified if multiracial adolescents discover that they are no longer welcome in certain peer groups because of racial issues (eg, family objections to interracial relationships[69,70]). Additionally, some peers, and even their own parents, may pressure the adolescent to identify with only one ethnic background,[71] prompting feelings of guilt or disloyalty.[68]

The authors find it useful to adopt a stance, first described by Root[69] and modified by Northrup and Bean,[66] that acknowledges that biracial youth can either adopt the label that society gives them; choose to identify with both racial groups or only one of those groups; or choose to be known as multiethnic (or perhaps choose another racial group altogether). The therapist should stress that the decision is the youth's alone and that parents should be consulted but cannot make this decision for the child. Clinicians should also explain that the decision need not be made immediately and that it is acceptable to change one's mind later. The therapist should also emphasize that this decision is not to be made quickly, but rather must be thought through. They should also address parents' fears and concerns sensitively, but stress that it is essential for the child's optimal development that they be accepting and patient toward their child regardless of their choice. This process can be complicated, given the high likelihood that both parents will tightly adhere to the values (cultural or otherwise) that have helped them develop as individuals.[66]

LaFromboise and colleagues[72] described some important psychological features of biculturalism. They cite Rashid,[73] who was among the first to define biculturalism more formally, who encouraged all Americans to strive for this attribute, "because it creates a sense of efficacy within the institutional structure of society along with a sense of pride and identification with one's ethnic roots."[73] LaFromboise and colleagues[72] also proposed the idea that bicultural efficacy (the belief that one can develop and maintain effective interpersonal relationships in two cultures) is directly related to one's ability to develop bicultural competence.

The authors believe it may also have much to do with parental modeling of this construct, and can be directly related to how well the parent has either accommodated the new culture (adopted certain aspects of the new culture, while still retaining important features of the root culture, or culture of origin) or assimilated the new culture (adopted most or all of the new culture, while having cast off the previous cultural values and belief system). A related term to accommodation, *acculturation*, is used to describe the specific changes that may occur among people of different cultures after contact with one another.[74] Bornstein and Cote[74] provide a fuller discussion of these issues related to their societal contexts.

LaFromboise and colleagues[72] further show that those who achieve this bicultural efficacy can live effectively and satisfactorily within two groups without compromising their sense of cultural identity, and furthermore, that they can also create and maintain support groups and connections to both minority and majority cultures. This bicultural efficacy may also allow the individuals to persist through periods when they may experience rejection from one or both cultures.[75] (According to the common vernacular for immigrant children and their families in the United States, *first-generation* refers to the immigrants themselves who arrived in the United States in their adulthood, *second-generation* to their children who were born and are being raised in the United States, and *generation 1.5* to the children who were born in the country of origin, usually parental, and are now being raised in the United States).

Culture and the Educational System

Another topic that has received attention in the literature is that of the culture of special education, a topic especially relevant to chronic mental health issues or behavioral problems of childhood. In a thought-provoking book on the topic, Kalyanpur and Harry[76] highlight the potential impact of unrecognized (or underrecognized) cultural assumptions that may influence family–professional staff interactions.

The pernicious effect of these assumptions becomes apparent when considering that the recognition of the cultural basis of one's actions, although a difficult process for service providers, is doubly so for parents who may be struggling with the maze of special education procedures, terminologies, and programs. Parent–professional discourse in special education requires a level of articulation and awareness that even middle-income parents, whose "language" may be similar to those of the professionals, find difficult to acquire[77]; families that do not share the same understandings are at a further disadvantage.[78(p83)]

That adolescents would choose to affiliate or identify with specific peer groupings is not surprising. What is curious is to see how frequently some teenagers will change peer groups during the course of a junior high or high-school career. Frequently, when racially mixed schools are examined for the degree of integration that actually occurs, it may be surprising to learn that self-segregation with racially and ethnically similar teens is more the rule than the exception.[79] Self-segregation in schools has been a topic that has caught the attention of the popular media, and has been studied formally and described recently by Rodkin and colleagues.[80]

In a study of approximately 750 mostly third and fourth graders in nine elementary schools in Illinois, African American children who self-segregated were more popular than African Americans who had Caucasian friends. For white children, in contrast, self-segregating seemed to hurt their popularity. The authors commented that 20 or 30 years ago, "no black kids would have been seen as popular by white kids—and few black kids would have had social influence. Black kids would not have been setting the social standard, schoolwide. [In this study] it appears that they are."[79]

Resilience

In an influential paper examining the cultural aspects of resilience, Cameron and colleagues[81] describe the "scaffolding" that characterizes successful adaptation to adversity across cultures, which includes familial, environmental, cultural, social, psychological, and physiologic processes. Using an attachment paradigm, the authors cite international data[82,83] supporting the idea that "children [and youth] seen by their communities as resilient demonstrate complexity in how they negotiate relational resources to protect themselves against personal and environmental stressors."[81(p296)] The authors identified seven "tensions" requiring resolution to achieve healthy psychosocial development by the end of adolescence[81(pp296–7)]:

1. Access to material resources: The availability of structural provisions, including financial assistance and education, and the provision of basic instrumental needs (eg, food, shelter, clothing, access to medical care, and employment) is a function of the security of family, peer, and community relationships. Although primary caregivers are key to ensuring availability, they are not able to provide everything engaged adolescents requires as their needs become more complex.
2. Relationships: Study participants used the matrix of their relationships to negotiate access to the resources necessary to cope with their surroundings. These relationships included networks of family members, peers, adults in their communities, teachers, mentors, role models, intimate partners, and even enemies who could be manipulated to achieve status-related goals, such as being perceived as powerful or empathetic.
3. Identity: A sense of individuality has to be negotiated through relationships with others. Assertions such as "I am," "I believe." and "I feel" are ways youth reify a bounded sense of self. The process of this identity formation, however, was described as one of co-construction through mutual discursive spaces.
4. Cohesion: In contrast to the theme of individuality, participants identified the need to balance one's sense of responsibility to self and duty to one's broader community as critical to healthy development. This construct of cohesion borrows theoretically from the social capital theory. The complexity of adolescent attachments that result from ecologic diversity demands attention to the needs of others in a reflexive process that nurtures the self.
5. Power and control: Attachments at multiple ecologic levels bring with them the basis for shared and agentic experiences of power to make decisions, and the control to enact them. These experiences, like those of the 2-year-old child who negotiates roots and wings, must be found through interactions in shared relational spaces.
6. Cultural adherence: Adherence, or standing in opposition to cultural norms, demands complex negotiations with caregivers and communities. Culture clashes between localized family and cultural norms and global culture (often synonymous with popular culture) is a function of the relationships experienced by the youth.
7. Social justice: In the expanding topography of children's relationships, they develop the capacity to individually and collectively assert their rights. Experiences of prejudice and dynamics of sociopolitical disenfranchisement that often come with exposure to risk (such as poverty, disability, or racial prejudice) can be catalysts for conscientization and resistance.

Other Influences on Development

According to a recent qualitative research review by Houskamp and colleagues,[84] most children in the United States consider themselves spiritual beings, and therefore clinicians should ask about a child's spiritual or religious life. Furthermore, families may benefit greatly when clinicians use spiritual or religious resources as adjuncts in treatment if these are perceived as helpful for the family or child in coping better with the current situation.

In a useful article on worldview in psychiatric practice,[85] Josephson and Wiesner[86] offer thoughtful and researched-based recommendations regarding the clinician's role. They highlight a brief screen to help structure questions better, with the acronym FICA—F represents the question, "is religious *faith* an important part of your day-to-day or weekly life?" This question could be followed by other questions about formal religious affiliation and level of spirituality. *I* represents the question, "How has faith *influenced* your life, past and present?" This question may uncover important spiritual experiences. *C* represents the question, "Are you currently (or is your family) a part of a religious or spiritual *community*?" This question can help clarify the role a spiritual community might play in treatment interventions. Finally, *A* represents the question, "What are the spiritual needs that you would like me to *address*?" This question allows the clinician to identify spiritual areas that may become part of a treatment plan.

Another approach involves the use of two screening questions developed by Matthews[87]: "Is religion or spirituality important to you (your child/teen)?" and "What can I do to support your faith or religious commitment?"

This attunement to worldview can be particularly important in the case of cross-cultural or international adoption, wherein the parents may be trying to raise a child with as much cultural adaptation as possible, but for whom familiarity with a child's ethnocultural origins may be limited. Recent investigation and policy statements in this area, although not without controversy, have kept the discussion of cultural attunement and sensitivity in cross-cultural parenting and adoption very active.[88–90]

From Vonk's comprehensive review,[91] three main principles that can lead to the most culturally effective parenting include:

1. Multicultural or racial awareness: Knowledge of how the variables of race, ethnicity, culture, language, and related power status operate in one's own and other's lives,[92] including an understanding of the dynamics of racism, oppression, and other forms of discrimination.[93]
2. Multicultural planning: Active pursuit of opportunities for transracially adopted children to learn about and participate in their culture of birth. Although socialization in the culture of one's racial group is generally congruent with the racial makeup of the family, this is not the case in families formed through transracial adoption. Furthermore, if the family is involved in other groups, such as neighborhoods, schools, and churches that are exclusively or primarily made up of European Americans, the child has no access to others of his or her birth culture. This dynamic seems to make it difficult for some adoptees to identify with and develop pride in their race, ethnicity, or culture of birth.[91]
3. Survival skills: The recognition of the need for parents to prepare their children to cope successfully with racism. This skill is as important for transracial adoptees as for children with same-race parents, but may be more difficult to learn from European American parents who have had little experience of racism directed toward them. Minimizing or ignoring racial incidents is insufficient for children who may find themselves at the receiving end of racially based prejudice or discrimination. These children need help to develop a strong self-images despite racism.[91]

RECOMMENDATIONS FOR PRACTICE

This article attempted to highlight some of the most important research in culture and child development. The recognition of diverse normative patterns of development and parenting in any clinical evaluation is a crucial finding in much cross-cultural work. Other areas in which the child and adolescent clinician can be especially useful include providing support for traditional patterns of parenting while informing parents when certain behaviors cross legal or moral boundaries established by the mainstream society, and engaging child-serving agencies (schools, youth organizations, child welfare, juvenile justice) around normative developmental differences to help these agencies' staffs serve youth in a more culturally attuned manner. Storck and Stoep,[6] in their paper on ecologic perspectives in child and adolescent psychiatry, sum up these clinicians' roles as advocates, pediatric ethnographers, and culturally curious clinicians:

> "The child psychiatrist's aim is to help a child successfully navigate his or her world. To accomplish this aim, we must ensure that our intervention strategies work effectively not only within the confines of our offices or hospital, but also in the child's real world zones [emphasis added]. In vivo observation of the adaptive repertoires of a young person in day-to-day realms broadens the provider's understanding of the variables (ecologic forces) that influence the patient's thoughts, emotions and behaviors. Observations made in family, treatment, and community settings can be the nutrients and fuel for clinicians as they build a professional repertoire of generalizable understandings, behavioral skills, and shareable vignettes that may be useful for decades to come. Helping patients to develop their own ethnographic skills also can improve their life navigation abilities."[6(p139)]

(Ethnopediatrics as a field represents the contribution of mental health clinicians and researchers, anthropologists, and pediatricians who engage in the comparative study of parents and infants across cultures to explore the way different caretaking styles affect the health, well-being, and survival of infants and children. Small provides a more detailed discussion of this topic in Our Babies, Ourselves: How Biology and Culture Shape the Way We Parent.[94])

FUTURE CONSIDERATIONS/AREAS FOR FURTHER RESEARCH

The developmental theories and constructs proposed by Vygotsky, Erikson, Montessori, Bandura, and Mead have stood the test of science particularly well, not only through field observational research with normal children but also more recently through research using neuroimaging and neuropsychological tools. However, a significant need still exists to integrate the perspectives of these theorists and to support or modify research findings into a unified theory of child and human development that truly integrates neurobiological, cultural, psychological, and social aspects and their interrelationships. Such a unifying theory would greatly facilitate cross-cultural and -national research on child development and also inform developmental aspects of psychopathology across different cultures and societies, while also helping to guide preventive and clinical interventions.

In addition to providing a more integrative conceptual foundation, a great need also exists for continued research on brain development and neural encoding of cultural patterns. Areas of important research include the role of critical periods in the development of language and cultural awareness, the role of culture and language in shaping cognitive and emotional constructs and functions, and the impact of a more heterogeneous cultural environment on development and the makeup of ethnic/racial identity and on cognitive development and its mapping. Research on the interface between culture and development has significant clinical applications in addressing the adverse consequences of cultural transition, geographic dislocation, trauma, and acculturation stress on the developing child. However, it has equally important value in helping develop the basis of effective preventive interventions to strengthen ethnic identity in diverse cultural groups of children and adolescents (thus enhancing their psychosocial resilience), and in preventing stereotypical patterns of thought that contribute to racism and xenophobia. These preventive approaches addressing the normal child's comfort with multicultural environments and diverse peers may need to be core elements of bully-prevention programs, as recent incidents involving the victimization of immigrant children (including white immigrants) and gay/lesbian children have illustrated.[95]

An added area of research is posed by the findings of the positive neurodevelopmental impact of bilingualism and multilingualism, suggesting that bilinguals have greater cognitive and neural flexibility.[48] This exploration has major implications for the United States, which is one of the few nations that emphasizes the learning of a single language in its educational system, and continually experiences public battles over the use of a single language in business transactions and day-to-day life. If the United States were to remain one of the few monolingual nations in a planet of polyglots, this may pose serious adverse consequences to the nation's intellectual and economic health, internal social harmony, international relations, and mental health. This possibility suggests the potential adaptive and preventive value of universal multilingual education in increasing multicultural effectiveness, including preventing prejudice, reducing the mental health risks associated with acculturation, and even enhancing the cognitive capabilities of the nation's children and youth in general.

REFERENCES

1. U.S. Census Bureau. American Community Survey (ACS). Available at: http://www.census.gov/acs/www/index.html. Accessed August 27, 2010.
2. Sholevar GP. Cultural child and adolescent psychiatry. In: Martin A, Volkmar F, editors. Lewis's child and adolescent psychiatry: a comprehensive textbook. Philadelphia: Lippincott, Williams and Wilkins; 2007. p. 57–65.
3. McLoyd VC. Socioeconomic disadvantage and child development. Am Psychol 1998;53(2):185–204.
4. McDermott JF. Effects of culture and ethnicity on child & adolescent development. In: Lewis M, editor. Child and adolescent psychiatry—a comprehensive textbook. 3rd edition. Philadelphia: Lippincott; 2002. p. 494–8.
5. Harkness S, Keefer CH, Super CM. Culture and ethnicity. In: Levine MD, Carey WB, Crocker AC, editors. Developmental-behavioral pediatrics. 4th edition. New York: W.B. Saunders; 2009. p. 182–91.
6. Storck MG, Vander Stoep A. Fostering ecologic perspectives in child psychiatry. Child Adolesc Psychiatric Clin N Am 2007;16:133–63.
7. Freud S. Civilization and its discontents. In: Freud S, Strachey J, Gay P, editors. Civilization and its discontents: the standard edition [with a biographical introduction by Peter Gay]. New York/London: W.W. Norton; 1989. p. 5–113.
8. James W. Principles of psychology. New York: Holt; 1890.
9. Vygotsky LS. Mind in society: the development of higher mental processes. Cambridge (MA): Harvard University Press; 1978.

10. Penuel W, Wertsch J. Vygotsky and identity formation: a sociocultural approach. Educ Psychol 1995;30:83–92.
11. Erikson E. Identity: youth and crisis. New York: Norton; 1968.
12. Haines A. Optimal outcomes along social, moral, cognitive, and emotional dimensions. North Am Montessori Teach Assoc J 2000;25:27–59.
13. Baker K. Optimal developmental outcomes for the child aged six to twelve: social, moral, cognitive, and emotional dimensions. NAMTA J 2001;26:71–93.
14. Kahn K. Philosophy, psychology, and educational goals for the Montessori adolescent, ages twelve to fifteen. NAMTA J 2003;28:107–22.
15. Bandura A. Social cognitive theory in cultural context. Applied Psychol Int Rev 2002;51:269–90.
16. Mead M. Coming of age in Samoa: a psychological study of primitive youth for western civilization. New York: William Morrow; 1928.
17. Moore J. Visions of culture: an introduction to anthropological theories and theorists. Walnut Creek (CA): AltaMira Press; 1997.
18. Pumariega AJ, Rothe E. Leaving no children or families behind: the challenges of immigration. Am J Orthopsychiat 2010;80(4):506–16.
19. Alvard M. The adaptive nature of culture. Evol Anthropol 2003;12:136–49.
20. Pachter L, Dworkin P. Maternal expectations about normal child development in 4 cultural groups. Arch Pediatr Adolesc Med 1997;151:1144–50.
21. Hopkins B, Westra T. Maternal expectations of their infants' development: some cultural differences. Dev Med Child Neurol 1989;31:384–90.
22. Klein M. Love, guilt, and reparation & other works, 1921–1945. New York: Free Press; 2002.
23. Winnicott D. Transitional objects and transitional phenomena—a study of the first not-me possession. Int J Psycho-Anal 1953;34:89–97.
24. Mahler M. On the first three subphases of the separation-individuation process. Psychoanal Contemp Sci 1974;3:295–306.
25. Bornstein M, Tamis-LeMonda C, Tal J, et al. Maternal responsiveness to infants in three societies: the United States, France, and Japan. Child Dev 1992;63:808–21.
26. Choi E. A contrast of mothering behaviors in women from Korea and the United States. J Obstet Gynecol Neonatal Nurs 1995;24:363–9.
27. Choi E, Hamilton R. The effects of culture on mother-infant interaction. J Obstet Gynecol Neonatal Nurs 1986;15:256–61.
28. Van Ijzendoorn M, Kroonenberg P. Cross-cultural patterns of attachment: a meta-analysts of the strange situation. Child Dev 1988;59:147–56.
29. Applegate J. The transitional object reconsidered: Some sociocultural variations and their implications. Child Adol Soc Work J 1989;6:38–51.
30. Rothbaum F, Rosen K, Ujiie T, et al. Family systems theory, attachment theory, and culture. Fam Process 2004;41:328–50.
31. Farver J, Kim Y, Lee Y. Cultural differences in Korean- and Anglo-American preschoolers' social interaction and play behaviors. Child Dev 2008;66:1088–99.
32. Cole P, Bruschi C, Tamang B. Cultural differences in children's emotional reactions to difficult situations. Child Dev 2003;73:983–96.
33. Lin C, Fu V. A comparison of child-rearing practices among Chinese. Immigrant Chinese, and Caucasian-American parents 2008;61:429–33.
34. Markstrom C, Iborra A. Adolescent identity formation and rites of passage: the Navajo Kinaaldá ceremony for girls. J Res Adolesc 2003;13(4):399–425.
35. Phinney J. Ethnic identity in adolescents and adults: review of research. Psychol Bull 1990;10:499–514.

36. American Psychiatric Association. Committee on black psychiatrists. Resolution against racism and racial discrimination and their adverse impacts on mental health. Available at: http://archive.psych.org/edu/other_res/lib_archives/archives/200603.pdf. Accessed July 11, 2010.

37. American Psychiatric Association. Committee on Hispanic psychiatrists. Position statement on xenophobia, immigration, and mental health. Am J Psychiatry 2010; 167:726.

38. Roberts R, Phinney J, Masse L, et al. The structure of ethnic identity of young adolescents from diverse ethnocultural groups. J Early Adolesc 1999;19:301–22.

39. Phinney J, Horenczyk G, Liebkind K, et al. Ethnic identity, immigration, and well being: an interactional perspective. J Soc Issues 2001;57:493–510.

40. Wellman H, Cross D, Watson J. Meta-analysis of theory-of-mind development: the truth about false belief. Child Dev 2001;72:655–84.

41. Vinden P. Children's understanding of mind and emotion: a multi-culture study. Available at: http://www.informaworld.com/smpp/title~db=all~content= t713682755~tab=issueslist~branches=13-v1313. Accessed August 11, 2010.

42. Lillard A. Developing a cultural theory of mind: the CIAO approach. Curr Dir Psychol Sci 1999;8:57–61.

43. Markus H, Kitayama S. Culture and the self: implications for cognition, emotion, and motivation. Psychol Rev 1991;98:224–53.

44. Ambady N, Bharucha J. Culture and the brain. Curr Dir Psychol Sci 2009;18: 342–5.

45. Tang Y, Zhang W, Chen K, et al. Arithmetic processing in the brain shaped by cultures. Proc Nat Acad Sci 2006;103:10775–80.

46. Gutchess A, Welsh R, Lu A, et al. Cultural differences in neural function associated with object processing. Cognit Affect Behav Neurosci 2006;6:102–9.

47. Zhu Y, Zhang L, Fan J, et al. Neural basis of cultural influence on self-representation. NeuroImage 2007;34:1310–6.

48. Chiao J, Harada T, Komeda H, et al. Dynamic cultural influences on neural representations of the self. J Cogn Neurosci 2009;22:1–11.

49. Pallier C, Dehaene S, Poline J, et al. Brain imaging of language plasticity in adopted adults: can a second language replace the first? Cereb Cortex 2003;13: 155–61.

50. Kovelman I, Shalinsky M, Berens M, et al. Shining new light on the brain's "bilingual signature": a functional near infrared spectroscopy investigation of semantic processing. NeuroImage 2008;39:1457–71.

51. Chiao J, Iidaka T, Gordon H, et al. Cultural specificity in amygdale response to fear faces. J Cogn Neurosc 2008;20:2167–74.

52. Adams R, Rule N, Franklin R, et al. Cross-cultural reading the mind in the eyes: an fMRI investigation. J Cogn Neurosc 2009;22:97–108.

53. Moriguchi Y, Ohnishi T, Kawachi T, et al. Specific brain activation in Japanese and Caucasian people to fearful faces. Neuroreport 2005;16:133–6.

54. Baron-Cohen S, Wheelwright S, Hill J, et al. The "Reading the Mind in the Eyes" test revised version: a study with normal adults, and adults with Asperger syndrome or high-functioning autism. J Child Psychol Psychiatry 2001;42: 241–51.

55. Kobayashia C, Gloverb G, Temple E. Cultural and linguistic effects on neural bases of 'Theory of Mind' in American and Japanese children. Brain Lang 2006;98:210–20.

56. Rajecki D, Ivins B, Kidd R. Affiliation, xenophobia, and the behavioral organization of the young domestic chicken. Behav Biol 1977;21:364–79.

57. Rajewski D, Lamb M, Suomi S. Effects of multiple peer separation in domestic chicks. Dev Psychol 1978;14:379–87.
58. Suomi S, Harlow H, Domek C. Effects of repetitive infant-infant separation of young monkeys. J Abnorm Psychol 1970;76:161–72.
59. Sackett G, Holm R, Ruppenthal G. Social isolation rearing: species differences in behavior of macaque monkeys. Dev Psychol 1976;12:283–8.
60. Brown R. Prejudice: its social psychology. London: Basil Blackwell; 1995.
61. Jones J. Prejudice and racism. 2nd edition;. New York: McGraw-Hill; 1997.
62. Brehm J. The intensity of emotion. Pers Soc Psychol Rev 1999;3:2–22.
63. Devine P. Stereotypes and prejudice: their automatic and controlled components. J Pers Soc Psychol 1989;44:20–33.
64. Bar-Haim Y, Ziv T, Lamy D, et al. Nature and nurture in own-race face processing. Psychol Sci 2006;17:159–63.
65. Pettigrew T, Meertens R. Subtle and blatant prejudice in Western Europe. Euro J Soc Psychol 1995;25:57–75.
66. Northrup JC, Bean RA. Culturally competent family therapy with Latino Anglo-American adolescents: facilitating identity formation. Am J Fam Ther 2007;35: 251–63.
67. Kerwin C, Ponterotto JG. Biracial identity development: theory and research. In: Ponterotto JP, Casas JM, Suzuki LA, et al, editors. Handbook of multicultural counseling. Thousand Oaks (CA): Sage; 1995. p. 199–217.
68. Wehrly B, Kenney KR, Kenney ME. Counseling multiracial families. Thousand Oaks (CA): Sage Publications; 1999.
69. Root MP. Resolving "other" status: identity development of biracial individuals. In: Brown LS, Root MP, editors. Diversity and complexity in feminist therapy. New York: Haworth; 1990. p. 185–205.
70. Diller JV. Cultural diversity: a primer for the human services. Toronto (ON): Wadsworth Publishing Company; 1999.
71. Cauce AM, Hiraga Y, Mason C, et al. Between a rock and a hard place: social adjustment of biracial youth. In: Root MP, editor. Racially mixed people in America. Newbury Park (CA): Sage; 1992. p. 207–22.
72. LaFromboise T, Coleman HLK, Gerton J. Psychological impact of biculturalism: evidence and theory. Psychol Bull 1993;114:395–412.
73. Rashid HM. Promoting biculturalism in young African-American children. Young Child 1984;39:13–23.
74. Bornstein MH, Cote LR. Introduction to acculturation and parent-child relationships. In: Bornstein MH, Cote LR, editors. Acculturation and parent-child relationships: measurement and development. Mahwah (NJ): Lawrence Erlbaum; 2006. p. 3–12.
75. Rozek F. The role of internal conflict in the successful acculturation of Russian Jewish immigrants. Dissertation Abstracts International 1980;41:2778 B. University Microfilms No. 8028799.
76. Kalyanpur M, Harry B. Culture in special education: building reciprocal family-professional relationships. Baltimore (MD): Paul H. Brookes Publishing, Inc; 1999.
77. Turnbull AP, Turnbull HR, Shank M, et al. Exceptional lives: special education in today's schools. 2nd edition. Upper Saddle River (NJ): Merrill/Prentice-Hall; 1999.
78. Harry B, Allen N, McLaughlin M. Communication versus compliance: African-American parents' involvement in special education. Exceptional Children 1995;61:364–77.
79. Bronson P, Merriman A. By third grade, Black students who self segregate are more popular. Newsweek, September 10th, 2009, Education Section. Available

at: http://www.newsweek.com/blogs/nurture-shock/2009/09/10.html. Accessed August 28, 2010.

80. Rodkin PC, Wilson T, Ahn HJ. Social integration between African American and European American children in majority black, majority white, and multicultural elementary classrooms. In: Rodkin PC, Hanish LD, editors. Social network analysis and children's peer relationships. San Francisco (CA): Jossey-Bass; 2007. p. 25–42.

81. Cameron CA, Ungar M, Liebenberg L. Cultural understandings of resilience: roots for wings in the development of affective resources for resilience. Child Adolesc Psychiatr Clin N Am 2007;16:285–301.

82. Ungar M, Lee AW, Callaghan T, et al. An international collaboration to study resilience in adolescents across cultures. J Soc Work Res 2005;6(1):5–24.

83. Ungar M, Liebenberg L. The international resilience project: a mixed methods approach to the study of resilience across cultures. In: Ungar M, editor. Handbook for working with children and youth: pathways to resilience across cultures and contexts. Thousand Oaks (CA): Sage Publications; 2005. p. 211–26.

84. Houskamp BM, Fisher LA, Stuber ML. Spirituality in children and adolescents: research findings and implications for clinicians and researchers. Child Adolesc Psychiatr Clin N Am 2004;13:221–30.

85. Josephson AM, Wiesner IS. Worldview in psychiatric assessment. In: Josephson AM, Peteet JR, editors. Handbook of spirituality and worldview in clinical practice. Washington, DC: American Psychiatric Press, Inc; 2004. p. 15–30.

86. Puchalski CM, Romer AL. Taking a spiritual history allows clinicians to understand patients more fully. J Palliat Med 2000;3:129–37.

87. Matthews D, McCullough M, Larson D, et al. Religious commitment and health status: a review of the research and implications for family medicine. Arch Fam Med 1998;7:118–24.

88. National Association of Black Social Workers. Preserving families of black ancestry. 2003. Available at: http://www.nabsw.org/mserver/PreservingFamilies.aspx. Accessed August 27, 2010.

89. Andujo E. Ethnic identity of transethnically adopted Hispanic adolescents. Social Work 1988;33:531–5.

90. Johnson PR, Shireman JF, Watson KW. Transracial adoption and the development of black identity at age eight. Child Welfare 1987;66:45–55.

91. Vonk ME. Cultural competence for transracial adoptive parents. Soc Work 2001; 46(3):246–55.

92. Greene RR, Watkins M, McNutt I, et al. Diversity defined. In: Greene RR, Watkins M, editors. Serving diverse constituencies. New York: Aldine de Gruyter; 1998. p. 29–57.

93. McPhatter AR. Cultural competence in child welfare: what is it? how do we achieve it? what happens without it? Child Welfare 1997;76:255–78.

94. Small M. Our babies, ourselves: how biology and culture shape the way we parent. New York: Anchor Books; 1998.

95. Eckholm E, Zezima K. 6 Teenagers are charged after classmate's suicide. New York Times. March 29, 2010; U.S. section. Available at: http://www.nytimes.com/2010/03/30/us/30bully.html?pagewanted=1. Accessed July 15, 2010.

Acculturation, Development, and Adaptation

Eugenio M. Rothe, MD[a],*, Dan Tzuang, MD[b],
Andres J. Pumariega, MD[c,d]

KEYWORDS

• Culture • Acculturation • Childhood • Development

Acculturation refers to the process that occurs when groups of individuals of different cultures come into continuous first-hand contact, which changes the original culture patterns of either or both groups. The encounter causes cultural diffusion of varying degrees and may have one of 3 possible outcomes: (1) acceptance, when there is assimilation of one group into the other; (2) adaptation, when there is a merger of the 2 cultures; and (3) reaction, which results in antagonistic contra-acculturative movements.[1] Acculturation is a concept that applies to individuals living in communities other than where they were born, such as immigrants, refugees, and asylum seekers. It does not apply to groups whose ancestors were subjected to involuntary subjugation in their own land, such as Native Americans, or to individuals whose ancestors were brought to the United States by force and subjugation, such as African Americans. Today more than ever before acculturation has become a relevant concept as a result of the phenomenon of globalization, which defines the sociocultural climate of the twenty-first century.

Globalization occurs when there is an acceleration of movement of people, products, and ideas between nations.[2] It is characterized by an increase in fluidity between the financial and political borders between countries, which in turn increases the complexity of the everyday problems that are faced by the inhabitants of the countries. Another important aspect of globalization has been the increase in large migrations in the last decades, predominantly from poor countries to more developed ones, like the United States.[3] Historically, federal legislation has played a significant role in this process. In 1965, President Lyndon Johnson signed the Hart-Celler Act, also known as the Immigration and Nationality Act, which abolished racial discrimination in

[a] Herbert Wertheim College of Medicine, Florida International University, Miami, FL, USA
[b] Child and Adolescent Psychiatry, Stanford University School of Medicine, Psychiatry and Behavioral Sciences Building, 401 Quarry Road, Stanford, CA 94305, USA
[c] Temple University School of Medicine, Philadelphia, PA, USA
[d] Department of Psychiatry, The Reading Hospital and Medical Center, Sixth Avenue & Spruce Street, West Reading, PA 19611, USA
* Corresponding author. 2199 Ponce de Leon Boulevard, Suite 304, Coral Gables, FL 33134.
E-mail address: erothe@fiu.edu

Child Adolesc Psychiatric Clin N Am 19 (2010) 681–696
doi:10.1016/j.chc.2010.07.002
1056-4993/10/$ – see front matter © 2010 Elsevier Inc. All rights reserved.
childpsych.theclinics.com

immigration law. As a result, each independent nation had a yearly quota of 20,000, whose children, parents, and spouses could enter as legal immigrants. This legislation had a significant effect in certain immigrant populations. For instance, the ethnic Chinese population in the United States almost doubled each decade after the act was passed, although Chinese people accounted for only one-tenth of 1% of the population in the 1960 census.[4]

As a result of their arrival and resettlement in the United States, immigrants usually undergo varying degrees of acculturation stress, which leads to alterations in the person's mental health status.[5] These alterations may improve or worsen with the person's later acculturation and adaptation to the United States.

THE NEW DEMOGRAPHICS OF THE UNITED STATES

Until the mid-twentieth century, the United States received predominantly European immigrants, whose racial and cultural characteristics allowed them to assimilate rapidly into the American social fabric. In the past 40 years, immigration from Europe and Canada has declined dramatically, and non-European immigration has increased faster.

The foreign-born population in the United States increased by 57% in the last decade, compared with only a 9.3% growth of the US native population. By the year 2050, European-origin Americans will no longer be the numerical majority; this will happen before 2030 among children younger than 18 years and is already true among 6-year-olds.[6] Most of the new immigrants to the United States describe themselves as nonwhite, and immigrants from the Caribbean and Central and South America are the most racially mixed, with less than 45% self-reporting as white. The United States faces a rapidly changing demographic landscape with an increasing multiracial and multicultural population. These changes largely result from 3 major factors: (1) progressive aging and low birth rate of its European-origin population; (2) lower mean ages and increasing birth rates in non-European minority groups; and (3) a significant increase in immigration from Latin America, Asia, and Africa. These growing populations of children are diverse in their racial, ethnic, national origin, immigration, and socioeconomic makeup. However, as a group, they are different from the older, European-origin, white, and higher socioeconomic mainstream population.

CULTURE AND IDENTITY

Hughes[7] defines culture as a socially transmitted system of ideas that: (1) shapes behavior, (2) categorizes perceptions, (3) gives names to selected aspects of experience, (4) is widely shared by members of a particular society or social group, (5) functions as an orientational framework to coordinate and sanction behavior, and (6 conveys values across the generations. Cultural process refers to the fluid and ever-changing characteristics of a culture that responds to changes in the historical and cultural contexts in which cultures are imbedded. Hughes[7] considers that it is more accurate to refer to a particular group's cultural process, rather than a group's culture, which implies that it is stationary. However, in this article the term culture is used, although what is implied is cultural context.

In childhood, from the age of 3 to 4 years old, children are already capable of detecting differences in language use, and between 4 and 8 years of age children develop a sense of ethnic identity. They identify as members of a particular ethnic group, they consolidate a sense of group identity, and they develop curiosity about other groups that are different from their own.[8]

Identity formation has been historically viewed as one of the principal tasks of the passage into adulthood. The concept of identity is composed of individual and social components and is closely related to the culture. Erikson[9] conceptualized identity as resulting from the dynamic interplay between the individual and his group and cultural context, and added that identity development is the central task of adolescence that (1) optimally results in a coherent and self-constructed dynamic organization of drives, abilities, beliefs, and personal history and that (2) functionally guides the life course.[10] However, this concept of the universality of development, representative of the modernist European tradition, has been vigorously challenged. It has been considered to be based on male oriented and Western values that are more descriptive of the white mainstream majority in the United States. The critics of this model postulate that it may not adequately represent the experiences of members of minority groups, such as adolescents born to immigrant families. The postmodernist tradition suggests the opposite. It argues that identity formation is idiosyncratic and that it is different each time, and particular to every individual. In a review of the literature, Schwartz and Montgomery[11] were unable to find any empiric studies supporting the postmodernist tradition; instead, their research supports a third alternative hypothesis, which argues that the fundamental structure of identity is consistent, but it is also influenced by variables that are particular to the individual and take into account the different styles of acculturation. Taking this third model into account, Schwartz and colleagues[12] regard identity as "the organization of self-understandings that define one's place in the world"[(p5)]. They conclude that identity is a synthesis of personal, social, and cultural self-conceptions. Identity has been divided into (1) personal identity, which refers to the goals, values, and beliefs that the individual adopts and holds, (2) social identity, which refers to the interaction between the personal identity and the group with which one identifies, and (3) cultural identity, which refers to the sense of solidarity with the ideas, attitudes, beliefs, and behaviors of the members of a particular cultural group. There is often confusion between the terms cultural identity and ethnic identity. Ethnicity refers to the cultural, racial, religious, and linguistic characteristics of a people,[13] and ethnic identity refers to the subjective meaning of one's ethnicity. Ethnic identity is contained within the broader concept of cultural identity, which refers to specific values, ideals, and beliefs belonging to the particular cultural group. Ethnic identity has always been a socially constructed product, which is affected by several variables. It can recede into the background, or it can become an engulfing concern.

Case 1

Ives, a 17-year-old Haitian adolescent, was sent away by his family to a prestigious boarding school in the midwest United States, to protect him from violence and the possibility of being kidnapped in Haiti. His father occupied an important government position on the island and the family belonged to the mulatto aristocratic class. Ives was unable to adapt or fit in at the school. He complained that his peers "were not used to dealing with an educated black person and didn't know what to do with me," and that they talked down to him and treated him with fear and contempt. He added that he could not find anything in common with the American blacks who attended the school, most of whom came from poor families, had come from the adjacent urban ghettos, and were studying on scholarship. Ives became depressed and suicidal at the school and eventually moved to Miami, where he began residing with extended family and attending day school. At this time, Ives was also seen in weekly psychotherapy. Immediately, he began to question his Hispanic male therapist about the perceptions his therapist had of him, given that both were of a different culture and race, and together they were able to explore his emotional pain, his sense of alien-ation, and his fears of rejection. Ives slowly became aware that sometimes he pre-sented with a hostile attitude toward others, which was a defense against the anticipation of being rejected, and realized that this attitude kept people away from him. Slowly, Ives became less defensive and together with his therapist began discus-sing Haitian culture and history. Ives also developed an interest in the short stories of Haitian folk author Edwidge Danticat, which he described and discussed during the therapy sessions. One day, after several months in psychotherapy, he told his thera-pist "I had never given much thought to the fact that I'm black until I came to the United States. I have now discovered that I am 'Black and Haitian'. I feel proud of my heritage, because Haiti was the first free Black Republic in the world. Now I feel more Haitian than ever, and in Miami I have found enough people that are like me. Yet, I am also beginning to feel like an 'American'. I consider that the United States is my home and I have no interest in ever going back to live in Haiti." In the therapy, and with the help of the supportive community of compatriots in Miami, Ives was able to discover new aspects of his ethnicity and culture of origin; these identity fragments became integrated into a new, richer, and more cohesive sense of self. In turn, this allowed him to successfully integrate to his new peer group, which included adoles-cents of various ethnic origins and nationalities.

The concept of identity functions as a regulatory social-psychological structure and is particularly pertinent to immigrant people, who are trying to locate themselves between the culture of origin and the host culture, and who are trying to maintain a sense of self-consistency and consider new possibilities.[12]

The Stresses of Immigration

DeVos[14] and Ogbu[15] describe 3 themes that have a determining effect on the adap-tation and identity formation of the immigrant child and his or her family.

1. Under what circumstances does the immigrant enter the host culture (voluntary migration vs forced migration, conqueror vs slave)?
2. Is there a structural ceiling (social hierarchy) above which the immigrant cannot rise, regardless of effort, talent, or achievement?
3. Is there a cultural ethos or stereotype that fits the immigrant, from which he or she cannot separate?

At times, a person who is regarded by the majority culture as a member of a partic-ular ethnic group or who regards himself or herself as of a particular ethnicity may find his or her identity changed by the immigration process.

Most immigrants that come to the United States are financial immigrants who have fled poverty in their country of origin in search for a better life. However, because of the changing immigration landscape influenced by federal law, there is tremendous diver-sity among immigrants and their levels of education. Amongst Asian Americans, first-generation experiences vary tremendously, ranging from initial penniless Chinese immigrants who came to work on America's railroads and gold mines in the 1800s, to more recent patterns of college-educated professionals from Taiwan, China, Korea, and India who came to pursue graduate degrees and stayed, versus the experiences of those in the Hmong, Laotian, and Cambodian populations who may have entered the United States to seek political asylum from their war-torn home countries. However, overall it can be said that the immigrant experience is one of the most stressful experiences a family can undergo. It removes the family from their relation-ships, friends, neighbors, and members of the extended family. It also removes the family from their community, jobs, customs, and sometimes language, placing them in a strange and unpredictable environment.[16]

Garza-Guerrero[17] constructed a theoretic model to understand culture shock, a phenomenon that immigrants experience when they first encounter the new culture. He describes 2 elements that are the hallmark of culture shock: (1) mourning, related to the loss of the culture, country, language, friends, and predictable environment; and (2) the vicissitudes of identity, in the face of the threat of a new culture. He divides culture shock into 3 phases: (1) the cultural encounter, (2) reorganization, and (3) a new identity. If completed successfully, this process leads to personal growth and an enrichment of the self. This process of culture shock closely resembles the process of adolescence itself, and presents a double developmental challenge to the immigrant adolescent.

Case 2

Juan, a 13-year-old adolescent arrived in Boston abruptly with his mother and 3 brothers following a marital dispute caused by his father's infidelity. The family began residing in the small one-bedroom apartment of his aunt and cousin, which soon led to tensions. Juan and his brothers struggled to fit into a multiethnic, inner-city school, where his difficulties were aggravated by his poor command of English. Juan became aggressive and joined a school gang. He was referred to therapy by his pediatrician, who believed that Juan was depressed and experiencing auditory and visual hallucinations. Juan presented as an angry and despondent adolescent, who missed his father and his home life in Puerto Rico. One day he told his psychiatrist about a dream he had had the night before: "I dreamt that my brothers and I were riding on a train, that we fell off and found ourselves trudging through a marsh that never seemed to end. Suddenly, we were attacked by three men that were wearing masks. We fought with them and their masks fell off. One man was blond, the other man was black, and the third one was Chinese."

Juan's dream is an example of the first phase of culture shock, the cultural encounter, which is characterized by a sense of confusion that results when aspects of the old culture are compared with aspects of the new, host culture. The discrepancy that results from the comparison may lead to feelings of disorientation, loss, mourning, and helplessness. Often in these situations, aggression becomes a defense against helplessness, which may explain Juan's acting-out behaviors. If these feelings of aggression are projected outwards, some aspects of the new, host culture may be perceived as persecutory. Juan's persecutory feelings and his feelings of helplessness and social alienation may serve to explain why he joined a gang. The gang provided him with a peer group that offered protection and also validated his feelings and his defensive acting-out behaviors.

ACCULTURATION ACROSS HISTORY: CHANGING VIEWS

The history of the United States is a history of immigration. The massive migrations that have shaped the identity of the United States throughout its history as a nation have often given rise to nativist movements, whose goal has been to stop or decrease immigration. They are led by the previously settled inhabitants, who perceive a threat to their established customs, or fear competition in their job markets. These fears are often enhanced by the high fertility rates found among immigrant minority groups and lower fertility rates found among the more established groups.[18] These historical events contributed to the notion that the best way to enter into the American culture was to assimilate, totally renouncing the culture of origin and immediately becoming

American. This model applied well to immigrants arriving from Europe in the 1800s and into the twentieth century. Most of these immigrants had similar ethnic characteristics and often Americanized their names, forming the American melting pot. The term acculturation was first used in 1936 by a group of anthropologists of the Social Sciences Research Council, and became an issue of wide discussion after the burgeoning refugee and immigrant resettlement crisis generated after World War II.[19] The acculturation process causes change not only in the immigrant but also in the receiving culture, leading to a process of interculturation. Immigrants often choose one of several acculturation strategies: (1) cultural maintenance (choosing to what extent cultural characteristics are important to maintain), (2) cultural participation (determining how they participate with members of the host culture, or remain among themselves), (3) integration (equivalent to assimilation), and (4) marginalization (choosing to segregate themselves from the host culture).[5] The United States is an ethnically complex society, so rather than understanding acculturation as a uniform and linear phenomenon, Portes and Rumbaut[20] have proposed the concept of segmented acculturation. Their research has mapped segments of immigrants with different patterns of acculturation in the United States, whose differences are determined by factors that are intrinsic to the immigrant, as well as factors that are intrinsic to the particular area of the host country to which the immigrant has arrived. For example, an immigrant from a rural area in Cambodia arriving in Oregon has a different acculturation experience to that of an Eastern European professional arriving in a northeastern American city to further his professional training.

Effects of Acculturation on Children, Adolescents and Their Families

The family is the primary context in which the child grows, develops an identity, is socialized, is hurt and healed, and struggles with powerful developmental issues.[21] There is an abundant literature describing how people of different cultures express their distress.[22,23] The process of immigration causes intrafamilial stressors that result from the process of acculturation, because family members frequently have different levels of acculturation and family bonds can be threatened by conflicting acculturation responses. In addition, sometimes even members of the third and fourth generation may still differ from the dominant culture in their customs, values, and behaviors. For example, Cespedes and Huey[24] found that Hispanic female adolescents experienced more discrepancy in gender roles between themselves and their parents than Hispanic male adolescents. These discrepancies led to increased levels of depression and poorer family functioning for Hispanic girls, but not for boys. Romero and colleagues[25] reported similar findings for Hispanic female adolescents, but found that bicultural stress and depression affected Asian female adolescents even more, when both groups were compared with European Americans.

For Asian Americans in particular, there is the added stress of being looked on as the model minority, which has progressively been debunked but still casts long shadows. Originally coined by sociologist William Peterson in the 1960s to describe Japanese Americans who had assimilated successfully into American culture, this catch phrase was reapplied by the media in the 1980s to expound on the educational triumphs of Asian Americans.[4] Although some Asian Americans may take pride in the model minority image, the general consensus in academia and Asian American studies is that this image is detrimental to Asian Americans because it can lead to stereotyping and to viewing Asian Americans as a uniform group. This may affect resources allotted by federal assistance programs to Asian ethnic subgroups in need. In addition, the model minority myth may play a significant role in Asian American mental health. Asian American scholars have postulated that the pressures exerted by Asian-American parents on their children, so they will do well in school can lead to increased suicide rates.[26] Among 15- to 24-year-old women, Asian Americans have the highest rates (14.1%) of suicide deaths compared with other racial groups in the United States. Asian American men of the same age have the second-highest rate of suicide deaths, at 12.7%.[27] Despite these alarming statistics and other mental health problems such as depression, there is still consistent underuse of mental health resources by Asian Americans across the United States.[28]

Case 3

Joann is a 17-year-old Asian American adolescent girl of Vietnamese descent who presented to the outpatient clinic after her mother brought her in for evaluation of "academic problems." Her mother was primarily concerned that Joann's grades had fallen from As to Bs and Cs during her junior year of high school, and that her poor performance would adversely affect her chances of entrance to a prestigious university and becoming a lawyer. Joann had been reporting problems concentrating and after some hesitation, her family decided that it was time to get her some help. She was seen by a psychiatrist and was diagnosed with clinical depression and eating disorder. She also had difficulty sleeping, decreased appetite, and had been exercising 2 to 3 hours a day in an effort to "look like Asian girls should." She reported passive suicidal ideations, with occasional cutting that was unknown to her parents. Joann came from a middle-class blended family, and her mother had recently given birth to a younger half-brother, who "is treated like a prince." She had limited knowledge of her biologic father until this past year, when he contacted her without her mother's knowledge, and she learned that he lived in a different part of the state and had difficulty maintaining consistent employment. Joann felt that she was not able to really talk to her parents about how sad and confused she felt in relation to her recent reconnection with her father. "All they want to talk about is grades, and how I need to do well on my SATs or I won't get accepted into UC Berkeley or Stanford." She felt the only person in whom she could confide was her boyfriend. Joann was sexually active with him and they practiced the rhythm method of contraception. She constantly felt insecure "because I just worry he's going to leave me for a hotter, skinnier Asian girl." Joann and her mother reluctantly engaged in therapy and were firmly against psychopharmacologic intervention. "I don't want to take medications just because I'm messed up. I should be able to handle this… and no way am I going to take medications. My parents are definitely against anything that's not 'natural'."

Several factors in Joann's case are commonly encountered by clinicians when treating Asian American teens: parental and societal pressures to succeed, in addition to parental focus on academic success, without attention to emotional well-being, compounded by stigma against mental health treatment. Clinicians treating Asian Americans should be aware of how these cultural demands may play an important role in the mental health of this population.

One of the functions of the parents in the family is to teach and to provide leadership and guidance in firm but loving ways. This capacity can be weakened by immigration. If there are disagreements between parents and children about the basic blueprint of how the family should operate, this can be destructive and may lead to triangulation among the different family members. Family factors have a direct effect on the development of adverse outcomes of children and adolescents, and exert a strong influence in which behaviors endure and are linked to adolescent substance-abuse disorders and delinquency.[29] Also, family functioning and acculturation often have a circular effect on one another. For example, Hovey and King[30] described how low levels of family functioning increase acculturative stress, which in turn leads to depressive symptoms in the adolescents of immigrant families. Also, Duarte and colleagues[31] found that low parental acculturation was associated with more antisocial behaviors in Puerto Rican adolescents living in New York City, as well as in Puerto Rico. Conversely, adaptive family processes can serve as a protective factor in high-risk environments and alleviate adolescent problems that have already surfaced. For example, Liu and colleagues[32] studied Chinese immigrant families residing in the United States and found that adolescents with Chinese mothers who were more acculturated, had higher levels of maternal monitoring of their children, and used less harsh discipline had lower levels of conduct problems. In a recent Harvard study of high-school students,[33] Asian American students who participated and reported symptoms of depression had higher grades than their peers but reported more concern about academic factors and also felt that their parents were not interested in their emotional lives.

Language barriers sometimes result in disempowering the parents of immigrant children. For example, parents of minority children are expected to advocate on behalf of their children in schools and in neighborhoods that are often filled with discrimination and prejudice. A good command of the English language is often necessary to undertake these tasks. Liu and colleagues[34] found that Chinese mothers who were more proficient in English tended to have children with higher academic scores and fewer depressive symptoms. In addition, these researchers found that proficiency in both English and the native Chinese language was a protective factor against depression for foreign-born young Chinese people, more than for young Chinese people born in the United States.

Among immigrant families, it is not unusual for a disciplinary meeting to take place at school in which the child serves as the translator between the parents and the school teacher or principal, thus undermining the hierarchical structure of the family and compromising the executive power of the parents in the eyes of the school authorities.

Parents of different cultures also relate differently to institutions. In some cultures, such as among members of the Asian cultures, institutions are greatly respected and considered sacred and never challenged. There are also countries, such as Haiti, where citizens have been subjected to centuries of abuse and persecution. It is not uncommon for psychiatrists to come into contact with Haitian immigrants who may initially perceive American institutions as potentially cruel and persecutory, and relate to them with fear and distrust. This fear and distrust also permeate the therapeutic relationship; the psychiatrist often has to use tact, empathy, patience, and perseverance to overcome this resistance. These distorted perceptions can undermine the parents' capacity to advocate for their children in the new, host culture. The family member with the greatest competence in the mainstream American culture is the best prepared to negotiate with powerful extrafamilial systems, such as courts, schools, and social agencies.[31]

Language and Ethnicity in the Second Generation

Acquisition of unaccented English has been, and continues to be, the litmus test of citizenship in the United States. In no other country are languages extinguished with such speed.[35] For immigrants, the switch to English is both an empiric fact and a cultural requirement demanded of those who have sought a new life in America. Kataoka and colleagues[36] found that in California, students with lower English-language proficiency had a disproportionate impairment in difficulties with grades. Outside the ethnic enclaves that exist in the United States, to speak English only is a prerequisite for social acceptance and integration, and those who try to educate their children in their mother tongue confront immense pressure for social conformity from peers, teachers, and the media. Portes and Rumbaut[20] explain that "In a country lacking centuries old traditions, and simultaneously receiving thousands of foreigners from the most diverse lands, language homogeneity has been seen as the bedrock of nationhood"[(p96)].

Several empiric studies highlight that the first generation of immigrants learns enough English to survive economically, the second generation (born in the United States to immigrant parents) may use the parental tongue at home but use English in school, and in the third generation, the home language and mother tongue shift to English.[35] Language use can also have subtle connotations in everyday life in America. Waters[37] studied first- and second-generation blacks in New York City and noted that middle-class blacks convey, through the use of mainstream English, verbal and nonverbal cues that they are not from the ghetto and that they disapprove of ghetto-specific behavior.

Language retention is closely related to socioeconomic variables. For example, immigrant children growing up in impoverished communities receive no encouragement to retain their parents' native language, because the native language is stigmatized as a symbol of lower status.[35] This is the case in second-generation Haitian young people in Miami, who rapidly shed Haitian Creole for English and prefer to be identified as African American, rather than Haitian American.

Portes and Stepic[38] studied language use in Miami, Florida. They found that Spanish was alive and well among first-generation Cuban immigrants, but that language retention decreased in proportion to the length of stay in the United States. They found that despite the economic prosperity, excellent self-esteem, and social support offered by the Cuban ethnic enclave in Miami, 90% of second-generation Cubans preferred to communicate in English.

The interplay between the immigrant parents and their children in the second generation also accounts for the type of "goodness of fit"[39] that occurs in the acculturation process into the United States. Generational consonance occurs when parents and children acculturate at the same rate, or when the parents encourage selective acculturation among the second generation, such that the cultural harmony between parents and children is maintained, allowing the children to adapt to their new American reality. Cultural dissonance occurs when the second generation is neither guided nor accompanied by the changes in the first generation. Consonant resistance to acculturation occurs among isolated immigrant groups that are strongly oriented toward return and view their presence in the host society as temporary, such as exiles.[20]

Case 4

Kathy (Ekaterina), an 18-year-old adolescent girl, emigrated from Russia to Miami with her family at the age of 7 years. Kathy was referred for psychotherapy because of oppositional-defiant behavior at home and difficulties getting along with her parents. Kathy shared with her Hispanic male therapist that she felt "very American," and added "I feel embarrassed to take anyone to visit my home, because my parents barely speak English and they insist on speaking to me in Russian in front of my friends. It makes me stand out and feel different and I don't like it. I just want to be a regular person, like everyone else. My parents don't make any effort to fit in, they just hang out with other Russian people and they don't understand anything about my life, it's like they live in another planet."

This case presents an example of how language use increases the cultural dissonance between 2 generations of an immigrant family. This dissonance leads to feelings of alienation in the adolescent, who lacks the necessary guidance and protection that parents are able to provide during the adolescent passage.

RESILIENCY AND RISK

Second-generation children (American-born offspring of immigrants) have been found to be at higher risk of more behavioral conditions, such as substance abuse, conduct disturbance, and eating disorders, than the first generation of immigrant young people.[31,40,41] In some groups, such higher risk may be a result of this group facing the chronic stresses created by poverty, marginalization, and discrimination without the secure identity and traditional values of their parents, when they do not yet have a secure bicultural identity and skills. Garcia and Lindgren[42] studied Hispanic families and found that adolescents boys reported that having to work in addition to or instead of going to school to provide financially for the family was the key stressor of immigration, whereas the girls complained about losing relationships and mothers spoke about the fears of deportation, listing names of friends who had been deported. Also, Pumariega and colleagues[43] found that second-generation Mexican Americans who had an overreliance on peers, were more exposed to the media, and spent less time with their families and in religious activities had a significantly higher risk of substance abuse and suicidality[44] than more traditional young people born and living in Mexico. Various studies have shown greater risk for eating disorders in more acculturated immigrant young people both in the United States and in Europe.[44] This situation may hold particularly true for Asian Americans, who face the double pressure of perfectionism brought on by the expectations of the model minority myth and the glorification of the perfect body image. Low self-esteem and personal identity confusion can result from feeling marginalized and discriminated against and often lead to substance abuse, increased sexual risk-taking behavior, conduct problems, and poor school performance[45]; acculturation orientation has been associated with prosocial behaviors.[46] Being the victim of racism has been associated with low self-esteem, depression, poor school performance, and poor school motivation, as well as increased parent-child conflicts.[47] Some second-generation immigrants seem to be more vulnerable to the effects of racism than those who were born outside the United States. For example, US-born Chinese people reported experiencing more discrimination than those who were born in Asia.[48] Yet, Chinese-Americans who remained close to the Chinese culture experienced less depressive symptoms than those who reported feeling more dissociated from the Chinese culture.[49] Also, self-esteem proved to be the most important protective factor against substance abuse among Hispanic adolescents who resided in monocultural Hispanic households.[50]

Racism, discrimination, and social marginalization among minority adolescents often lead to the development of adversarial identities, such as affiliation with gangs. The adolescent who feels marginalized and discriminated, lacking opportunities for upward mobility and who belongs to a racially unmeltable minority group, seeks validation from peers, standing in defiance of the values of the mainstream majority culture.[51]

Adolescent refugees have also been found to be at high risk for mental health problems, especially posttraumatic stress disorder and depression. These problems are often unrecognized by parents and teachers, and culturally competent mental health services for refugees are often lacking.[52,53]

The degree of closeness among family members varies according to whether the family functions as a nuclear or extended network system. Some Hispanic and Asian families function as extended families, and thus mothers and grandmothers act as coparents to the children. In these families, the failure to involve key family members in therapy, such as grandmothers, can lead to sabotage of the therapy by the excluded member. Also, the degree of closeness among family members and the sense of filial duty tend to be greater in extended families. Rodriguez and Weisburd[54] reported that adolescents who are closer to their families are also less reliant on their peers. When the level of family bonding is high, adolescents tend to find peers whose values and beliefs are similar to those of their families. This tendency can serve as a protective factor, but may also slow down acculturation. A greater degree of acculturation is also inversely related to family obligations, because immigrants frequently transition from an extended family network system more commonly found in developing countries, to a nuclear family, which is more commonly found in industrialized societies.

Loyalty and conformity are also influenced by how authority is handled in the family. Some cultures have families in which authority is linear and hierarchical, maintaining traditional gender roles, whereas others are more egalitarian and emphasize negotiation. Sometimes, immigration-related changes in parental authority and communication can undermine the traditional family structure and lead to family deterioration. For example, language can present a concrete obstacle to communication among the members of different generations within the immigrant family. If well-acculturated adolescents speak only English and parents and grandparents speak only the language of the country of origin, this diminishes the amount of communication. Interests and shared experiences decrease, and the parents and children may feel a sense of distancing that makes them believe that they are living in different worlds. Szapozc-nik and colleagues[29] studied Cuban families with poorly acculturated parents who spoke little English and with well-acculturated adolescents who spoke little Spanish. They found that these adolescents felt alienated from their parents, had an overreliance on their peer group, and gravitated toward peers who felt equally alienated. These adolescents were found to be more at risk for depression, substance abuse, and delinquent acting-out behaviors. In contrast, German and colleagues[55] found that among Mexican American adolescents, higher levels of family involvement acted as a protective factor against deviant peer affiliation, and accounted for lower levels of conduct problems and externalizing behaviors. Zayas and colleagues[56] reported that among Hispanic adolescent females who attempted suicide, less mutuality between mothers and daughters increased suicide risk, whereas increased communication between mothers and daughters served as a protective factor against suicide. In addition, McHale and collegues[57] reported less depression and involvement in risky behaviors among Mexican American adolescents who were well supervised by their parents, as well as more involvement in academic activities when the parents valued the importance of education.

In addition to family integrity, love, and supportive communities, school has been found to play an important role in the resiliency of immigrant and second-generation adolescents in the United States. The Longitudinal Immigrant Student Adaptation Project (LISA)[58] showed that immigrant families place their hopes of improvement on providing a better education for their children. Dominican immigrants in New York City have the third-lowest level of educational attainment of all immigrants to the United States. However, in less than one generation, their children accomplish the highest level of school retention and the highest percentage of high-school completion of all the immigrant groups in the New York public school system.[59] This "Dominican miracle in New York"[60] supports the finding that success in school is one of the most important predictors of psychosocial adaptation for first- and second-generation immigrant children to American society. Immigrant children who succeeded in school also became more connected to their ethnic communities.

Rather than shamefully distancing themselves from the cultural heritage of their parents, these children saw success in school as payback for their parents' efforts and sacrifices, and as a way to make their community proud of their success.[58]

MEASURING ACCULTURATION

Acculturation is a complex construct that presents a challenge to investigators because it encompasses socioeconomic, historical, political, and psychodynamic variables. For this reason, the study of acculturation has become of interest to the fields of sociology, political science, economics, and the mental health sciences. The inherent complexity of how culture influences cognitive mechanisms and human behavior may help to explain the proliferation of acculturation measures and the lack of substantive reviews of the literature that evaluate the specificity and validity of these measures. The understanding of acculturation has evolved from a linear concept to a multidimensional process of confluence between the cultural-heritage community and the cultural-receiving community. In the linear model of acculturation, the components of acculturation that are assumed to change are (1) language and (2) cultural practices. In most of these studies, greater acculturation is associated with negative outcomes, a concept known as the immigrant paradox.[61,62] However, Schwartz and colleagues[63] highlight that it is not clear whether the negative outcomes that appear with progressive acculturation are caused by acquiring new practices, or to losing the practices of the heritage culture. These investigators add that it is also not clear whether immigrants should be discouraged from acquiring new practices, or encouraged to preserve the old ones. Escobar and Vega[19] have concluded that little explanatory power is added to psychiatric epidemiologic studies by the inclusion of multidimensional acculturation scales. Instead, when conducting epidemiologic studies, the preferred language, the person's place of birth, and number of years residing in the United States are frequently used as proxies for acculturation. They are used as dependent variables that have consistent main effects on problems such as drug use and psychiatric disorders. Preferred language and place of birth are also stronger predictors when using multivariate models to predict health outcomes. However, Schwartz and colleagues[63] argue that the linear model of studying acculturation misses multiple dimensions that are involved in acculturation. In terms of language use, these investigators propose that some immigrants may identify with their culture of origin, yet not be proficient in their heritage language, such as many Asians in the United States. In terms of ethnic identification, traditionally most white non-Hispanics have identified themselves as American. However, with the changing racial composition of the United States, it is unclear whether in the future people who reside in the United States will continue to equate American with white. Cultural values are assumed to change when the person acculturates. Some of the values that have been attributed to certain immigrant groups are also common to other groups. Schwartz and colleagues[63] argue that more than being characteristic of any ethnic group in particular, these values may be common to people who emigrate from collectivist, agricultural societies to individualistic, industrialized societies, and that it is important for acculturation measures to take into account the context of reception of the host country, for example, if the immigrant is arriving in a rural, possibly more closed community versus an urban, possibly more open community, the economic characteristics of the community and of the host country at the time of the immigrant's arrival and whether the skills that the immigrant possesses or lacks are valued in the host community at the time of the immigrant's arrival. Biculturalism can vary from a model that involves synthesizing the elements of both cultures to the point at which the separation of the elements of each culture sometimes becomes indistinct, to a model of blended biculturalism, in which the immigrant keeps the cultural values, practices, and identifications of the heritage culture separate from the new influences. Schwartz and colleagues[63] propose that in future studies, to accurately understand and measure acculturation, 6 processes need to be taken into account: (1) the practices, (2) values, and (3) cultural identifications of the receiving culture; and the (1) practices, (2) values, and (3) cultural identifications of the heritage culture.

SUMMARY AND RECOMMENDATIONS

The process of immigration and acculturation often leads to a fluidity of household compositions that may generate distancing and conflicts among the different family members and result in adverse mental health outcomes. Clinicians treating immigrant children, adolescents, and their families must be prepared to understand divergent, and often well-hidden, world views, as well as difficulties with acculturation that may cause intrafamilial conflicts and that interfere with the completion of the child's developmental process. Most important is to keep in mind that the children of today's immigrants are a generation oriented not to their parents' immigrant pasts, but to their own American futures.

REFERENCES

1. Redfield R, Linton R, Herskovits M. Memorandum on the study of acculturation. Am Anthropol 1936;38:149–52.
2. Coatsworth JH. Globalization, growth and welfare in history. In: Suarez-Orozco MM, Baolian Qin-Hilliard D, editors. Globalization, culture and education in the new millennium. Berkeley (CA): University of California Press; 2004. p. 1.
3. Suarez-Orozco MM, Baolian Quin-Hilliard D. Globalization, culture and education in the new millennium. Berkeley (CA): University of California Press; 2004.
4. Chang I. The Chinese in America, a narrative history. New York: The Penguin Group; 2003.
5. Berry JW. Immigration, acculturation and adaptation. Appl Psychol 1997; 46(1):5–68.
6. US Census. Population reports. Available at: http://www.census.gov/population/www/index.html. Accessed June 1, 2003.
7. Hughes CC. Culture in clinical psychiatry. In: Gaw AC, editor. Culture ethnicity and mental illness. Washington, DC: American Psychiatric Press; 1993. p. 3–42.
8. Porter JW. Black child-white child: the development of racial attitudes. Cambridge (MA): Harvard University Press; 1971.
9. Erikson EH. Childhood and society. New York: Norton; 1950.
10. Erikson EH. Identity: youth and crisis. New York: Norton; 1968.
11. Schwartz SJ, Montgomery MJ. Similarities or differences in identity development? The impact of acculturation and gender identity in process and outcome. J Youth Adolesc 2002;31(5):359–72.
12. Schwartz SJ, Montgomery MJ, Briones E. The role of identity and acculturation among immigrant people: theoretical propositions, empirical questions, and applied recommendations. Hum Dev 2005;304:1–30.
13. Stein J, Urdang L, editors. Random House dictionary of the English language: the unabridged edition. New York: Random House; 1966.
14. DeVos G. Ethnic adaptation and minority status. J Cross Cult Psychol 1980;11: 101–12.

15. Ogbu JU. Minority education and caste: the American system in cross-cultural perspective. New York: Academic Press; 1978.
16. Ticho G. Cultural aspects of transference and countertransference. Bull Menninger Clin 1971;35:313–34.
17. Garza-Guerrero AC. Culture shock: its mourning and the vicissitudes of identity. J Am Psychoanal Assoc 1977;2:408–31.
18. Pedraza S. Origins and destinies: immigration, race and ethnicity in contemporary American history. In: Pedraza S, Rumbaut RG, editors. Origins and destines: immigration, race and ethnicity in America. Belmont (CA): Wadsworth Press; 1996. p. 1–20.
19. Escobar JI, Vega WA. Mental health and immigration's three AAA's: Where are we and where do we go from here? J Nerv Ment Dis 2000;188(11):736–40.
20. Portes A, Rumbaut RG. Immigrant America: a portrait. 2nd edition. Berkeley (CA): University of California Press; 1997.
21. Santiesteban DA, Mitrani VB. The influence of acculturation process on the family. In: Chun KM, Organista PB, Marin G, editors. Acculturation: advances in the theory, measurement, and applied research. Washington, DC: American Psychological Association; 2003. p. 121–35.
22. Rogler LH. International migrations: a framework for directing research. Am Psychol 1994;49:701–8.
23. Saldana DH. Acculturative stress and minority status. Hispanic Journal of Behavioral Health Sciences 1994;16:117–25.
24. Cespedes YM, Huey SJ Jr. Depression in Latino adolescents: a cultural discrepancy perspective. Cultur Divers Ethnic Minor Psychol 2008;14(2):168–72.
25. Romero AJ, Carvajal SC, Valle F, et al. Adolescent bicultural stress and its impact on mental well-being among Latinos, Asian Americans, and European Americans. J Community Psychol 2007;35(4):519–34.
26. Leong F, Leach M, Yeh C, et al. Suicide among Asian Americans: what do we know? what do we need to know? Death Stud 2007;31:417–34.
27. Lee S, Juon HS, Martinez G, et al. Model minority at risk: expressed needs of mental health by Asian American young adults. J Community Health 2008; 34(2):144–52.
28. Durvasula R, Sue S. Severity of disturbance among Asian American outpatients. Cult Divers Ment Health 1996;2:43–51.
29. Szapocznik J, Ladner S, Scopetta MA. Youth, drug abuse and subjective distress in the Hispanic population. In: Beschner L, Friedman L, editors. Youth and drug abuse. Lexington (KY): Lexington Books; 1979. p. 197–209.
30. Hovey J, King C. Acculturative stress, depression and suicidal ideation among immigrant and second generation Latino adolescents. J Am Acad Child Adolesc Psychiatry 1996;35:1183–92.
31. Pumariega A, Rothe EM, Pumariega J. Mental health of immigrants and refugees. Community Ment Health J 2005;45(5):581–97.
32. Liu LL, Lau AS, Chia-Chen Chen A, et al. The influence of maternal acculturation, neighborhood disadvantage, and parenting on Chinese American adolescents' conduct problems: testing the segmented assimilation hypothesis. J Youth Adolesc 2009;38:691–702.
33. Song S. Presentation to the Northern California Psychiatric Society Asian American Issues Committee, Fall 2009.
34. Liu LL, Benner AD, Lau AS, et al. Mother-adolescent language proficiency and adolescent academic and emotional adjustment among Chinese American families. J Youth Adolesc 2009;38:572–86.

35. Portes A, Schlauffer R. Language and the second generation: bilingualism yesterday and today. In: Portes A, editor. The new second generation. New York: Russel-Sage; 1996. p. 28.
36. Kataoka S, Langley A, Stein B, et al. Violence exposure and PTSD: the role of English language fluency in Latino youth. J Child Fam Stud 2009;18:334–41.
37. Waters MC. Ethnic and racial identities of second-generation black immigrants in New York City. In: Portes A, editor. The new second generation. New York: Russel-Sage; 1996. p. 177.
38. Portes A, Stepic A. City on the edge: the transformation of Miami. Berkeley (CA): University of California Press; 1993.
39. Winnicott DW. The maturational processes and the facilitating environment. 11th edition. Madison (WI): International Universities Press; 1988.
40. Almqvist K, Broberg A. Mental health and social adjustment in young refugee children 3 1/2 years after their arrival in Sweden. J Am Acad Child Adolesc Psychiatry 1999;38(6):723–30.
41. Fox P, Burns K, Popovich J, et al. Southeast Asian refugee children: self-esteem as a predictor of depression and scholastic achievement in the U.S. Int J Psychiatr Nurs Res 2004;9(2):1063–72.
42. Garcia C, Lindgren S. Life grows between the rocks: Latino adolescents' and parents' perspectives on mental health stressors. Res Nurs Health 2009;32: 148–62.
43. Pumariega A, Swanson JW, Holzer C, et al. Cultural context and substance abuse in Hispanic adolescents. J Child Fam Stud 1992;1(1):75–92.
44. Miller M, Pumariega AJ. Eating disorders: a historical and cross-cultural review. Psychiatry 2001;64(2):93–110.
45. Schwartz SJ, Mason CA, Pantin H, et al. Relationships of social context and identity to problem behavior among high-risk Hispanic adolescents. Youth Soc 2009;40:541–70.
46. Schwartz SJ, Zamboanga BL, Hernandez Jarvis L. Ethnic identity and acculturation in Hispanic early adolescents: mediated relationships to academic grades, prosocial behaviors, and externalizing symptoms. Cultur Divers Ethnic Minor Psychol 2007;13(4):364–73.
47. Portes PR, Zady MF. Self-esteem in the adaptation of Spanish-speaking adolescents: the role of immigration, family conflict, and depression. Hisp J Behav Sci 2002;24:296–318.
48. Yoo HC, Lee RM. Does ethnic identity buffer or exacerbate the effects of frequent racial discrimination on situational well-being of Asian-Americans? Asian American Journal of Psychology 2009;S(1):70–87.
49. Juang LP, Cookston JT. Acculturation, discrimination, and depressive symptoms among Chinese American adolescents: a longitudinal study. J Primary Prevent 2009;30:475–96.
50. Zamboanga BL, Schwartz SJ, Hernandez Jarvis L, et al. Acculturation and substance use among Hispanic early adolescents: investigating the mediating roles of acculturative stress and self-esteem. J Primary Prevent 2009;30:315–33.
51. Vigil D. Barrio gangs: street life and identity in Southern California. Austin (TX): University of Texas; 1988.
52. Lustig SL, Kia-Keating M, Grant-Knight W, et al. Review of child and adolescent psychiatry refugee mental health. J Am Acad Child Adolesc Psychiatry 2004; 43(1):24–36.
53. Rothe EM. Post-traumatic stress symptoms in Cuban children and adolescents during and after refugee camp confinement. In: Corales TA, editor. Trends in

post-traumatic stress disorder research. New York: Nova Science Publishers; 2005. p. 101–27.

54. Rodriguez O, Weisburd D. The integrated social control model and ethnicity: the case of Puerto Rican-American delinquency. Crim Justice Behav 1991;18:464–9.

55. Germán M, Gonzales NA, Dumka L. Familism values as a protective factor for Mexican-origin adolescents exposed to deviant peers. J Early Adolesc 2009; 29:16–42.

56. Zayas LH, Bright CL, Alvarez-Sanchez T, et al. Acculturation, familism and mother–daughter relations among suicidal and non-suicidal adolescent Latinas. J Primary Prevent 2009;30:351–69.

57. McHale SM, Updegraff KA, Kim JY, et al. Cultural orientations, daily activities, and adjustment in Mexican American youth. J Youth Adolesc 2009;38:627–41.

58. Suarez-Orozco C, Suarez-Orozco MM. Children of immigration. Cambridge (MA): Harvard University Press; 2001.

59. Pew Hispanic Center. Available at: http://www.pewhispanic.org; 2007. Accessed, November 20, 2009.

60. Rothe EM. La Salud Mental de los Inmigrantes Latinoamericanos en los Estados Unidos. Revista Latinoamericana de Psiquiatria 2006;6:46–57 [in Spanish].

61. Alegria M, Canino G, Shrout P, et al. Prevalence of mental illness in immigrant and non-immigrant U.S. groups. Am J Psychiatry 2008;165:359–69.

62. Alegria M, Shrout P, Sribney W, et al. Understanding differences in past year mental health disorders for Latinos living in the U.S. Soc Sci Med 2007;65: 214–30.

63. Schwartz SJ, Unger JB, Zamboaga BL, et al. Rethinking the concept of acculturation: implications for theory, measurement and health research. Am Psychol 2010;65(4):237–51.

Language, Culture, and Adaptation in Immigrant Children

Claudio O. Toppelberg, MD[a,b,c,]*, Brian A. Collins, PhD[d]

KEYWORDS
- Dual language • Minority • Immigrant • Bilingual
- Psychopathology • Development

OVERVIEW

In this article the authors first discuss why it is crucial, from a clinical and public health perspective, to better understand the development as well as risk and protection processes for the mental health of immigrant children. This article focuses on Latino immigrant children because they represent the majority of immigrant children in America and it is a way to illustrate the risks and circumstances that are potentially shared by other immigrant groups. The authors then shift focus to the main tenet of this article, namely, that specific aspects of the dual language development of immigrant children are highly relevant to their mental health and adaptation. This argument is illustrated with the case of Latino immigrant children. Finally, the authors differentiate dual language development and its mental health impact from the dual-culture (bicultural) development and circumstance of immigrant children.

BACKGROUND: LATINO CHILD IMMIGRATION TO THE UNITED STATES
Demographic Significance of Child Immigration

America is currently experiencing the largest wave of child immigration in its history. Children of immigrants constitute the largest minority and the fastest growing segment of the US child population.[1,2] One out of 7 children was from an immigrant family in 1990, more than 1 out of 5 children has such a background in 2010, and it is estimated

This study was supported primarily by National Institute of Mental Health grant number K01 MH01947-01A2 and by an Early Investigator Grant from the American Academy of Child and Adolescent Psychiatry.

a Child Language & Developmental Psychiatry Research Lab, Judge Baker Children's Center, 53 Parker Hill Avenue, Boston, MA 02120-3225, USA
b Manville School, Judge Baker Children's Center, 53 Parker Hill Avenue, Boston, MA 02120-3225, USA
c Harvard Medical School, 25 Shattuck Street, Boston, MA 02115, USA
d Hunter College, 695 Park Avenue, W1023, New York, NY 10065, USA
* Corresponding author. Child Language & Developmental Psychiatry Research Lab, Judge Baker Children's Center, 53 Parker Hill Avenue, Boston, MA 02120-3225.
E-mail address: topi@hms.harvard.edu

Child Adolesc Psychiatric Clin N Am 19 (2010) 697–717
doi:10.1016/j.chc.2010.07.003
1056-4993/10/$ – see front matter © 2010 Elsevier Inc. All rights reserved.

childpsych.theclinics.com

that these figures will rise to 1 out of 3 children by the year 2020.[3] There is a significant 3-way overlap between Latino, dual language, and immigrant children in the United States. The majority of Latino children come from immigrant families, and most immigrant families and children in the United States are Latino.[4] Most immigrant families speak a language other than English at home (most commonly Spanish) and a large proportion of children in America grow up using 2 languages. The past 3 decades have seen a rapid increase in Latinos in the United States with their numbers more than tripling from 1970 (10 million) to 2000 (35 million).[4] Latino children are already the largest minority group in schools.[5]

The majority of children from immigrant families are second-generation immigrants, that is, born in the United States to 1 or 2 foreign-born parents; most US Latino youth are young (median age 12.8) and from the second generation (52%).[6,7] Despite their young age and growing numbers, empirical research addressing the development, wellbeing, and mental health of children of immigrants is lacking, with most of the work focused on adolescents and adults.[8]

Public Health Significance: Risk of Depression, Suicidality, and School Failure in Latino Children

Many children of immigrants, including Latinos, live in families exposed to multiple risk factors, such as poverty; poor schools; neighborhood violence; discrimination; and disparities in access to health care, education, and jobs.[9–11] All these factors are strongly associated with low performance at school and poor psychosocial adaptation, as well as negative economic and health outcomes.[3,12,13] Most of these factors have been found to be associated with high prevalence of mental disorders. In several important areas, Latino youth are at a higher emotional, behavioral, and academic risk than European American and other minority youth.[14,15]

Depression, violence, and substance abuse risk indicators

When compared with European Americans and African Americans, Latino youth (both boys and girls) present the highest prevalence of indicators of depression (36%)[14] and suicidality, including having made a suicide plan (14.5%) or attempt (11%), with this risk being *astonishingly high* among Latino girls.[14,16] Most indicators of violence (being threatened with a weapon or being in a physical fight while on school property, missing school because of safety concerns, carrying a gun or weapon) are higher in Latino than in white and black youth.[14] Latino teenagers have the highest rates of illegal injection drug abuse, methamphetamine, ecstasy, and cocaine.[14] US-born Latinos may have higher behavioral problem prevalence[17] and, in large epidemiologic studies, higher lifetime prevalence of mental disorders (32% to 24%)[18] than foreign-born Latinos (see the later discussion about the immigrant paradox). This prevalence has led 2 prominent Latino researchers to ask the question: "What is it about living in the US that may place Latinos at risk for psychological disorders and suicidal behaviors?"[19]

Educational risk indicators

Latinos as a group have extremely low high school graduation rates (53%),[20] college graduation rates, and achievement and reading scores[21,22] (at grade 11, they average grade 8 achievement levels), but the causes of such alarming educational outcomes are not fully understood. Latino children are 6 times more likely to be placed in special education services. They lag behind African Americans, European Americans, and Asian Americans in high school completion, high-technology education, and college admission. As a consequence, Latino children as a group are more likely to become or remain poor. Educational and socioeconomic status are linked to health in general and to mental health in particular.[9] Although there is important overlap between psychopathology and negative educational outcomes (for instance, depression, conduct, and antisocial disorders are associated with low educational achievement), the extent to which mental health factors contribute to high-school dropout rates and educational failure in Latino youth is unknown.

Protective Processes and Resilience in Children of Immigrants: the Immigrant Paradox

A multidimensional perspective on psychosocial strengths, rather than a narrow, exclusive focus on deficit and pathology, is fundamental in gaining a deeper understanding of the mental health and functioning of Latino children of immigrants. Although many immigrant families and their children face the multiple risk factors already discussed, they also bring with them several characteristics that may serve as protective factors, such as religion, community, optimism, dual frame of reference, and high valuing of education.[23] Many children of immigrants have shown to be extremely resilient despite risk and adversity.[24] Latino parents frequently share the goal to have their children develop instrumental competences and to preserve values related to intrapersonal (*personalismo*) and interpersonal (*respeto*) skills, family connections (*familismo*), the expression of affection (*cariños*), and the value of education (*educación*).[25] These types of strengths are an important part of the traditions and values of Latinos and other immigrant groups and are widely cited in the literature.[2,8,26,27]

For a long time and based on a deficit model, it had been assumed that recent immigrants would have less favorable outcomes than their US-born immigrant and nonimmigrant peers. However, recent empirical work strongly suggests exactly the opposite, namely, that recent immigrants fare better in many areas of health, a phenomenon that has come to be known as *the immigrant paradox*.[12,28,29] Better physical and mental health as well as educational achievement are being documented in foreign-born Latino immigrants (first generation) compared with their US-born counterparts (second and later generations).[9,30] The first generation has lower levels of depression, anxiety, and substance abuse, and higher positive adjustment than their US-born peers,[31–33] in particular in those of Mexican and, to some extent, Cuban descent.[34] As stated before, this raises the question of what it is about living in the United States that may place Latinos at higher risk.[19]

The knowledge base on Latino and other dual language immigrant children is limited and needs to be significantly expanded. For important clinical, public health, and educational reasons, it is critical to understand risk and protective domains specific to the development of these children. Further research expanding evidence-based understanding, and leading to interventions and policy directed at young children of immigrants are critically needed. One specific area that is poorly understood is the impact of these children's developing linguistic competence in 2 languages on their emotional/behavioral functioning and mental health.

THE DEVELOPMENT OF DUAL LANGUAGE (BILINGUAL) COMPETENCE

Most of the research on language development has centered on monolingual children. Although the study of children acquiring 2 or more languages is still in its early stages, significant progress made in the last 3 decades is reviewed in the section that follows.

The Development of Dual Language Linguistic Competence

Domains of language development

Language competence is composed of competences in specific domains of language development, such as phonology (the sound system), syntax and morphology (principles that govern word order and word formation), and lexicon/semantics (vocabulary, meaning), all of which interface with language usage (pragmatics, discourse).[35–37] Although first-language acquisition is a lifelong process, the majority takes place during early childhood.[35,38,39] Language competence is not a stable construct[40] but, rather, a fluctuating, dynamic, multidomain capacity.[41,42]

The influence of the environments of the child on dual language development

Dual language development is dependent, among other factors, on the type and amount of exposure and the age at which children begin acquiring their second language. Sequential bilinguals acquire their first language (L1) during the period of rapid language acquisition before 3 years of age and a second language (L2) later. Simultaneous bilinguals acquire both languages as first languages (2 L1s). Because Latino children in the United States typically acquire Spanish as an L1 and English as an L2, most are sequential bilinguals. The term *dual language* children has become favored over *bilingual* more recently, because it does not presuppose full proficiency in both languages and it allows for the reality of individual differences in bilingual development, with wide variability of L1 and L2 competences.[43,44]

Sequential bilinguals have their language competences distributed across languages, with varying degrees of skills in each language, particularly in those domains highly dependent upon language exposure, such as semantics.[45,46] In this way, it would be natural to find, in Spanish/English dual language children, that vocabulary related to the school context is stronger in English, whereas that related to the home context is stronger in Spanish. This situation presents unique complexities in the mental processing of their language systems, and how these relate to their adaptational functioning and their ability to tap into protective resources.

Although it is rare for anyone to be equally proficient across all linguistic contexts and domains, high competence in both languages is possible.[47] Also common is for bilinguals to be dominant in 1 language, but the particular configuration of language dominance varies widely.[48] The dominant language of an individual often fluctuates over time and across contexts,[49] so that language dominance is not stable.

Because of the assimilative forces that propel children of immigrants to learn English quickly, language shift or loss starts occurring as soon as they begin school. Second-generation immigrants are more likely to lose their first language than to remain bilingual.[50] Contrary to the popularized (but inaccurate) belief that immigrant children are not learning English, this process of L1 loss is occurring much sooner than in prior waves of immigration, when it was more typical for the second generation to remain bilingual, and only for the third generation to become English dominant.[51–53] Outside of the home, children of immigrants often start using English exclusively, and in the home, as much as they can,[33] even when they have only learned barely enough to muddle through communication.[54] Considering the frequent discrimination and stigmas associated with speaking a language other than English in the United States,[55] it is understandable that children will prefer to speak the dominant, community language. This result of societal and school pressures, combined with a devalued view of the minority language, is truly unfortunate, as there is wide consensus among dual language acquisition researchers that it is not necessary for children to have to abandon their home language to develop strong competences in the second, majority language[56] and that proficient bilingualism, a normative developmental outcome, often results in academic, cognitive, and social benefits.[43,45,57–59]

The development of both the L1 and L2 is to a good extent dependent upon the level of language support and language exposure. *Subtractive* bilingualism tends to occur when L2 acquisition comes at the cost of the loss of the L1, when children are submersed in a majority language with limited support and exposure to their home language (subtractive bilingual settings).[51,60–62] *Additive* bilingualism, in contrast, is common in settings where substantial support for the L1 is offered as the L2 is acquired,[51] which leads to the well-documented benefits of proficiency in 2 languages.[38,57,63,64] Research from 2 decades ago[65] suggested that increased movement toward English-language use among children of immigrants occurs primarily during the adolescent years as youths spend more time in contexts outside of the home. However, more recent research is showing a similar shift much earlier, when children first begin schooling and develop proficiency and general preference for the English language. Language shift has been evidenced as early as preschool or kindergarten, and through the elementary grades.[66] Wong-Fillmore[62] found that early exposure to English leads to first-language loss. The younger children are when they learn English, the greater the effect; children attending L2 preschools were subsequently more likely to be unable to speak the home language than children who attended L1 preschools. For all children, there is an established relationship between the linguistic environment at home and children's later language competence.[67,68] Children in stimulating environments show more rapid language development[69] and maternal language abilities contribute to large variation in children's vocabulary growth.[70] Children from lower socioeconomic status (SES) have lower language skills and smaller vocabularies than children from higher SES.[71,72] For dual language children, the linguistic environment at home is closely associated with children's language preference, dominance, competence, and usage.[43,73] It is therefore clear that the environments at home and school are influential in language development and, more specifically, the maintenance and loss of first and second languages. Societal and school pressures to lose L1 raise serious ethical concerns. Ethical concerns arise because pressing children into losing their first language and the chance of proficiency in their 2 languages means, in an increasingly globalized economy and diverse society, "to deprive them of access to important job- and life-related skills."[74]

The development of children's home language may associate with strengthening of family cohesion and intimacy, parental authority, and transmission of cultural norms, all of which can lead to healthy adjustment and a strong identification and internalization of the social values of the family.[75–79] Developing L2 skills is crucial for academic success and long-term social and economic well-being[80,81] because children's ability to function within the school context influences school retention, graduation rates, and continuation into higher education.

For adolescents, the wide range of media increasingly available in immigrants' L1s (radio, television, and the Internet) may help immigrants maintain a meaningful connection to their heritage, culture, and language, but also allows increased access to aspects of American society.[82] Likewise, prior exposure to the destination language before migration contributes to better skills in the host language upon immigration.[83]

Contextualized interpersonal communication skills versus decontextualized academic language proficiency

All children typically move between language environments throughout the day, as the characteristics of language spoken differs from the classroom to other environments, with a remarkable contrast in the quality of language competences required. Language at home and the playground tends to be *contextualized* (ie, it contains multiple references to shared physical, family, social, affective, and communicative contexts), relying on shared knowledge (long-term memory). It is individualized for the listener, who can ask for clarification.[84–86] Contextualized language thus minimizes the linguistic and cognitive processing demands. In contrast, language in the classroom tends to be *decontextualized*; that is, it is abstract, relies heavily on linguistic and cognitive processing, and is detached from a common outside reference. The message is self-contained, to be decoded by any unknown listener without reference or assistance.[87] Cummins[88] formally distinguished the 2 types of language competences as *basic interpersonal communicative skills* (BICS; the more context rich, less cognitively complex areas of language use, common in the home and the playground) and *cognitive academic linguistic proficiency* (CALP; the more content specific, cognitively demanding areas of language, typical in the classroom). The specific relevance of this to the dual language child is that acquiring CALP in a second language, a prerequisite for academic achievement, generally takes an extended time (5–7 years). BICS in a second language takes much less time to develop (2–3 years) and this superficial communicative ability may mislead adults and teachers into thinking that the child is ready for English-only classroom placement, when in fact the child only has interpersonal fluency, but not enough academic proficiency in English.

Dual language profiles and low language competence

The language profiles of dual language children can be characterized, at a given developmental point, based on whether they have age-appropriate competence in both languages (balanced bilinguals), age-appropriate competence in one language and low competence the other (typically, children who are L1 or L2 dominant), or low competence in both (low L1/L2 competence).[47,49,89–92] The low L1/L2 profile is considered here a low language competence (low LC) group, while it is also hypothesized that when children dominant in one language have low LC in the other language, they may be at risk as well. Although these children's low LC profiles may represent, in many cases, a stepping stone toward established balanced bilingualism or functional language dominance, in other cases they may arguably be an early risk indicator for persistently low LC associated with adaptational and mental health problems. The low L1/L2 profile group likely includes children with true language impairments and delays, which are certainly possible in bilingual (as they are in monolingual) children.

DUAL LANGUAGE (BILINGUAL) LINGUISTIC COMPETENCE AND THE MENTAL HEALTH OF CHILDREN OF IMMIGRANTS

Association of Language Competence and Psychosocial Adaptation

It has been well documented that language competence is a critical contributor to the emotional and behavioral development of monolingual children.[37,93] However, less is known about how this contribution is represented for children who speak multiple languages. The empirical research focusing on the association between dual language linguistic competence and mental health and emotional/behavioral functioning is limited.[94] Thus, the authors will first review the related research in monolingual children and then extend the discussion to dual language children. Language competence is related to mental health in children. On the one hand, low language competence accompanies poor adaptation and psychopathology. On the other, good language skills are the substrate of many protective factors, such as IQ, and communicative, social, and school competences. Low language competence has been conventionally and operationally defined in research in monolinguals as language delays and disorders. Empirical studies in monolinguals published in the last decade have shown the high true comorbidity of childhood language disorders and psychiatric disorders.[95–99] Longitudinal studies show that the presence of a language disorder predicts greater severity or prevalence of (1) attention-deficit/hyperactivity disorder (ADHD) and externalizing disorders, (2) learning disorders, and (3) internalizing disorders (anxiety and depression).[97] A systematic review[37] indicates that language deficits forecast both externalizing and internalizing problems, but that the risk for externalizing problems is significantly higher. Moreover, receptive deficits are considered to be the most potent risk factors and specifically associated with diminished social competence, and aggressive and disruptive behavior outcomes.[96] To be sure, nonpathologic psychosocial outcomes are of importance in understanding the impact of language in children. Language competence predicts social competence, literacy skills, and school achievement.

Some pathways from language competence to adaptation and maladaptation
Child language competence has internal and interpersonal functions relevant for adaptation. In the internal sphere, language competence is a major tool for emotional, behavioral and cognitive self-regulation.[100] For instance, private speech, the subvocalized transition from external speech to internal speech, proposed by Vygotsky as helpful to promote task-related behavior, seems to play an ample role in cognitive, behavioral, and emotional self-regulation.[101–103] Semantic competence in labeling of emotions plays an important role in the regulation of emotional and affective states, as well as in practical tasks and schoolwork. Basic language processes underlie literacy and math, and subsequent school achievement. Narrative competences participate in self-image regulation and in the organization of a personal history as continuous and meaningful. A solid inner narrative can be used as a template to forecast and lend cohesion to one's future states and reactions. Specific aspects of language, such as the development of a theory of the mind (as indicated by the emergence of narratives containing evaluative references to others), help the child to predict others' reactions and to anticipate consequences. Similarly, certain language domain competences (for instance, grammatical development of verb tenses, lexical acquisition of categories or superordinates, narrative development of temporal anchoring and sequence chaining, and conversational skills that initiate and maintain topics) help move beyond the here and now, aiding with gratification and impulse delay.

In the interpersonal sphere, language competence is a major tool for social communication, crucial for the social navigation of the outside world, school, friendships, and family life.[104] Pragmatic language skills allow for better gauging and fine tuning of the exchange with the environment. Verbal humor and verbal aggression are a constant of child language used to negotiate hierarchies and other roles with peers.[104] The ability to narrate is a basic substrate of many other social skills, such as the ability to make new friends. Communicative competence is also necessary for self-agency within the family system, to negotiate with the parent and within the sibling subsystems. Communicative competence is also essential to elicit emotional responses, praise and useful feedback, to defend one's viewpoint, and to help in processing stressful and pathogenic events. In summary, theoretical and empirical consideration point to ways specific aspects of language may underlie enhanced attentional, emotional, cognitive, affective, and behavioral functioning.

Low language competence: mechanisms and pathways to psychopathology and adaptation in bilingual children
Some intrapsychic and interpersonal implications of language for adaptation are specific to dual language children. Proficiency in 2 languages can be a promoter of cognitive and other development. Balanced bilingualism (defined as age-appropriate competences of 2 languages) and successful L2 acquisition are associated with, and may be determinants of, growth in a host of verbal and nonverbal cognitive skills, such

as metalinguistic awareness, concept formation, creativity, and cognitive flexibility (intrapsychic aspects).[105,106] Balanced bilingualism is also associated with sociocultural (interpersonal) and linguistic advantages.[107] The cognitive and other advantages may, in turn, result in increased adaptation and low risk for psychopathology. L1 competence plays an important role in internal labeling of emotions, regulation of inner states, and family functioning. According to a rich case study literature, each language has a differential emotional valence, and the first language (mother's tongue) encodes and labels the first emotions and regulates early mental states.[108] In this way, poor L1 may lead to emotional dysregulation (internal sphere). At home, intact interpersonal communication modulates behavior and emotions[109]; hence, poor L1 may result in difficulties in family communication and loss of its protective functions,[100] which in turn may add to maladaptation. As Wong Fillmore states "When parents are unable to talk to their children, they cannot easily convey to them their values, beliefs, understandings, or wisdom about how to cope with their experiences."[62]

Language competence is also a predictor of social competence and school achievement. Interpersonally, poor language skills often predict poor social skills in monolinguals as well as in bilinguals. Social competence and communicative competence are correlated.[110] Language-delayed children are often poorly socialized,[111] shy, aloof, or less outgoing.[112] Their peer interactions are shorter and they infrequently initiate them.[113] Their peers do not accept them well.[114] Longitudinal studies confirm these same links.[115] Communicative competence and social competence are also correlated in L2-learning children; children with poor L2 mastery are treated as babies, not spoken to and often ignored by their peers.[113,116] In turn, social incompetence may lead to behavioral, mood, and anxiety problems. Moreover, L2 competence supports the child's intrapsychic emotional/behavioral regulation and access to interpersonal resources (eg, praise by teachers and understanding rules, schoolwork, and expectations). Communication rendered ineffectual by low second-language skills may lead to the unmasking or emergence of psychopathology. The authors argue that good language skills predict growth in social adaptation and low risk of psychopathology. In addition, poor L2 skills interfere with academic performance and predict poor educational outcomes, which, in turn, feed into a cycle of maladjustment and poor behavioral/emotional outcomes. In a clinical study of psychiatrically referred Latino bilingual children, levels of academic language proficiency were extremely low, with classroom language demands considered to be extremely difficult to impossible for 40% of the children in at least 1 language, and for 19% in either language.[117]

Empirical evidence for an association between low dual language competence and psychopathology
A basic question is whether language disorders are associated with psychopathology in bilingual children as they are in monolingual children. In a study of Latino dual-language children consecutively referred to a child psychiatry clinic, estimated prevalence of language deficits (48%) and disorders (41%) was high, with most cases being of the mixed receptive-expressive type.[94] These prevalences were found to be comparable to prior studies in monolingual children.[98] A second question is whether levels of dual language competence are associated with psychiatric symptom severity. Several analyses of the same sample addressed this question. In a subgroup of children with clinically significant emotional/behavioral problems, the correlations between a composite of dual language competences and psychiatric scores explained 45% of the variance in total, delinquency, and social problems, and approximately 20% to 33% in externalizing, aggression, thought, and attention problems, with most associations remaining significant after controlling for the most relevant

confounds.[94] In a different set of analyses, levels of language competence in both languages correlated to psychiatric symptom severity, explaining an average of 38% (range 28%–46%) of the variance in total, social, thought, attentional, delinquency, and aggression problems, with no significant decrease when adjusted for relevant control variables. A third set of related questions is (1) whether the language competences in each language act as a unit or independently when it comes to their associations with psychopathology and (2) whether one language is more important than the other when it comes to the relation of language competence and psychopathology. In the previous clinical study, the associations between psychopathology and language competence in each language were independent from each other, so that each language explained, overall, as much variance in psychopathology as the other, but the variances explained did not overlap, suggesting that each language plays an important role, but that the roles are differentiable, and that low competence in one language only (eg, English dominance) would be associated with psychiatric severity in this clinical sample.[118] To avoid the impact of selection bias in a clinically referred sample, these relations were studied in a community-based study of young Latino, dual language children recruited from urban public schools (n = 228; mean age: 6 years). Unpublished preliminary analyses of this cohort suggest the same findings of independent and robust negative associations of language competences in each language with levels of psychiatric symptoms; associations remained significant after relevant controls.[119] In this same community cohort, Spanish and English language competences also accounted for moderate to large portions of variance in multiple dimensions of emotional and behavioral wellbeing.[120]

In terms of other linguistic communities, adjusting to a new culture and developing English language skills is significantly and substantially associated to immigrants' home country of origin, even after controlling for factors related to SES.[83] One potential reason is the linguistic distance between immigrants' first language and English,[121] affecting the time it takes to learn the new language as a function of the distance between the language structure of L1 and L2. One could speculate that higher demands are present for languages that are more distant, in turn affecting adaptation, although no empirical studies have, to the authors' knowledge, explored this question.

DIFFERENCES BETWEEN DUAL-CULTURE ACQUISITION AND DUAL LANGUAGE ACQUISITION

Second culture contact may result in challenging or overwhelming demands, known as *acculturative stress*. Second culture contact and second language contact often co-occur, so that acculturative demands overlap with language demands. However, each one sets in motion different specialized responses. Acculturative demands are met by the immigrant's varying degrees of bicultural competence, resulting in bicultural or monocultural adaptation (or maladaptation) with their mental health implications.[122,123] Monocultural adaptation results from the immigrant's exclusive adoption of the second, mainstream culture (assimilation) or of the ethnic, home culture (ethnic monocultural affiliation). Of the various proposed models of second culture acquisition, bicultural adaptation is considered, by the literature on minority children and adults, the healthiest and most successful overall outcome, resulting from the ability to develop and maintain competence in both cultures.[122–124] In contrast, language demand is met by the child's current dual language competence, his capacity to acquire languages, and specific protective resources supporting the child (linguistically and emotionally) in the process of second-language acquisition.

Cross-cultural research on immigrants documents large contributions of language competence to variance in acculturation[123] and low language competence as a determinant of acculturative stress[122] and poor social and educational outcomes.[30] Acculturative stress appears to be associated with psychopathology in Latino youth,[19] and language conflict may explain a good portion of the impact of acculturative stress.[125] Bicultural competence of the child and family may have a protective effect, favoring bicultural adaptation. In the discussion that follows, the authors justify their particular focus on dual language competence by viewing it as closely connected to but differentiable from other components of bicultural competence.

Cultural Competence in Bicultural Individuals

Bicultural competence is considered the optimal outcome of the acculturation/dual culture acquisition process and is conceptualized as a multidimensional, heterogeneous construct.[124] The following component dimensions of bicultural competence have been proposed: (1) language competence, (2) knowledge of cultural beliefs and values, (3) positive attitudes toward both majority and minority groups, (4) bicultural efficacy, (5) role repertoire, and (6) a sense of being grounded (ie, having support networks in both cultures).[124] Thus, language competence is considered a major building block of bicultural competence; when L2 acquisition is accompanied by support of L1 maintenance, as shown by the research on bilingual programs, bicultural competence is promoted. Other research suggests that language competence explains most of the variance in acculturation,[123] and views its deficits as strong determinant of acculturative stress[122] and as a risk factor.[30] In the authors' conceptualization, being able to communicate in the language of both worlds maximizes the child's capacity to draw upon available protective resources, while at the same time it enables an adaptive response to the language demand. Conversely, nonlinguistic aspects of bicultural competence in the child, family, and extended social environment have an important protective role in Latino children of immigrants, supporting language and cultural acquisition and minimizing distress.

Dual language competence can and should be explicitly differentiated from other nonlinguistic components of cultural competence, since it has a unique and central role within the broader construct, and its own constraints, qualities, and complexities that set it apart from other dimensions in the bicultural competence construct. Dual-language competence is differentiable from other elements of bicultural competence in at least the following 5 ways. First, the linguistic systems mobilized in L2 and bilingual acquisition are independent and involve specific strategies. Second, acculturative stress is fully conceivable and observed even in the absence of language barriers, such as in the case of nonimmigrant minorities. Third, although bicultural adaptation may ideally tend to compromise as a way of resolving cultural conflict, the conflicts between discrepant linguistic systems (eg, Spanish allows flexibility in subject-verb-object order, whereas English is rather rigid) are ideally resolved by fully differentiating the 2 languages. In bilingual acquisition, solutions of compromise are only transient, intermediate steps. In other words, bicultural adaptation tends toward synthesis and compromise as an end result, while bilingual acquisition progresses toward language-system independence, albeit often incomplete. Fourth, immigrants can gain knowledge of target cultural beliefs and values or a positive attitude more easily and quickly than they can gain the experiences that support L2 acquisition and L1 maintenance. Because of globalization and penetration of American mainstream culture in Latin America, many nonimmigrant Latin Americans develop knowledge of American cultural beliefs without ever setting foot on American soil. Fifth, although positive attitudes toward American culture are part of the motivation behind voluntary immigration to the United States, few adult and adolescent first-generation immigrants (including highly motivated ones) become nativelike speakers of English. Group analyses show associations among various component bicultural dimensions, but stratification will likely show individual differences, such as a strong monocultural identity with high bilingual competence, or strong bicultural knowledge of cultural beliefs without accompanying bilingual competence.

CLINICAL AND POLICY IMPLICATIONS

Dual language children often enter school with a wide variability of competences in their L1 and L2, and a large proportion of these children have low competences in 1 or both languages. However, many are able to meet developmental expectations during the first 2 years of school. Latino children of immigrants often grow up in linguistic isolation, enter school at a disadvantage, and experience increasing academic achievement gaps and mental health disparities over time. From a developmental perspective, the authors can suggest that supporting the development of both L1 and L2, especially during the transition from home to school, is developmentally beneficial.

It is imperative that clinicians and specialists understand the importance of recognizing the wide range of language competences young children of immigrants have in their L1 and L2. By better understanding normal and abnormal dual language development, we can develop intervention strategies to target language delays as soon as possible while also supporting the development of both languages.

Maintaining (or not) the Two Languages in Children with Language and Other Deficits

Maintaining the first language is important for guaranteeing access to family and community supports and protective factors. There has been a poorly substantiated but unfortunately common practice of recommending to parents that they discontinue exposure to one of the languages (typically the home language) when a child is facing cognitive, language, or learning delays, without consideration of the social and family consequences of this recommendation. This practice has little or no empirical support, and some research suggests that children with language impairment can be healthily exposed to and learn 2 languages,[43] even with benign manifestations of language impairment in both languages. It may be true, nonetheless, that for individual children with language deficits or disorders, the additional cognitive and linguistic demands of dual language learning may become overwhelming. A clinical recommendation to discontinue exposure to one of the languages in children who are struggling with language learning or learning in general, or who express distress or overload on exposure to a language may then be necessary, but it is nonetheless a serious decision that, because of its lasting consequences, should not be made lightly.[126] Such decisions should ideally involve a speech/language pathologist with expertise in assessing dual language children, consultation with the parents and others who know the child well, and an informed decision process by the parents with consideration to the family's plans for the future.[126] For instance, it may be crucial to maintain Spanish, for a child whose immigrant family maintains firm ties with the home country or older members of the family, or as a way to prevent family distancing caused by poor communication.[127] When recommendations are made about abandoning one of the languages, the linguistic ability of the parents and family should be considered. It is important to maintain the richness of the linguistic environments of the child.[128]

Instructing parents to switch to English at home, when they do not master this language, is ill advised and possibly counterproductive in most situations.

Suspecting and Diagnosing Language Disorders in Dual Language Children

Of considerable concern with the large and growing dual language population is how to properly recognize normal and abnormal dual language development. Both the overdiagnosis as well as the underdiagnosis of language delays of English-language learners is a persistent problem.[129–132] There is a pressing need for standard guidelines in understanding normal and abnormal dual language development when using the current tests and norms recommended for assessing oral-language competence.[133] An ongoing problem with the diagnosis of language delays in dual language children is that children's English competences are often the only ones assessed. This practice renders it impossible to differentiate children who have not yet had the opportunity or the time to learn English (eg, Spanish dominant) from those that are not making significant gains despite adequate exposure because of impairments in their language-acquisition ability. A language disorder should be suspected in a dual language child, when the child is reported to be significantly behind in the understanding of both languages, when there has been significant exposure to both languages, and when there are language-based learning problems. Although it has been clearly documented that bilingualism does not cause language delay or language disorder,[128] language disorders are certainly possible in bilingual children and such possibility should not be easily dismissed, and apparent delays should not instead be misattributed to the child's bilingual condition. Auditory-verbal working memory deficits associated with ADHD[134] or a language disorder[135] may slow down the acquisition of a second language.

Dual Language Assessment

Dual language assessment is a complex task and some important conceptual and empirical progress has occurred in the last years[92,93,136] to distinguish between language delays and normal dual language developmental variability.[136,137] The field of language pathology has made headway in the area of determining dual language competence.[133,136,138] Although research on the normal dual language development has used normed standardized measures of language competence developed for monolinguals,[139–141] there are no widely accepted, normed standardized assessments of dual language competence exclusively for bilingual children. Instead, parallel measures of language competence available in multiple languages have been used. Dual language children with a regular and rich exposure to both languages exhibit similar developmental patterns and milestones as monolinguals in terms of the order of acquisition of linguistic structures.[58,142,143] The interpretation of normed standardized scores of language assessments with monolingual populations can be used cautiously as a reference point in the assessment of dual language children and as an indicator of reasonable approximation of age-appropriate language competence.[133] Dual language children in the transitional process of language acquisition typically fall short of the monolingual normal[48,144,145] because of the distributive nature of dual language acquisition (eg, vocabulary related to school is stronger in English, whereas that related to home is stronger in Spanish).[46] Grammatical and other language errors made by a child learning a second language or a second English dialect (such as standard American English) should not be confused with the grammatical or lexical abnormalities of language disorders. Specialized early speech/language assessment in 2 languages is often necessary to differentiate normal dual language acquisition from language disorder.[136,146]

Silent Period and Selective Mutism

Children who are suddenly immersed in a second-language environment with no knowledge of the language, particularly young children, will normally go through a nonverbal period limited to the second language,[116] which should not be confused with selective mutism.[147] Although sudden immersion and its nonverbal period can be stressful depending on environmental support and the temperamental characteristics of the child, selective mutism typically lasts longer, appears in both languages and unfamiliar situations, and tends to be disproportionate in relation to the child's language exposure and competence.[147] The prevalence of selective mutism appears to be, however, higher among immigrant dual language children, and it is thus important that the clinician be familiar with features that differentiate selective mutism from the normal nonverbal period.[147]

Educational Implications

It is important that educational approaches and policies recognize the increasing diversity in today's schools and establish a connection between home and school by incorporating aspects of the home and community into the curriculum. For dual-language children of immigrants, adequately functioning in 2 languages at home and school may be associated with their wellbeing.[120] Supporting the development of both L1 and L2 at school may prove to be beneficial to children's linguistic, psychosocial, and academic development. Future policy decisions and educational practice should reflect the importance of the development of L1 and L2 competences in multiple domains of children's wellbeing and academic progress.

SUMMARY

The study of dual language acquisition and how its developmental trajectories impacts the overall wellbeing and mental health of the immigrant child is in its early stages,[148] requiring further major empirical and theoretical work. Nonetheless, several important implications can be derived from extant developmental and clinical research: (1) Decisions about discontinuing learning or exposure to one of the languages should not be made lightly and should consider the personal and family circumstances of the child; (2) Delays in language acquisition can be formally evaluated without prematurely dismissing them as normal in bilingual children. Assessments are available that allow for evaluation of bilingual children; (3) A complete language assessment will often require testing in both languages; (4) The brief, normal, nonverbal period in second-language acquisition can and should be differentiated form selective mutism; and (5) Educational, clinical, and family efforts to maintain and support the development of competence in the 2 languages of the dual language child may prove rewarding in terms of long-term wellbeing and mental health, and educational and cognitive benefits. These considerations are critical for clinicians and practitioners working with the most rapidly growing segment of the US child population, dual language children of immigrants.

ACKNOWLEDGMENTS

The first author expresses his special gratitude to his late mentor, Stuart Hauser, MD, PhD, who provided him with inspiration, insight, and support over many years of working together.

REFERENCES

1. Capps R, Capps R, Fix ME, et al. The health and well-being of young children of immigrants. Washington, DC: The Urban Institute; 2005.
2. Suárez-Orozco C, Suárez-Orozco MM. Children of immigration. Cambridge (MA): Harvard University Press; 2001.
3. Mather M. Children in immigrant families chart new path. PRB Reports on America. Washington, DC: Population Reference Bureau; 2009.
4. U.S. Census: The 2002, 2003, and 2005 U.S. Current Population Survey, Annual Demographic and Economic Supplement, March: 2006. Washington, DC: Census of Population; 2006.
5. Zehler AM, Fleischman HL, Hopstock PJ, et al. Descriptive Study of Services to Limited English Proficient (LEP) Students and LEP Students with Disabilities, vol. I. Research Report. Arlington (VA): Development Associates, Inc; 2003.
6. Fry R, Passel J. Latino children: a majority are US-born offspring of immigrants. Washington, DC: Pew Research Center; 2009.
7. Suro R, Passel JS. The rise of the second generation: changing patterns in Hispanic population growth. Washington, DC: Pew Hispanic Center; 2003.
8. Flores G, Fuentes-Afflick E, Barbot O, et al. The health of Latino children: urgent priorities, unanswered questions, and a research agenda. JAMA 2002;288:82.
9. Adelman L. Unnatural causes: is inequality making us sick? Prev Chronic Dis 2007;4(4). Available at: http://www.cdc.gov/pcd/issues/2007/oct/07_0144.htm. Accessed March 5, 2010.
10. Hernandez DJ. Child development and the social demography of childhood. Child Dev 1997;68:149.
11. Hernandez DJ, Denton NA, Macartney SE. Children in immigrant families —the U.S. and 50 States: national origins, language, and early education. Albany (NY): University at Albany, SUNY; 2007.
12. Perreira K, Harris K, Lee D. Making it in America: high school completion by immigrant and native youth. Demography 2006;43:511.
13. Suárez-Orozco C, Suárez-Orozco MM, Todorova I. Learning a new land: immigrant students in American Society. Cambridge (MA): Harvard University Press; 2008.
14. Eaton DK, Kann L, Kinchen S, et al. Youth risk behavior surveillance–United States, 2005. MMWR Surveill Summ 2006;55:1.
15. Grunbaum JA, Kann L, Kinchen SA, et al. Youth risk behavior surveillance–United States, 2001. J Sch Health 2002;72:313.
16. Zayas L, Lester R, Cabassa L, et al. Why do so many latina teens attempt suicide? A conceptual model for research. Am J Orthop 2005;75:275.
17. Reardon-Anderson J, Capps R, Fix ME. The health and well-being of children in immigrant families, in "new federalism: national survey of america's families. Washington, DC: Urban Institute; 2002. p. 1.
18. Alegría M, Mulvaney-Day N, Torres M, et al. Prevalence of psychiatric disorders across latino subgroups in the United States. Am J Public Health 2007; 97:68.
19. Canino G, Roberts RE. Suicidal behavior among Latino youth. Suicide Life Threat Behav 2001;31:122.
20. Orfield G, Losen D, Wald J, et al. Losing our future: how minority youth are being left behind by the graduation rate crisis. The Civil Rights Project at Harvard University. Contributors: advocates for children of New York. Cambridge (MA): The Civil Society Institute; 2004.

21. President's Advisory Commission on Educational Excellence for Hispanic Americans. Final report: from risk to opportunity: fulfilling the educational needs of hispanic americans in the 21st century. Washington DC: White House Initiative on Educational Excellence for Hispanic Americans; 2003.

22. Villarruel FA, Walker NE. "Donde esta la justicia?" A call to action on behalf of Latino and Latina youth in the U.S. justice system. Building blocks for youth. San Francisco (CA): Center on Juvenile & Criminal Justice; 2002.

23. Fuligni AJ. A comparative longitudinal approach to acculturation. Harv Educ Rev 2001;71:566.

24. Masten AS. Resilience in individual development: Successful adaptation despite risk and adversity. In: Wang MC, Gordon EW, editors. Educational resilience in inner-city America: challenges and prospects. Hillsdale (NJ): Lawrence Erlbaum Associates; 1994. p. 3.

25. Suárez-Orozco C. Commentary. In: Suárez-Orozco MM, Paez MM, editors. Latinos: remaking America. London (England): University of California Press; 2002. p. 302.

26. Perez M, Rodriguez J, Wisdom JP, et al. Trauma treatment outcome among culturally diverse Latino children and adolescents. Paper presented at Critical issues in Latino mental health. New Brunswick (NJ), June 9, 2009.

27. Pumariega A. Acculturation and mental health in adolescents. Paper presented at AACAP Annual Meeting. Honolulu, Hawaii, October 31, 2009.

28. Alegria M, Sribney W, Woo M, et al. Looking beyond nativity: the relation of age of immigration, length of residence, and birth cohorts to the risk of onset of psychiatric disorders for Latinos. Res Hum Dev 2007;4:19.

29. Garcia-Coll C. The immigrant paradox in child and adolescent development. Paper presented at CUNY Graduate Center Latino/a and Caribbean Psychology Colloquium. New York (NY), 2008.

30. Hernandez DJ, Charney E, editors. From generation to generation: the health and well-being of children in immigrant families. National Research Council and Institute of Medicine: Committee on the Health and adjustment of immigrant children and families; board on children, Youth and families. Washington, DC: National Academy Press; 1998. p. xvii.

31. Bankston CL, Zhou M. Being well us. doing well: self-esteem and school performance among immigrant and nonimmigrant racial and ethnic groups. Int Migr Rev 2002;36:389.

32. Kao G, Thompson JS. Racial and ethnic stratification in educational achievement and attainment. Annu Rev Sociol 2003;29:417.

33. Portes A, Rumbaut RG. Legacies: the story of the immigrant second generation. Berkeley: University of California Press; 2001.

34. Alegria M, Canino G, Shrout PE, et al. Prevalence of mental illness in immigrant and non-immigrant U.S. latino groups. Am J Psychiatry 2008;165:359.

35. Berko GJ. The development of language. 3rd edition. New York: Macmillan; 1993.

36. Hymes D. On communicative competence. Hammondsworth (UK): Penguin; 1972.

37. Toppelberg CO, Shapiro T. Language disorders: a 10-year research update review. J Am Acad Child Adolesc Psychiatry 2000;39:143.

38. Collier V. Acquiring a second language for school, vol. 1. Washington, DC: National Clearinghouse for Bilingual Education; 1995

39. Pan BA. Semantic development: learning the meaning of words. In: Berko Gleason J, editor. The development of language. 3rd edition. New York: Macmillan; 1993. p. 302.

40. Kopke B. Neurolinguistic aspects of attrition. J Neurol 2004;17:3.
41. Cook V. Effects of the second language on the first. Clevedon (UK): Multilingual Matters; 2003.
42. Cook V. Evidence for multicompetence. Lang Learn 1992;42:557.
43. Genesee F, Paradis J, Crago M. Dual language development and disorders: a handbook on bilingualism and second language learning. Baltimore (MD): Brookes Publishing Company; 2004.
44. Gutiérrez KD, Zepeda M, Castro DC. Advancing early literacy learning for all children: Implications of the NELP report for dual language learners. Educat Res 2010;39:334.
45. Hakuta K. Mirror of language: the debate of bilingualism. New York: Basic Books; 1986.
46. Oller DK, Pearson BZ, Cobo-Lewis AB. Profile effects in early bilingual language and literacy. Appl Psycholinguist 2007;28:191.
47. Rosenberg M. Raising bilingual children. Internet TESL J 1996;2.
48. Valdes G, Figueroa RA. Bilingualism and testing: a special case of Bias. Norwood (NJ): Ablex Publishing Corporation; 1994.
49. Baker C. Foundations of bilingual education and bilingualism. Multilingual Matters; 2006.
50. Portes A. Lost in translation: language acquisition and loss in the United States. Paper presented at Spanish in the US Biannual Conference. Washington, DC, March, 2007.
51. Hakuta K, D'Andrea D. Some properties of bilingual maintenance and loss in Mexican background high school students. Appl Ling 1992;13:72.
52. Portes A, Hao L. E. Pluribus Unum: bilingualism and loss of language in the second generation. Sociol Educ 1998;71:269.
53. Portes A, Schauffler R. Language and the second generation: bilingualism yesterday and today. Int Migr Rev 1994;28:640.
54. Wong FL. Loss of family languages: should educators be concerned? Theory into practice 2000;39:4.
55. Deaux K. To be an immigrant: psychological design and social fabric. New York: Russell Sage; 2006.
56. Winsler A, Diaz RM, Espinosa L, et al. When learning a second language does not mean losing the first: bilingual language development in low-income, Spanish-speaking children attending bilingual preschool. Child Dev 1997;70:349.
57. Cummins J. Linguistic interdependence and the educational development of bilingual children. Rev Educ Res 1979;49:222.
58. Lambert WE, Tucker GR. Bilingual education of children: the St. Lambert experiment. Rowley (MA): Newbury House Publishers, Inc; 1972.
59. Swain M. Home-school language switching. In: Richards JC, editor, Understanding second language learning: issues and approaches, vol. 34. Rowley (MA): Newbury House; 1978. p. 557.
60. Pease-Alvarez L, Vasquez O. Language socialization in ethnic minority communities. In: Genesee F, editor. Educating second language children. Cambridge (UK): Cambridge University Press; 1994. p. 82.
61. Tse L. Resisting and reversing language shift: heritage-language resilience among U.S. Native biliterates. Harv Educ Rev 2001;71:676.
62. Wong Fillmore L. When learning a second language means losing the first. Early Child Res Q 1991;6:323.
63. Ben-Zeev S. The effect of bilingualism in children from Spanish-English low economic neighborhoods on cognitive development and cognitive strategy.

Working Papers on Bilingualism, Institute for Studies in Education. Toronto, Ontario, Canada, 1977.

64. Cummins J. Bilingual children's mother tongue: why is it important for education? SprogForum 2001;19:15–21.
65. Veltman C. Language Shift in the United States. Berlin: Mouton Publishers; 1983.
66. Pease-Alvarez L, Winsler A. Cuando el maestro no habla español: children's bilingual language practices in the classroom. TESOL Quarterly 1994;28:507.
67. Bradley RH, Caldwell BM, Rock SL, et al. Home environment and cognitive development in the first 3 years of life: a collaborative study involving six sites and three ethnic groups in North America. Development 1989;25:217.
68. Snow C. Beginning from baby talk: twenty years of research on input and interaction. In: Galloway C, Richards B, editors. Input and interaction in language acquisition. London: Cambridge University Press; 1994. p. 3.
69. Tamis-LeMonda CS, Bornstein MH, Baumwell L. Maternal responsiveness and children's achievement of language milestones. Child Dev 2001;72:748.
70. Pan BA, Rowe ML, Singer JD, et al. Maternal correlates of growth in toddler vocabulary production in low-income families. Child Dev 2005;76:763.
71. Arriaga RI, Fenson L, Cronan T, et al. Scores on the macarthur communicative development inventory of children from low- and middle-income families. Appl Psycholinguist 1998;19:209.
72. Hoff E. The specificity of environmental influence: socioeconomic status affects early vocabulary development via maternal speech. Child Dev 2003;74:1368.
73. Hakuta K, Pease-Alvarez L. Proficiency, choice and attitudes in bilingual Mexican-American children. In: Extra G, Verhoeven LT, editors. The cross-linguistic study of bilingual development. Amsterdam (The Netherlands): North-Holland; 1994.
74. Genesee F. The suitability of French immersion for students who are at-risk: a review of the research evidence. Canadian Modern Language Review 2007;63(5):655–87.
75. Fishman JA. Reversing language shift: theoretical and empirical foundations of assistance to threatened languages. Clevedon (UK); Philadelphia: Multilingual Matters; 1991.
76. Hamers JF, Blanc M. Cultural identity and bilinguality. Foreign Language Teaching and Cultural Identity 1982;35.
77. Koplow L, Messinger E. Developmental dilemmas of young children of immigrant parents. Child Adolesc Soc Work 1990;7:121.
78. Pease-Alvarez L, Hakuta K. Perspectives on language maintenance and shift in Mexican-origin students. In: Phelan P, Davidson AL, editors. Renegotiating cultural diversity in American schools. New York: Teachers College Press; 1993. p. 302.
79. Tseng V, Fuligni AJ. Parent-adolescent language use and relationships among immigrant families with east Asian, Filipino, and Latin American backgrounds. J Marriage Fam 2000;62:465.
80. Bianchi SM. Children's progress through school: a research note. Sociol Educ 1984;57:184.
81. Suárez-Orozco C, Carhill A. Afterword: new directions in research with immigrant families and their children. In: Yoshikawa H, Way N, editors. Beyond the family: contexts of immigrant children's development, vol. 121. San Francisco (CA): Jossey-Bass; 2008. p. 87.
82. Zhou M, Cai G. Chinese language media in the United States: immigration and assimilation in American life. Qual Sociol 2002;25:419.

83. Van Tubergen F, Kalmijn M. Destination language proficiency in cross national perspective: a study of immigrant groups in nine western countries. Am J Sociol 2005;110:1412.

84. Cummins J. BICS and CALP. Clarifying the distinction. New York (NY): ERIC Clearinghouse on Urban Education; 1999.

85. Cummins J. Primary language instruction and the education of language minority students. Schooling and language minority students: a theoretical framework. Los Angeles (CA): California State University; 1994. p. 3–49.

86. Snow CE. The theoretical basis for relationships between language and literacy development. J Res Child Educ 1991;6(Fal).

87. Westby CE. Culture and literacy: frameworks for understanding. Top Lang Disord 1995;16:50.

88. Cummins J. Wanted: a theoretical framework for relating language proficiency to academic achievement among bilingual students. In: Rivera C, editor. Language proficiency and academic achievement. Clevedon (England): Multilingual Matters; 1984. p. 2–19.

89. Cummins J. Cognitive factors associated with the attainment of intermediate levels of bilingual skills. Mod Lang J 1977;61:1977.

90. Peal E, Lambert WE. The relation of bilingualism to intelligence. Psychol Monogr 1962;76:23.

91. Tabors PO, Páez MM, López LM. Early childhood study of language and literacy development of Spanish-speaking children: theoretical background and preliminary results. Paper presented at Annual Meeting National Association for Bilingual Education. Philadelphia (PA), 2002.

92. Verhoeven L. Early bilingualism, language transfer, and phonological awareness. Appl Psycholinguist 2007;28:425.

93. Beitchman JH, Cohen NJ, Konstantareas MM, et al, editors. Language, learning, and behavior disorders: developmental, biological, and clinical perspectives. New York: Cambridge University Press; 1996. p. xv.

94. Toppelberg CO, Medrano L, Peña Morgens L, et al. Bilingual children referred for psychiatric services: associations of language disorders, language skills, and psychopathology. J Am Acad Child Psychiatry 2002;41:712.

95. Baker L, Cantwell DP. Attention deficit disorder and speech/language disorders. Comprehensive Mental Health Care 1992;2:3.

96. Beitchman JH, Brownlie EB, Inglis A, et al. Seven-year follow-up of speech/ language impaired and control children: psychiatric outcome. J Child Psychol Psychiatry 1996;37:961.

97. Cantwell DP, Baker L. Psychiatric and developmental disorders in children with communication disorders. Washington, DC: American Psychiatric Press, Inc; 1991.

98. Cohen NJ, Davine M, Horodezky N, et al. Unsuspected language impairment in psychiatrically disturbed children: prevalence and language and behavioral characteristics. J Am Acad Child Adolesc Psychiatry 1993;32:595.

99. Giddan JJ. Communication issues in attention-deficit hyperactivity disorder. Child Psychiatry Hum Dev 1991;22:45.

100. Dale PS. Language and emotion: a development perspective. In: Beitchman JH, Cohen NJ, Konstantareas MM, et al, editors. Language, learning, and behavior disorders: developmental, biological, and clinical perspectives. New York: Cambridge University Press; 1996. p. 5.

101. Berk L, Landau S. Private speech in the face of academic challenge: the failure of impulsive children to "get their act together." Paper presented at Society for Research in Child Development Annual Meeting. Washington, DC, 2009.

102. Bivens JA, Berk LE. A longitudinal study of the development of elementary school children's private speech. Merrill Palmer Q 1990;36.
103. Goodman SH, Gotlib IH. Risk for psychopathology in the children of depressed mothers: a developmental model for understanding mechanisms of transmission. Psychol Rev 1999;106:458.
104. Gleason JB, editor. The development of language. 4th edition. Needham Heights (MA): Allyn & Bacon; 1997.
105. Diaz R. Bilingual cognitive development: addressing three gaps in current research. Child Dev 1985;56:1376.
106. Diaz R. The intellectual power of bilingualism. The Quarterly Newsletter of the Laboratory of Comparative Human Cognition 1985;7:15.
107. Grosjean F. Life with two languages. 1st edition. Cambridge: Harvard University Press; 1982.
108. Aragno A, Schlachet PJ. Accessibility of early experience through the language of origin: a theoretical integration. Psychoanal Psychol 1996;13:23.
109. Crittenden PM. Language and psychopathology: an attachment perspective. In: Beitchman JH, Cohen NJ, Konstantareas MM, et al, editors. Language, learning, and behavior disorders: developmental, biological, and clinical perspectives. New York: Cambridge University Press; 1996. p. 59.
110. Farmer M. Exploring the links between communication skills and social competence. Educ Child Psychol 1997;14:38.
111. Paul R, Shiffer ME. Communicative initiations in normal and late-talking toddlers. Appl Psycholinguist 1991;12:419.
112. Paul R, Kellogg L. Temperament in late talkers. J Child Psychol Psychiatry 1997; 38:803.
113. Rice ML, Sell MA, Hadley PA. Social interactions of speech- and language-impaired children. J Speech Lang Hear Res 1991;34:1299.
114. Craig HK, Washington JA. Access behaviors of children with specific language impairment. J Speech Lang Hear Res 1993;36:322.
115. Beitchman JH, Wilson B, Brownlie EB, et al. Long-term consistency in speech/language profiles: II. Behavioral, emotional, and social outcomes. J Am Acad Child Adolesc Psychiatry 1996;35:815.
116. Tabors PO. One child, two languages: a guide for preschool educators of children learning English as a second language. Baltimore (MD): Brookes Pub. Co; 1997.
117. Toppelberg CO, Munir K, Nieto-Castañon A. Spanish-English bilingual children with psychopathology: language deficits and academic language proficiency. Child Adolesc Ment Health 2006;11:156.
118. Toppelberg CO, Nieto-Castañon A, Hauser ST. Bilingual children: cross-sectional relations of psychiatric syndrome severity and dual language proficiency. Harv Rev Psychiatry 2006;14:15.
119. Collins B, Toppelberg CO, Katz-Gershon S, et al. Cross-sectional associations of low Spanish and English language competence and psychopathology in young Latino boys and girls. Poster presented at Critical Research Issues in Latino Mental Health, Robert Wood Johnson Medical School. New Brunswick (NJ), 2009.
120. Collins BA. Dual language competences and psychosocial wellbeing of children of immigrants [dissertation]. New York (NY): New York University; 2010
121. Chiswick BR, Miller PW. Language skill definition: a study of legalized aliens. Int Migr Rev 1998;32:877.
122. Garcia CC, Magnuson K. The psychological experience of immigration: A developmental perspective. In: Booth A, Crouter AC, Nancy L, et al, editors.

Immigration and the family: research and policy on U.S. immigrants. Hillsdale (NJ): Lawrence Erlbaum Associates, Inc; 1997. p. viii, 91–131, 307.

123. Rogler LH, Cortes DE, Malgady RG. Acculturation and mental health status among Hispanics: Convergence and new directions for research. Am Psychol 1991;46:585.

124. LaFromboise T, Coleman HL, Gerton J. Psychological impact of biculturalism: evidence and theory. Psychol Bull 1993;114:395.

125. Vega WA, Khoury EL, Zimmerman RS, et al. Cultural conflicts and problem behaviors of Latino adolescents in home and school environments. J Community Psychol 1995;23:1995.

126. Toppelberg CO, Snow CE, Tager-Flusberg H. Severe developmental disorders and bilingualism. J Am Acad Child Adolesc Psychiatry 1999;38:1197.

127. Hwang W, Wood J. Acculturative family distancing: links with self-reported symptomatology among Asian Americans and Latinos. Child Psychiatry Hum Dev 2009;40:123.

128. King K, Fogle L. Raising bilingual children: common parental concerns and current research. Washington, DC: Center for Applied Linguistics; 2006.

129. Artiles AJ, Rueda R, Salazar JJ, et al. Within-group diversity in minority disproportionate representation: english language learners in urban school districts. Except Child 2005;71:283.

130. Gutierrez-Clellen VF. Language diversity: implications for assessment. Assessment 1996;6:29.

131. Restrepo MA. Identifiers of predominantly Spanish-speaking children with language impairment. J Speech Lang Hear Res 1998;41:1398.

132. Tomblin JB, Smith E, Zhang X. Epidemiology of specific language impairment: prenatal and perinatal risk factors. J Commun Dis 1997;30:325.

133. Thordardottir E, Rothenberg A, Rivard ME, et al. Bilingual assessment: can overall proficiency be estimated from separate measurement of two languages? J Multiling Commun Disord 2006;4:1.

134. McInnes A, Humphries T, Hogg-Johnson S, et al. Listening comprehension and working memory are impaired in attention-deficit hyperactivity disorder irrespective of language impairment. J Abnorm Child Psychol 2003;31:427.

135. Gathercole SE. Word learning in language-impaired children. Child Lang Teach Ther 1993;9:187.

136. Bedore LM, Pena ED. Assessment of bilingual children for identification of language impairment: current findings and implications for practice. Int J Bilingual Educ 2008;11:1.

137. Kritikos EP. Speech-language pathologists' beliefs about language assessment of bilingual/bicultural individuals. Am J Speech Lang Pathol 2003;12:73.

138. Gutierrez-Clellen VF, Restrepo MA, Simon-Cereijido G. Evaluating the discriminant accuracy of a grammatical measure with Spanish-speaking children. J Speech Lang Hear Res 2006;49:1209.

139. Oller DK, Eilers RE, editors. Language and literacy in bilingual children. Child language and child development. New York: Multilingual Matters; 2002.

140. Páez MM, Tabors PO, López LM. Dual language and literacy development of Spanish-speaking preschool children. J Appl Dev Psychol 2007;28:85.

141. Proctor CP, Carlo M, August D, et al. Native Spanish-speaking children reading in English: toward a model of comprehension. J Educ Psychol 2005;97:246.

142. Döpke S. Is simultaneous acquisition of two languages in early childhood equal to acquiring each of the two languages individually? Paper presented at Proceedings of the 28th Annual Child Language Research Forum. Boston (MA), 1996.

143. Genesee F. Early bilingual development: one language or two? J Child Lang 1989;16:161.
144. Junker DA, Stockman IJ. Expressive vocabulary of German-English bilingual toddlers. Am J Speech Lang Pathol 2002;11:381.
145. Pearson BZ, Fernandez SC, Oller DK. Lexical development in bilingual infants and toddlers: comparison to monolingual norms. Lang Learn 1993;43:93.
146. Lidz CS, Pena ED. Dynamic assessment: the model, its relevance as a non-biased approach, and its application to Latino American preschool children. Lang Speech Hear Serv Schools 1996;27:367.
147. Toppelberg CO, Tabors P, Coggins A, et al. Differential diagnosis of selective mutism in bilingual children. J Am Acad Child Adolesc Psychiatry 2005;44: 592–5.
148. Abbeduto L, Benson G, Short K, et al. Effects of sampling context on the expressive language of children and adolescents with mental retardation. Ment Retard 1995;33:279.

The Cultural Sensibility Model: A Process-Oriented Approach for Children and Adolescents

Niranjan S. Karnik, MD, PhD[a],*,
Nisha Dogra, BM, DCH, MA, PhD, FRCPsych[b]

KEYWORDS

- Cultural sensibility model • Psychiatry • Adolescents
- Children • Cultural expertise

A BRIEF HISTORY OF CULTURAL PARADIGMS IN PSYCHIATRY

The history of the inclusion of culture within child and adolescent psychiatry is a limited one, and until recently has not attracted particular attention. This history is in many regards a modification of the broader trends set in general psychiatry and pediatrics that child and adolescent psychiatry has tended to follow. It has only more recently established itself as a specialty within its own right. Reviewing this history briefly helps provide a background for the model that this article proposes, and also highlights potential directions for future research and practice in child and adolescent psychiatry.

The First Moment: Recognition of Cultural Difference

Research on culture as a domain within medicine and psychiatry came into focus after World War II. Although the earlier psychoanalytic era often paid attention to aspects of culture within individual cases, the recognition of the multiple facets and complexity of culture can be most clearly linked to the rise of the disciplines of sociology and anthropology in the post-war era. This period was marked by a large number of United States soldiers who had fought across the globe, from Europe to Africa and the Pacific

---

The authors have nothing to disclose.
[a] Department of Psychiatry, The University of Chicago, Pritzker School of Medicine, 5841 South Maryland, 5841 South Maryland, MC 3077, Chicago, IL 60637, USA
[b] Greenwood Institute of Child Health, University of Leicester, Westcotes House, Westcotes Drive, Leicester LE3 0QU, UK
* Corresponding author.
E-mail address: nskarnik@uchicago.edu

Child Adolesc Psychiatric Clin N Am 19 (2010) 719–737
doi:10.1016/j.chc.2010.07.006
1056-4993/10/$ – see front matter

Islands. These soldiers returned to the United States and took advantage of the GI Bill to obtain access to higher education in the 1950s and 1960s. The modern faculties in the social sciences became led partly by professors who came through these pathways of education.

Among the many areas of interest to social scientists of this era were the cultural experiences of health and illness. It was during this post war era that the interdisciplinary behavioral science research and teaching programs established by the U.S. National Institute of Mental Health had a major impact on the social sciences. Harvard's Department of Social Relations, an interdisciplinary program led by the distinguished sociologist Talcott Parsons, brought together doctoral students such as Robert K. Merton, Clifford Geertz, Harold Garfinkel, and Renée C. Fox; scholars who would later change the fields of anthropology and sociology. Parsons himself was influenced by the work of Sigmund Freud, but extended his scholarship beyond psychopathology to seek structural models that would explain various aspects of the social system.

In the United States, these broader trends in the social sciences came to have their most significant impact on medical education through the publication of two key works in the late 1950s and early 1960s. The first was *The Student Physician*, edited by Robert K. Merton[1] in 1957, and *Boys in White*, by Howard Becker[2] in 1961. Both of these books showed that social factors not only were a part of the medical education process but also profoundly shaped the nature and attitudes of the students who were training to become physicians. These works linked to a broader reformist movement within medical education that sought to bring the social sciences to bear on the study of health and illness as a way to address factors that seemed to impact health care, and also as a means to train doctors to be more humane and empathic in their approach to care.

Notably in the field of psychology, Mary Ainsworth[3] published her studies of Ugandan childrearing practices in 1967. The volume was published several years after she completed her studies, but it shows a growing interest in trying to ascertain universal phenomena and patterns of child development. Ainsworth studied under John Bowlby[4–6] and was clearly influenced by his thinking and the conceptualization of attachment as a central point of childhood development. Both Bowlby and Ainsworth were attentive to the social environment but did not necessarily focus on culture as a key factor. Their studies sought to define general patterns of attachment and childhood development, and the research that they undertook beyond the Euro-American context was framed by this approach.

The Second Moment: Cultural Psychiatry Emerges

Despite this attention to social and cultural elements, very little of the research from this era focused on children or adolescents. Primarily in the 1970s and 1980s in the United States, a corpus of research began to emerge that examined ethnic differences of psychiatric illnesses for children and adolescents. Much of this research was driven by a small number of individuals in child psychiatric clinics who focused their efforts on the experiences of minority youth and families.

Jeanne Spurlock, for example, served as the chair of psychiatry at Meharry Medical College in the early 1970s, and thereafter moved to positions at the National Institute of Mental Health and the American Psychiatric Association in the 1980s. From these locations, she forwarded an agenda that illuminated the different experiences of ethnic minority youth, particularly African American children and adolescents.[7] In parallel, in the 1980s Hector Bird launched a series of studies, initially psychoanalytically focused and then epidemiologically, that examined the experiences of Hispanic and Puerto

Rican youth and the differential presentation of psychiatric disorders and their particular cultural manifestations.[8,9] Other scholars[10–17] could easily be cited to show this trend further, but space limitations do not allow a full explication on this period.

Family therapy, which is a widely used modality of intervention in child psychiatry, also began examining the meaning of culture for families and its impact on their development and functioning. During this period, the field of child and adolescent psychiatry also became more international, and studies from parts of the world other than Europe and North America were added to the literature. Child psychiatrists from non-European and American backgrounds clearly also began training in these contexts and added different perspectives to the clinical experience.

The Third Moment: Cultural Competence in Medical Education

During the 1980s and 1990s, the American Association of Medical Colleges (AAMC), and accreditation bodies in the both the United States and United Kingdom began pushing to include more teaching about ethnic and cultural issues as they pertain to medical education into the curricula of all educational institutions.[18] Much of this was driven by the growing recognition that health disparities existed between different groups in society and that ethnicity, culture, gender, and socioeconomic status may all be relevant variables. This model posited that the practice of medicine was influenced by these factors and that disparities were recognized as having roots in the racial biases of individual practitioners and broader structural, economic, and social trends that entrench patterns of behavior and risk that differentially affect minority populations.

In the United States, the cultural competence model became the accepted mode for teaching about these topics. The general pattern of these courses focused on first defining the fact that culture (usually used interchangeably with ethnicity and race, and seen as being the indicator of culture) has an impact on practice and that health disparities exist, and then presenting a series of lectures or units that covered the health attitudes, beliefs, or experiences of various minority groups. Culture, in this way, was presented as being primarily defined by ethnicity and little attention seems to have been paid to the complex interplay between the different factors. Groups were also presented as relatively homogenous. Typically, the groups would include the dominant minorities in the United States, such as African Americans, Latino/as, Asian Americans, and Native Americans. Many courses would recruit lecturers from specific backgrounds to teach on each of these groups, and would sometimes draw on local sociologists or anthropologists to provide the necessary teaching. In less-ideal situations, clinicians would do their best to cover this material by drawing on the limited teaching resources available. The cultural competence model emphasized a notion that clinicians and trainees need to develop expertise in particular cultures to be effective providers.

In 1994, the Fourth Revision of the *Diagnostic and Statistical Manual of Mental Disorders* (DSM) included as Appendix I an "Outline for Cultural Formulation" (the Outline) for the first time.[19] This shift was prompted by the actions of many advocates for ethnic and minority issues who had pushed for greater inclusion of these concepts in the DSM. The placement of the Outline in the appendix was seen as recognition of the importance of these topics, whereas the relegation of it to the end of the DSM seemed to minimize some of its potential impact. The Outline, along with the accompanying "Glossary of Culture-Bound Syndromes," are bridges from the expertise model to a more process-oriented approach. It recognizes the need to create a space for understanding the individual's cultural experience of health and illness, and does so in ways that are highly pragmatic. The inclusion of the concept of culture-bound syndromes creates a differentiation between a mainstream experience of psychiatric illness and other or external cultural experiences.

In many respects, the Outline creates the potential for a process-oriented framework. In practice, the current trends in medical education tend to focus on teaching content about culture based on a single narrative or broad generalizations. Current research in the social sciences has, in some fundamental ways, abandoned the concept of master narratives with the postcolonial and postmodern turn.[20–22] For example, the limitations imposed by creating a list of culture-bound syndromes are many. Such a list is necessarily incomplete and also represents a fixed notion of these experiences. The need to generalize for expediency of teaching faces a challenge because of a lack of specificity and inclusivity of the vast range of cultures present in the world.

The final major challenge facing the Outline is that it is not written with a focus on child and adolescent psychiatry. This fact is especially problematic because a distinct lack of acknowledgment of developmental process exists within the DSM as a whole. Although the experts who developed the outline were clearly aware of the differential nature of family structures and influences on the psychiatric experience of illness, the overall structure of the DSM necessitates a more individualistic and targeted framework that is reflected in the Outline. Francis Lu, one of the pioneers of the cultural formulation, and others attempt to address this gap elsewhere in this issue, and readers are encouraged to look for insights into their approach as complement to the model proposed herein. Although this article does not wish to classify having expertise as a problem per se, in the current multiethnic, increasingly diverse world, having a dynamic and process-oriented approach seems to make sense, and is likely necessary given the simultaneously globalizing and differentiating local cultures.

The model proposed by Dogra[23] examined the extremes of potential cultural education models. The reality is that most programs likely incorporate aspects of both models. However, unless educators are explicit about their philosophic base, the models developed are unlikely to be coherent. It is also important to stress context: the cultural competence type models arose at a particular time when ideas were relatively new and less debated than currently. The authors recognize the importance of the cultural expertise type programs in having created the groundwork for other models to be developed, and that at the time they were developed they challenged the status quo and identified that culture was an important factor to consider when looking at health matters.

THE NEXT MOMENT: THE CULTURAL SENSIBILITY MODEL

The authors propose that the field of child and adolescent psychiatry needs to move to a more fully developed process-oriented approach to culture and diversity issues. This framework must be designed to guide the practitioner into discovering and learning about the child, adolescent, and family's culture. It also must recognize that developmentally, adolescents and teens may begin to define their own self-definition of culture as being different from that of their family of origin.

This framework also must recognize that an individual's, family's, and society's culture is not fixed and is a dynamic process that changes over time. Individuals likely change faster than families, who in turn change faster than society. Nevertheless, inferring that culture is a constant would be a mistake, and practitioners may need to revisit cultural elements repeatedly over the course of a therapeutic relationship.

Development of the Cultural Sensibility Model

The cultural sensibility model was developed by one of the authors as part of research that investigated the learning and teaching of cultural diversity to medical students in the United Kingdom.[23] It arose because at that time few clear educational models or processes existed in the field for educators to follow. The model has since been applied in training in several contexts. The authors also suggest that the framework can be used without necessarily arriving at the same programs they might devise.

Educational Models: Ideal Types of "Cultural Expertise" and "Cultural Sensibility"

Using Weber's construct of ideal types,[24] Dogra[25] compared several characteristics of the concepts of *cultural expertise* and *cultural sensibility*. These characteristics are grouped into four major areas of course development:

1. Educational philosophy and policy
2. Educational process
3. Educational content
4. Educational and clinical outcomes.

Educational philosophy and policy usually inform all stages of course development and also affect the educational process, educational content, and outcomes. When discussing the educational process, the way that the educational philosophy is translated into practice is an important guiding principle. The question is how the values and ideologies of the course directors are used to develop the course. Some course designers may, of course, not recognize that their underlying beliefs about the merits or disadvantages of certain approaches influence their choices. In considering educational content, the very nature of the material is under review. This stage involves identifying the key areas that the teaching will emphasize and whether the programs will focus on the attainment of knowledge, skills, or attitudinal outcomes. Assessment is often perceived to be the major educational outcome measure, but there will be other outcomes, with some more explicit than others.

Cultural Expertise and Cultural Sensibility

A dictionary definition of *expertise*[26] is expert skill, knowledge, or judgment, with *expert* being defined as having special skill at a task or knowledge in a subject. A view exists that through learning knowledge about other cultures, one can develop cultural expertise and that much of this knowledge can be learned through didactic teaching. *Cultural expertise* is having facts about other cultures. The concept of cultural expertise encompasses the well-established model of cultural competence.

Cultural sensibility is proposed to broaden the concept of cultural sensitivity, which generally has been a tentative alternative to the idea of cultural expertise. A dictionary definition[26] of *sensibility* is an openness to emotional impressions, susceptibility, and sensitiveness. It relates to a person's moral, emotional, or aesthetic ideas or standards. Cultural sensitivity is not the same as cultural sensibility. Cultural sensitivity is the quality or degree of being sensitive, which is more limited than sensibility and does not take into account the interactional nature of sensibility. If one is open to the outside, one might reflect and change because of that experience; this is not necessarily the case with sensitivity.

The approach of cultural sensibility arose from the author Nisha Dogra's work in cultural diversity and medical education, and an experience that the cultural expertise model potentially limits the benefits of cultural diversity teaching.

The different underlying philosophies of the cultural expertise and cultural sensibility models result in differing educational processes, contents, and assessments (**Table 1**). Using the cultural expertise model, the following outcomes in each of the learning domains might be used:

Knowledge: history and culture of country of origin; pertinent psychosocial stressors, family life, and intergenerational issues; culturally acceptable behaviors versus psychopathology; role of religion; cultural beliefs about causes and treatments of disease; and differences in disease prevalence and response to medicine and other treatments.

Skills: interview and assess patients in the target language (or via translator); communicate with sensitivity to cross-cultural issues; avoid under-/overdiagnosing disease states; understand the patient's perspective; formulate culturally sensitive treatment plans; effectively use community resources; and act as a role model and advocate for bilingual/bicultural staff and patients.

Attitudes: as evidence of understanding, acknowledge the degree of difference between patient and physician; to demonstrate empathy, recall the patient's history of suffering; allow for a shift away from the Western view of time and immediacy; respect the importance of culture as a determinant of health, the existence of other world views regarding health and illness, the adaptability and survival skills of patients, the influence of religious beliefs on health, and the role of bilingual/bicultural staff; and show humor by having the ability to laugh with oneself and others.[27]

By comparison, possible learning outcomes for using the cultural sensibility model might be:

Knowledge: the focus of cultural sensibility is not strictly knowledge about groups. Students are expected to be aware of broad psychosocial issues that can affect the way individuals perceive health and access health services. A need exists to have knowledge of the contexts in which information is presented or received.

Skills: the greater focus on this model is the acquisition of a method for acknowledging difference, and working with it in a constructive and positive way. Difference between the doctor and patient is potentially present in all encounters and not just those in which ethnicity differs.

Attitude: the focus is on self-reflection and awareness; the interaction between two individuals, which generates effective, shared understanding and dialog. The dialog has the potential to change either, both, or neither of the participants. It is built on a transformative learning approach.

The previous comparison focused on the conceptual differences between the two models at their purest. Cultural expertise models arose from the recognition that cultural influences impact on health care provision and use. The approach of cultural sensibility is presented as an evolution of the cultural expertise approach, which potentially limits the benefits of cultural diversity teaching. In an environment that demands increasingly evidence-based approaches, tighter teaching models may need to be developed that have clear conceptual frameworks and can evaluate more effectively whether the teaching meets its objectives. This concept is revisited later when the impact of educational programs is considered.

Why Use a Cultural Sensibility Approach?

The justification for any approach is ideally based on both best practices and firmest evidence. No major research has been published regarding the outcomes of any particular approach over another. Various programs have shown benefits, but little long-term follow-up has been conducted, and comparison is difficult across different programs because the material covered varies considerably. A description of the range of programs that have been used is beyond the scope of this article. Beach and colleagues[28] reviewed many cultural diversity education programs and concluded that cultural competence training shows promise as a strategy for improving the knowledge, skills, and attitudes of health professionals. The review from which the paper was generated is useful, because it identifies programs that are well described and may therefore be useful to other educators.

The cultural sensibility approach is advocated for the following reasons:

As an educational model it is explicit about all stages of the educational process, from educational philosophy to learning outcomes.

The position and perspectives of the authors are transparent.

The meanings of key terms are described and the definition of *culture* that is used to show the model is justified.

The model shows that everyone, and not just those from minority ethnic groups, have "culture."

The approach supports the development of skills that can be attained through practice and self-reflection.

It highlights that relationships are dynamic in their nature and that changes across one system may lead to changes in another connected system.

Hobgood and colleagues[29] describe different methods to teach cultural competency, and provide examples of each. Dogra[23,25] looked at the various programs described (with some of the examples those used by Hobgood and colleagues) and tried to ascertain which educational model they fit in with best. Most models tend to be a combination of cultural expertise and cultural sensibility. Methods such as portfolios, case studies, and cultural immersion can seem very appealing initially but may also encourage students to develop stereotypical representations based on "ethnicity" alone. The models may fail to acknowledge that individuals are more than just their ethnicity. For example, to learn about gay Hispanic men, would students immerse themselves in "gay" or "Hispanic" or "male" culture? In reality, the intersection of these groups is far more complex, and resists the notion that simply studying each specific culture can yield the necessary information to treat the individual at this intersection.

Another common approach is to focus on communication and give students useful checklists to attempt to understand the patient perspective, such as those developed by Berlin and Fowkes.[30] They recommended the LEARN model: *Listen* with sympathy and understanding to the patient's perception of the problem, *Explain* your perceptions, *Acknowledge* and discuss the differences and similarities, *Recommend* treatment and *Negotiate* treatment. Kleinman's questions,[31] which are a range of questions exploring the patients perspective on the causes of their problems and their hopes and expectations of treatment, can also be used.

The difficulty with the focus on communication is that students may fail to consider their own biases and prejudices that may influence how they can effectively apply these strategies. Communication is at the core of the clinical consultation, but so too is the impression patients and family gather of their doctors' genuineness and respect for them.

Table 1
Summary of comparison between the different educational components of cultural expertise and cultural sensibility

Item	Cultural Expertise	Cultural Sensibility
Educational philosophy		
Epistemology (ie, the theory of knowledge)	Knowledge exists independently	Knowledge is contextual to one's environment
Categorization of knowledge	Core competency is about categorizing groups of people and that these categories can be learned (ie, knowledge can be categorized)	Knowledge does not need to be categorized
Use of categorization	Categorization is helpful	Categorization may be unhelpful
Ontology (the nature of being)	Positivist (a view that one single empirically testable reality exists)	Social constructivist (a view that we live in a reality that is created by socially driven meanings and that this reality is framed by the standpoint of the observer)
Conception of reality	Objective reality to be revealed or discovered Structuralist Modern	No single objective reality to be discovered Nonstructuralist Postmodern
Analytical perspective	Reductionist	Holistic
Historical connection	Rooted in historical context of minority disadvantage and white domination	Steps outside of the historical context of race
Politics of institutions	Improve competence of providers and/or users to improve access to care/services	Proposes that competence, as a static concept, does not encompass the dynamic nature of clinical relationship
Relation to inequalities	Attempts to change and reduce health care inequalities	Acknowledges inequalities but as such does not directly attempt to change them
Role of teacher	Teacher sets the agenda	Teacher introduces the agenda
Role of learner	Primarily as receiver	Student contributes to the dialog and receives information
Conceptions of culture		
Conceptions of culture	Culture is an externally recognized characteristic Static One-dimensional Race/ethnicity emphasized Unitary	Culture is an internally constructed sense of self Dynamic/fluid Multidimensional Race is but one aspect Diverse/differentiated

Perception of individual's relationship to society

Conception of difference	Generalizes the differences between individuals	Sensitive to differences
Identity formation	Individuals are shaped by their social world	Individuals construct and accomplish their own social world
Conception of individual identity	An individual is defined by their culture	An individual defines their culture
Individual's relationship with society (relationship of self with society)	In defining culture, relationship is between groups	In defining culture, relationship is between an individual and others
	Dialog about culture takes place between groups	Dialog about culture takes place between individuals
	Individuals remain as defined by their culture, irrespective of the context	Individuals bring their own meanings and histories to different contexts (ie, the meanings may change dependent on the context)
Educational process		
Learning process	Acquisition of knowledge	Acquisition of principles (method)
Learning outcomes	Command of body of information and facts	Command of mode of respectful questioning
Expression of learning goals	In terms of skill and competence	In terms of attitudes and self-reflection
Content	Certain Dichotomous Right or wrong	Acknowledge uncertainty Mostly gray areas Not always right or wrong
Cultural focus	Majority view of other cultures dominant Majority whites must consider needs of minorities	No focus on particular groups, all individuals must consider needs of others
Cybernetics theory	First order (ie, the teacher teaches the student)	Second order (ie, the student and teacher learn together)
Pedagogic approach	Didactic	Directed self-learning
Role of experts	There are those who are experts on understanding cultural perspectives of certain groups	No one individual has ownership of expertise of others with respect to identification of cultural belonging
Educational content		
Curriculum type (as relating to Bernstein, 1973)[43]	Collection type	Integrated type
Nature of content	Parochial Specific	Global Nonspecific

(continued on next page)

Table 1
(continued)

Item	Cultural Expertise	Cultural Sensibility
Organization of content	To meet demands of local need	To maximize student self-learning
Curriculum	Fact acquisition to gain a body of knowledge	Self-reflection and self-awareness of students
Teaching focus	Groups (treats people as groups) More service-centered	Individuals (views individuals as potentially parts of different groups in different contexts) More patient-centered
Focus of content	Students learn about others	Students learn as much about themselves as about others
Outcomes		
What purpose does the assessment serve?	Demonstrates knowledge of other cultures	Demonstrates some understanding of self and ability to evaluate their own learning
Which methods are used?	Paper and pencil tests ranging from multiple- choice questions and short answers to long essays	Reflective journals, project work (usually experientially based)
Results of assessment	Norm-referenced (ie, students ranked against peers)	Not norm-referenced
Who leads the assessment process?	Teacher assessment	Student self-assessment
Measures to check outcomes	Checklists	Self-assessment
Outcome in clinical practice	Practical in that learner has facts about other cultures	Practical in that learner has a method of inquiry to be aware that others may have different perspectives More critical and self-reflective Greater capacity for dialog
Applicability	Learning can only be used for cultural issues	Learning can apply to any context in which differences exist between the doctor and patient, whether they are cultural-, gender-, or education-based
Patient centeredness	Doctor has position of expert	Doctor and patient are active partners in care
Definition of successful course	Students learn competence regarding other cultures, and bonus if students learn about themselves	Course is only successful if students learn about themselves, because this is necessary before they can relate to other perspectives

ADAPTING THE MODEL TO CHILD AND ADOLESCENT PSYCHIATRY

Psychiatry has been at the forefront of developing training in culture, because it has been long recognized that culture plays a part in how mental health is understood, how treatment of mental health problems are sought, and who is consulted about them (for example, transcultural psychiatry has been established for many years, as have journals such as *Transcultural Psychiatry, Culture, Psychiatry and Medicine* and, more recently, *The International Journal of Culture and Mental Health*, even while the understanding of culture has continued to develop). In the United States, the accrediting organizations for both undergraduate (Liaison Committee on Medical Education for medical school) and graduate medical education (Accreditation Council for Graduate Medical Education for residency and fellowship) have made this training mandatory across all medical specialties. In the United Kingdom, however, mental health is the only clinical specialty in which training in cultural issues is mandatory. Other specialties may then consider that these issues are not as relevant for them.

In the United States, psychiatry has strived to move away from its exclusive focus on psychoanalytic principles to become more biologic in focus and join other medical disciplines in having what is believed to be a rigorous and standardized approach to diagnosis and treatment. Although this move can be debated, the reality is that the "softer sciences" of anthropology and sociology were marginalized in the discipline just when cultural competence arose as a requirement from the medical education accreditation authorities. Furthermore, significant changes occurred over the past 20 years in the way culture is viewed, with essentialist perspectives being increasingly challenged. In trying to adapt any model to clinical context, it is useful to consider what implications diversity issues have on the practice of a particular medical specialty. In doing this, educators can identify the factors that may be specialty-specific.

Dogra and Karnik[32] argue that a cultural sensibility approach within the AAMC definitions places the practitioner in a position of learning about the unique cultural situation of a particular child and his or her family, allowing the assessment process to be used to gain information that will ensure any management plan incorporates the cultural perspective of the family, and thereby having the most potential acceptability to them.[33,34]

Clinicians must also identify their own biases about specific children and families. These assumptions constitute the "baggage" taken into the clinical or consultation context. Conscious awareness of bias is important not only because it may lead to suboptimal care toward those toward whom prejudice exists but also because overcompensation may occur from a sense of guilt. For example, if clinicians are uncomfortable dealing with a particular cultural subgroup but do not acknowledge this, they may be overly sympathetic and supportive in a context in which the more appropriate response may be to expect more responsibility from the young person or family. In training, this is often glossed over as "awareness" of the problem. However, the authors believe this approach must be more rigorous, and clinicians' assumptions must be challenged as routine practice.

The findings of Garland and colleagues[35] that adolescents, caregivers, and therapists have different expectations for outcomes of the consultation can also highlight how culture might influence who is allowed to express themselves at meetings. Family expectations may mean that the therapist is not supposed to give as much weight to the young person's perspective as to that of adults, or that the father's view may override the maternal perspective. All of these dynamics require careful negotiation and sensitivity, yet cannot be ignored. It is arguable that anyone working with patients and their families must be aware of these issues. However, effective child and adolescent psychiatry practice cannot be achieved without them.

The Cultural Sensibility Approach in Everyday Practice

The authors favor an approach that uses the clinical encounter as the beginning for the development of the cultural sensibility view. When engaging with their patients, they not only elicit important information about history and symptoms but also ask about elements of culture as these arise naturalistically in the encounter. The authors resist making assumptions about beliefs and instead tend to ask what the patients think about, how the symptoms began, what medicines mean, how the patients view psychiatry, and what the patients are hoping to achieve today. Superficially, these questions seem like standard open-ended clinical history questions, but when taking into consideration the culture of the individual and family, they take on a very different tone and focus.

Case Example

A 16-year-old woman with cystic fibrosis living in the San Francisco Bay Area was hospitalized because of disease exacerbation , and reported on several elements of her history and overall physical functioning. Her father was her only immediate family; her mother had died of a drug overdose several years earlier and her brother no longer lived in the household and had severed contact with the father, although he continued to keep in touch with the patient through phone calls. The patient herself used cannabis and alcohol, and smoked cigarettes regularly, causing regular flares of her cystic fibrosis. On interview, the child psychiatrist asked follow-up questions about her life, school, and home situation. It became apparent that although her father as a single parent was doing his best to provide for her, she spent large amounts of time without adult supervision. Her self-defined culture revolved around Facebook, her basketball-playing friends, and a series of unsupervised parties. The tobacco, drugs, and alcohol were elements of this culture and were partly the driving forces at the parties that she attended. This patient knew the calculus that she was engaged in: she was sacrificing her future health to have fun in the present. Her father's culture, in contrast, was framed by the blue-collar job he held as a truck driver and his constant efforts to make financial ends meet to support himself and his daughter. He recognized the destructive pattern that his daughter was on but felt powerless to prevent it, and they argued regularly.

The intervention in this case became one of reconciling the two cultures. The process began in eliciting the cultural perspectives. The reconciliation began by having the father understand his daughter's perspective that she was going to die despite whether she continued a clean-and-sober approach; that it was simply a matter of time. The father then decided to approach two of his daughter's friends and talk with them about their mutual partying and substance use. These friends knew about the patient's cystic fibrosis, but were unaware of the impact smoking had on her health. They cared deeply for their friend, and elected to change their patterns and try to get the patient to quit smoking. These friends also began to effect a change in their local cultural milieu by convincing many of their friends to start to have substance-free parties. Initially, the patient was upset about her father's interventions in her local world, but as her friends helped normalize the changes, she gradually came to accept them as a process of growing up and becoming more like an adult.

The cultural sensibility approach incorporates a developmental perspective through its very nature. It recognizes that culture is one of several elements, such as morality, spirituality, and personal beliefs, that evolve and emerge over time. Ward Goodenough[36] defined culture as "whatever it is one has to know or believe to operate in a manner acceptable to its members." For children, the members could be family, friends, or other social circles. Adolescents may identify with (and even define themselves in) different cultures at different points in time and depending on whom they are interacting with at the moment. This behavior is particularly true for teens who want to keep their family from understanding the other cultures to which they ascribe. For example, a gay teen might ascribe to views of other gay teens he spends time with at school or in other settings, but if he has not yet "come out" to his parents, he may present himself in an entirely different cultural light when he is with his family.

The process approach takes time for therapists to develop in a relationship with the patient and family, and also allows for cultural understandings to dynamically change over the course of treatment. Providers who want to use this approach can begin with some of the questions in the Outline,[19] and then continue to process and investigate the deeper aspects of cultural experience that emerge during treatment. The authors believe that culture is at the very heart of the therapeutic alliance in child and adolescent psychiatry: from the family's views about medications to the experience of psychiatric symptoms and their meaning in the social world.

Developmentally, cultural understanding may change and shift rapidly. Generally, toddlers and school-aged children share most of their culture with their parents or guardians. At these ages, the understandings of culture may be expressed by the child neither as a set of understandings nor as an overall system. It is more likely to emerge as a series of individual elements. For example, the child might describe the type of foods that she likes and how her mother prepares particular dishes that are unique and different from the foods that her friends and their families eat. The school-aged child can certainly appreciate difference but may not have the broader context within which to place these differences.

As the child grows and enters the middle school–aged years, she will begin to formulate more of a system. She will then likely have developed particular opinions and thoughts about music, movies, popular culture, and style that she sees reflected around her. At this point, the (now) teen may begin the process of differentiating from the parent's or family's cultural view. At this stage, young adolescents begin to identify with increasingly specific peer groups, and these groups begin to influence teens' perception of their own selves and consequently their culture.

In middle to older adolescence, as with many other developmental milestones, youth begin to differentiate from their families. This developmental period is characterized by elements of resistance and self-discovery. Cultural self-identification is one aspect of this process. Youths may see their parents as having outmoded beliefs, and not truly understanding the world as they know it. First relationships, an increasing reliance on peers, and greater immersion in popular culture and media may lead to a higher likelihood of cultural differentiation.

All of these cultural developmental processes are themselves ensconced in larger cultural frames. For some youths, this process will move rapidly, with a high degree of differentiation from their families of origin, whereas others will move along this continuum slowly and only marginally differentiate themselves. Thus, in practice, the child and adolescent psychiatrist must be sensitive to the developmental stages of their patients to accurately gauge their culture and the degree of relationship to the family.

TEACHING THE MODEL TO STUDENTS AND TRAINEES

It is arguable that diversity issues should be addressed during basic medical undergraduate education (before residency or fellowship). During child and adolescent training, the skills learned at medical school should be refined and honed in a practice context. However, directors of training programs must be aware that, despite the fact that the bodies governing medical school curricula mandate its inclusion, great variability exists in what is actually covered.[18] It can be erroneous to assume that trainees have the skills or confidence required to deliver culturally appropriate care to patients who may come from a wide range of sociodemographic backgrounds and communities.

In this section, the authors first propose what should be taught, and then describe a method for teaching it. Dogra and colleagues[37] suggest the following as essential and core:

> Curriculum planners should focus on educational policies to ensure that there is institutional ownership of cultural diversity education and to create a safe learning environment. The learning outcomes must be clear and achievable. The following learning outcomes are suggested as a minimum requirement:
> Define *cultural diversity* and apply this definition with respect to clinical practice.
> Critically appraise the use of key terms, such as race, ethnicity, culture, multiculturalism, and inequalities of access to health care.
> Acknowledge that bias and assumptions are a normal part of intersubjective experience, and then evaluate your own attitudes and perceptions (including personal bias) regarding different groups within society.
> Evaluate institutional prejudices and how these relate to your own perspectives.
> Identify strategies to challenge prejudice effectively and identify local policy in this area to ensure robustness.
> Evaluate and justify the approaches used in your own clinical practice.
> Assess the impact (both positive and negative) of your attitudes on your clinical practice and show respect for patients and colleagues who encompass diversity of background, opportunity, language, culture, and way of life.
> List the different approaches to developing skills in meeting the needs of diverse populations, and compare and contrast these.
> Describe existing equal opportunity legislation.
> Explain how you would apply the legislation to your practice as a health care provider and an employer.
> Evaluate the relevance of cultural diversity training in health care.

The rationale for these objectives comes from extensive research and teaching in this area. The authors suggest that a need exists to promote all aspects of human diversity (using broad definitions, such as that provided by the AAMC). Finally, culture must not be equated with merely ethnic, racial, or religious difference.

Methods for Teaching Cultural Sensibility

To meet the suggested outcomes, programs must use a range of methods. Whatever approaches are used, most of the teaching will need to allow students to discuss issues, reflect on their perspectives, and relate these to delivering high-quality care that is equitable irrespective of patient background, indicating that seminars allowing discussion should be an integral part of any program.

Selection of readings is particularly important in this type of classroom setting. Readings about particular cultures can be helpful, especially if trainees are able to ascertain broader principles regarding how to engage in dialog with patients and families about cultural views and practices, rather than relying on the learning of simple facts about cultures. Role-playing can be especially useful in this instance because it allows trainees to practice asking open-ended questions and allows them to become comfortable in bringing these questions to the foreground while also distilling this information from the basic clinical interview. Role-playing also allows interaction by the other trainees observing the situation, and critical feedback on the ways that questions can be either enabling or limiting. The cultural sensibility approach also allows trainees to use role-playing as a means to examine their own biases and prejudices, and bring these forward in a way that is productive and explorative.

The authors find it easiest for the instructor to begin the role-playing exercise as the patient and break from character as needed to facilitate points and discussion. As trainees grow more comfortable with this format, they should begin to play the patient role on a rotating basis. It is also helpful for the instructor to prepare character outlines for the trainees to play as a means to prompt discussion and interaction.

Online educational programs undertaken in groups may be a way of using education tools in the face of limited resources, but educators must be aware of some potential problems. Two major limitations are that students may not really challenge themselves or be challenged in a way that is possible in a more interpersonal learning context. Also, students may go through the motions of an online program but not really engage with the material; this is even more likely if students are resistant or dismissive to the idea of diversity education. Ideally, online programs can serve as an introductory guide that is then followed up with a group activity, during which views can be challenged or modified in response to discussion and reflection. However, some students may find it more comfortable (and perhaps not be challenged enough) to begin these programs alone before engaging in group activity.

Platt and colleagues[38] write about the key aspects of patient-centered interviewing. The key areas that require exploration are:

1. Who is this person? What constitutes that person's life? What are the patient's interests, work, important relationships, and main concerns?
2. What does the patient want from the physician? What are his/her values and fears? What does he/she hope to accomplish in the visit or over the longer term?
3. How does the patient experience the illness or problems?
4. What are the patient's ideas about the illness/problem?
5. What are the patient's main feelings about the illness?

It is arguable that this is nothing more than good psychiatric interviewing and part of a comprehensive assessment, just as are the questions suggested by Kleinman.[31] However, providing culturally appropriate care involves taking these questions and the answers to them one step further. The clinician must consider how the responses to the above questions fit in with the wider world and also with the provider's own perspective. Appendix 1 provides a sample curriculum used by one of the authors.

Whatever method is used to deliver the program, lectures, didactic teaching, and information about specific cultures should constitute very little of the curriculum. Students may find uncertainty uncomfortable,[39] but merely giving them information may provide a false sense of security. Culhane-Pera and colleagues[40] found that residents also preferred receiving information, and there can be a tendency to focus on learning information rather than engaging with one's own world views and how subjective it really is.

Faculty Support and Development

Dogra and colleagues[18] argue that faculty development is an essential component to consider, and evidence suggests that staff do not feel well supported in this area. Senior faculty and staff may also feel less comfortable with this issue.[41] Child and

adolescent psychiatrists will generally be familiar with managing different perspectives, but may still be less comfortable in owning their biases and considering the
potential impact of these on their practice. Although most psychiatrists are familiar
with the notion of transference and countertransference, blind spots may exist around
issues of diversity, with regard to members of cultural groups similar to one's own and
others'. Program directors may want to consider how the trainers they manage or
coordinate view these issues, and also how they think their trainees might best
develop their skills.

Whatever educational programs are developed, the education philosophy, process,
contents, and outcomes must be systematically considered. Clarity about the philosophy and outcomes should enable development of a coherent program. All programs
should include an expectation that clinicians identify their own biases and assumptions about the patients and families they are likely to encounter. Personal perspectives are crucial to recognize because they impact the clinical consultation.

SUMMARY: FUTURE DIRECTIONS AND RESEARCH AGENDA

The field of cultural child and adolescent psychiatry is a relatively new one, and treatment models and approaches have yet to develop consensus and an evidence base.
The cultural sensibility approach builds on present approaches to culture and medical
education. It can enable psychiatry trainees to develop a skill set that allows for the
interactive gathering of information in a culturally sensitive and open-minded way
that recognizes that patients, family members, and clinicians alike must develop an
understanding of each other's perspectives.

The future development of child and adolescent psychiatry depends on it being
a flexible and adaptable specialty that is able to meet the needs of diverse communities with coherence and integrity. To do so, it must address cultural issues with greater
sophistication than earlier models suggest. Cultural sensibility as a model may help
provide the field with the essential tools for meeting the needs of changing generations
and cultures of patients and families. The authors believe the field must begin to (1)
develop more pedagogic techniques to give trainees the tools to meet the needs of
their patients, (2) consider the generalizability of this model to other areas of medical
education and to the teaching of other health professionals, and (3) develop better
methods to assess the technical skills of trainees to effectively practice culturally
sensible child and adolescent psychiatry.

A need also exists to test the models and develop better evidence to ensure that
they can be modified and adapted to remain dynamic. Recent changes to the structure of the specialty board examinations in psychiatry training programs in the United
States have created an opportunity for the faculty to more directly assess a trainee's
clinical skill set. This change should include evaluation of the degree to which culture is
addressed in the clinical encounter, and also assessment of how this information can
be synthesized and used effectively in treatment planning.

Culture may uniquely influence the practice of child psychiatry compared with
other disciplines, given that how a society views children is to a lesser or greater
extent culturally influenced, as is the behavior they present with. Children are
dependent on their families, and the meaning of family and how families respond
to children's emotions and behaviors is a complex relationship between the wider
culture and the microfamilial culture. This fact has several implications for the field.
A need exists to strike a balance between understanding parental concerns and
perspectives and those of the child, which are no less important. In trying to
balance the wider culture and the culture of their family, young people may

face challenges that lead them to mental health services. To initiate appropriate interventions, clinicians must ensure that they are mindful of their own perspectives and how these interplay with those of the family and the young person. Only if these issues are acknowledged and addressed will it be possible to devise management plans that are clinically sound and also acceptable to the whole family. Any program that purports to teach trainees about providing culturally appropriate care to diverse communities should show that it enables trainees to take into account all perspectives and also the medicolegal contexts the field works in to deliver high-quality clinical care.

APPENDIX 1: SAMPLE CURRICULUM: TEACHING CULTURAL PSYCHIATRY

The approach to teaching cultural psychiatry will be defined by several factors: Is the course free-standing or part of other courses? How many hours are devoted to this topic? How many students are in the course? And, what is the level of experience for the trainees in the course? One example is provided of a small (6–8 students) postgraduate seminar that was 1 hour per week for 6 weeks and taught by one of the authors.

Trainees were assigned to read *The Spirit Catches You and You Fall Down* by Anne Fadiman.[42] This book is an excellent touchstone for discussion because it details the actual events of a young girl in the Hmong community who had epilepsy. The book is useful as a teaching tool because Fadiman carefully weaves the story by presenting both the biomedical perspective of the physicians along with the cultural story of the Hmong family. The clash of cultures emerges over time, and neither perspective ultimately gains primacy; both are given a degree of respect and a degree of criticism.

Through using this book as the focal point of discussion in the first class, students begin to discuss their cultural assumptions and beliefs, especially during the clinical encounter. In this first session, it is important to create a safe classroom space where trainees feel free to express their beliefs without fear of recrimination or retribution. It is also reasonable to set ground rules for the discussion that include a degree of group confidentiality, so that trainees can express their feelings openly and honestly.

The next 3 weeks of the course introduce the cultural sensibility framework using a case-based approach. Trainees are encouraged to bring active cases to the class to discuss and consider. Throughout this section of the course, definitions and readings drawn heavily from anthropology and sociology emphasize the core definitions of concepts while also presenting a model for trainees to incorporate into the clinical encounter. Trainees practice phrasing open-ended questions in nondirective ways to elicit the cultural, spiritual, and identity issues that are key to the patient. In addition, because of the child and adolescent subspecialty training in this class, the trainees are exposed to ways of thinking about the questions they raise in developmentally appropriate ways, and also to differentiate between the culture of the child or adolescent and that of the family and broader society.

The final 2 weeks of the class serve as an opportunity to bring closure to the course. Discussion focuses on transference and countertransference through the lens of culture, and the ways that trainees can establish ways to continue to explore their own biases and lifelong learning patterns.

The structure of this course is just one way of reflecting this material, but it allows trainees and faculty an opportunity for self-reflection and for building a durable framework from which to approach culture in the psychiatric context. This structure can be adapted depending on the size of the class and number of contact hours.

REFERENCES

1. Merton RK. Columbia University. Bureau of Applied Social Research. The student-physician; introductory studies in the sociology of medical education. Cambridge (UK): Published for the Commonwealth Fund by Harvard University Press; 1957.
2. Becker HS. Boys in white; student culture in medical school. Chicago: University of Chicago Press; 1961.
3. Ainsworth MD. Infancy in Uganda; infant care and the growth of love. Baltimore (MD): Johns Hopkins Press; 1967.
4. Bowlby J. A secure base: parent-child attachment and healthy human development. New York: Basic Books; 1988.
5. Bowlby J. The making & breaking of affectional bonds. London: Tavistock Publications; 1979.
6. Bowlby J. Institute of Psycho-analysis (Great Britain). Attachment and loss. London: Hogarth P; Institute of Psycho-Analysis; 1969.
7. Canino IA, Spurlock J. Culturally diverse children and adolescents: assessment, diagnosis, and treatment. New York: Guilford Press; 1994.
8. Bird HR, Canino GJ, Davies M, et al. Prevalence and correlates of antisocial behaviors among three ethnic groups. J Abnorm Child Psychol 2001;29(6): 465–78.
9. Bird HR. Epidemiology of childhood disorders in a cross-cultural context. J Child Psychol Psychiatry 1996;37(1):35–49.
10. Canino GJ, Bird HR, Rubio-Stipec M, et al. Reliability of child diagnosis in a Hispanic sample. J Am Acad Child Adolesc Psychiatry 1987;26(4):560–5.
11. Comer JP. Black children and child psychiatry. J Am Acad Child Psychiatry 1985; 24(2):129–33.
12. Lidz T. A psychosocial orientation to schizophrenic disorders. Yale J Biol Med 1985;58(3):209–17.
13. McClure M, Shirataki S. Child psychiatry in Japan [review]. J Am Acad Child Adolesc Psychiatry 1989;28(4):488–92.
14. Offord DR, Boyle MH, Jones BR. Psychiatric disorder and poor school performance among welfare children in Ontario. Can J Psychiatry 1987;32(7):518–25.
15. Rotheram-Borus MJ. Ethnic differences in adolescents' identity status and associated behavior problems. J Adolesc 1989;12(4):361–74.
16. Tseng WS, McDermott JF Jr, Ogino K, et al. Cross-cultural differences in parent-child assessment: U.S.A. and Japan. Int J Soc Psychiatry 1982;28(4):305–17.
17. Westermeyer J. Prevention of mental disorder among Hmong refugees in the U.S.: lessons from the period 1976-1986. Soc Sci Med 1987;25(8):941–7.
18. Dogra N, Reitmanova S, Carter-Pokras O. Teaching cultural diversity: current status in U.K., U.S., and Canadian medical schools. J Gen Intern Med 2010;25(Suppl 2):S164–8.
19. American Psychiatric Association, APA Task Force on DSM-IV. Diagnostic and statistical manual of mental disorders: DSM-IV-TR. 4th edition. Washington, DC: American Psychiatric Association; 2000.
20. Grossberg L, Nelson C, Treichler PA. Cultural studies. New York: Routledge; 1992.
21. Johnson AG. The Blackwell dictionary of sociology: a user's guide to sociological language. 2nd edition. Oxford (UK); Malden (MA): Blackwell Publishers; 2000.
22. Mulholland J, Dyson S. Sociological theories of "race" and ethnicity. In: Culley L, Dyson S, editors. Ethnicity and nursing practice. London: Palgrave; 2001. p. 17–37.

23. Dogra N. The learning and teaching of cultural diversity in undergraduate medical education in the UK. Leicester (UK): University of Leicester; 2004.
24. Giddens A. Capitalism and modern social theory; an analysis of the writings of Marx, Durkheim and Max Weber. Cambridge (UK): University Press; 1971.
25. Dogra N. Cultural competence or cultural sensibility? A comparison of two ideal type models to teach cultural diversity to medical students. International Journal of Medicine 2003;5(4):223–31.
26. Fowler HW, Fowler FG, Thompson D. The concise Oxford dictionary of current English. 9th edition. New York: Clarendon Press; 1995.
27. American Medical Association. Enhancing the cultural competence of physicians. In: American Medical Association, editor. Cultural competence compendium. Chicago: American Medical Association; 1999. Report 5-A-98 [online].
28. Beach MC, Price EG, Gary TL, et al. Cultural competence: a systematic review of health care provider educational interventions. Med Care 2005;43(4):356–73.
29. Hobgood C, Sawning S, Bowen J, et al. Teaching culturally appropriate care: a review of educational models and methods. Acad Emerg Med 2006;13(12):1288–95.
30. Berlin EA, Fowkes WC Jr. A teaching framework for cross-cultural health care. Application in family practice. West J Med 1983;139(6):934–8.
31. Kleinman A. Patients and healers in the context of culture: an exploration of the borderland between anthropology, medicine, and psychiatry. Berkeley (CA): University of California Press; 1980.
32. Dogra N, Karnik N. Teaching cultural diversity to medical students. Med Teach 2004;26(8):677–80.
33. Dogra N. Culture and child psychiatry. In: Bhattacharya R, Cross S, Bhugra D, editors. Clinical topics in cultural psychiatry. London: Royal College of Psychiatrists Press; 2010.
34. Dogra N. Ethnicity and culture and their relationship to health care. InnovAIT 2010;3(6):366–72.
35. Garland AF, Lewczyk-Boxmeyer CM, Gabayan EN, et al. Multiple stakeholder agreement on desired outcomes for adolescents' mental health services. Psychiatr Serv 2004;55(6):671–6.
36. Goodenough WH. Cultural anthropology and linguistics. In: Gavin PL, editor. Report of the 7th Annual Round Table Meeting on linguistics and language study. Washington, DC: Georgetown University Press; 1957. p. 167–73.
37. Dogra N, Reitmanova S, Carter-Pokras O. Twelve tips for teaching diversity and embedding it in the medical curriculum. Med Teach 2009;31(11):990–3.
38. Platt FW, Gaspar DL, Coulehan JL, et al. "Tell me about yourself": the patient-centered interview. Ann Intern Med 2001;134(11):1079–85.
39. Dogra N, Giordano J, France N. Cultural diversity teaching and issues of uncertainty: the findings of a qualitative study. BMC Med Educ 2007;7:8. PMCID: PMC1871589.
40. Culhane-Pera KA, Reif C, Egli E, et al. A curriculum for multicultural education in family medicine. Fam Med 1997;29(10):719–23.
41. Tang TS, Bozynski ME, Mitchell JM, et al. Are residents more comfortable than faculty members when addressing sociocultural diversity in medicine? Acad Med 2003;78(6):629–33.
42. Fadiman A. The spirit catches you and you fall down. New York: Farrar, Strauss & Giroux; 1989.
43. Bernstein B. On the classification and framing of educational knowledge. In: Young MFD, editor. Knowledge and control: new directions for the sociology of education. London: Collier MacMillan; 1971. p. 47–69.

Culturally Informed Child Psychiatric Practice

Andres J. Pumariega, MD[a,b,*], Eugenio M. Rothe, MD[c],
SuZan Song, MD[d], Francis G. Lu, MD[e]

KEYWORDS

- Culture • Psychiatry • Assessment • Treatment • Children
- Adolescents

As a result of the major demographic changes the United States is currently undergoing, there will no longer be a numeric majority of European-origin children and youth by 2030, and this is already the case among those 7 years old or younger.[1] Therefore, the patients treated by child and adolescent psychiatrists and child mental health professionals comprise an increasingly diverse group with unique and diverse needs. The acceptability of children's mental health services are highly influenced by attitudes, beliefs, and practices from their families' cultures of origin. The current science based around diagnosis and treatments, largely derived from research primarily with European-origin populations, has increasingly questionable validity for these emerging populations. At the same time, these new diverse populations face many different and at times increasing challenges regarding mental illness and emotional disturbances, including higher risks for certain forms of psychopathology, lower access to treatment services and evidence-based treatments, and higher burdens of morbidity and possibly mortality than Euro-Americans. For example, Latino and African American youth now have significantly higher rates of depression and suicidal

Disclosure: A.J.P. received access to data and data analysis support from Lilly Pharmaceuticals for 2 articles with his coauthorship cited in this article. E.R., S.S., and F.L. report no conflicts of interest.

[a] Child & Adolescent Psychiatry, The Reading Hospital and Medical Center, Sixth Avenue and Spruce Street, Reading, PA 19612, USA

[b] Temple University, Department of Psychiatry and Behavioral Sciences, Temple Episcopal Campus, 100 East Lehigh Avenue, Philadelphia, PA 19125, USA

[c] Herbert Wertheim College of Medicine, Florida International University, Modesto A. Maidique Campus, UHSC 270, 11200 SW 8th Street, Miami, FL 33199, USA

[d] Lucille Packard Children's Hospital, Stanford University School of Medicine, 725 Welch Road, Palo Alto, CA 94304, USA

[e] University of California-Davis, Department of Psychiatry and Behavioral Sciences, 2230 Stockton Boulevard, Sacramento, CA 95817, USA

* Corresponding author. Child & Adolescent Psychiatry, The Reading Hospital and Medical Center, Sixth Avenue and Spruce Street, Reading, PA 19612.

E-mail address: pumarieg@verizon.net

ideation and attempts than Euro-Americans, as highlighted by the most recent Youth Risk Behavior Survey by the US Centers for Disease Control and Prevention.[2]

Cultural, ethnic, and racial factors relating to mental illness, emotional disturbances, and their treatment deserve closer attention and consideration. However, our health care system, including our mental health system, has not been effective in addressing the needs of culturally diverse populations, resulting in racial/ethnic disparities in health associated with higher morbidity and even mortality among minorities. This outcome has led to the increasing recognition of racial and ethnic disparities in mental health care (see the article by Alegria and colleagues elsewhere in this issue for further exploration of this topic). In this article, the authors outline the practical application of cultural competence principles in day-to-day clinical work by child and adolescent psychiatrists and other mental health professionals.

CULTURAL COMPETENCE MODEL

In response to these mounting clinical and service delivery challenges, cultural competence became one of the core principles of the children's community-based systems of care movement from its outset. Cross and colleagues[3] defined cultural competence within the context of serving children with serious emotional disturbances as a "set of congruent behaviors, attitudes, and policies found in a system, agency, or a group of professionals that enables them to work effectively in a context of cultural difference." These investigators identified a spectrum of cultural competence that has been demonstrated by societies and their institutions over centuries, ranging from cultural destructiveness (genocide, lynching, ethnic cleansing), cultural incapacity (segregation, discrimination, immigration quotas, services that break up families), cultural blindness ("equal" treatment for all, but not making distinctions in services offered on differences in values or beliefs), cultural pre-competency (realization of differences but insufficient provision of services), to cultural competence. Few societies have achieved the last stage, cultural proficiency (provision of innovative culturally specific services and research).

Cross and colleagues[3] went on to define characteristics that culturally competent clinicians and organizations represented. For clinicians, they cited the key elements awareness/acceptance of difference, awareness of own cultural values, understanding dynamics of difference in the clinical encounter, the development of clinically relevant cultural knowledge, and the ability to adapt practice to cultural context of the patient. For the organization, they cited valuing diversity, the performance of cultural self-assessments, management of the dynamics of difference, institutionalization of cultural knowledge, and the adaptation to cultural diversity (including policies, values, structure, and services), accounting for unique characteristics such as their socioeconomic level, level of acculturation, and experience with the service system. Cross and colleagues asserted that it was difficult for clinicians to practice in a culturally competent fashion without the support from a culturally competent organization.

CULTURAL CHALLENGES TO DIAGNOSIS AND TREATMENT

Diagnosing culturally diverse children can be challenging to unfamiliar clinicians. Children from diverse populations can demonstrate different symptomatology compared with Euro-Americans, with misdiagnosis being a significant challenge.[4,5] One cause of misdiagnosis is different symptom expression as compared with European-origin populations for common forms of psychopathology. For example, somatization and anger are symptoms more frequently associated with depression and anxiety in minority youth, leading to underdiagnosis.[6,7] African American and Hispanic children who show anger or disruptive behaviors may have underlying internalizing disorders, but clinicians may focus on their externalizing symptoms.[8] Thresholds of distress are also different, as exemplified by differences in the degree of emotional reactivity seen during illness episodes. For example, depressed Asian-origin individuals show heightened reactivity during depression whereas Caucasians show less reactivity when depressed.[9] Similarly, Caribbean-origin Latinos can demonstrate more dramatic expressions of distress than Latinos originating from mainland Latin America and from European-origin populations.

Even normative affective expressiveness can vary greatly among and within cultural groups, and can similarly be misinterpreted as abnormal. For example, subdued expressiveness in Asian and American Indian children and adolescents, or aversion of eye contact with adults in Asian, African Americans, or mainland Latino children and adolescents, are signs of respect for elders. Native American culture emphasizes nonverbal communication, and feelings, particularly anger, are not to be expressed openly or verbally.

Diverse cultural groups' understanding of emotional distress and even mental illness can vary significantly, and can influence their expressions of distress and help-seeking behaviors. Idioms of distress are linguistic or somatic patterns of experiencing and expressing illness, affliction, or general stress. These idioms vary significantly among different ethnic/cultural groups; at times they may not even be indicators of psychopathology but of normal emotional distress, and as such can be misdiagnosed. For example, Latinos have specific cultural idioms of distress to describe the somatization process, such as *nervios* (nerves), anger-related illnesses such as *bilis* (bile) or *cólera* (rage), conditions associated with the hot-cold theory of disease such as *pasmo* (spasm of muscles), or afflictions attributed to the abnormal circulation of air in the body, such as *mal aire* (bad air) or *gases*. Some of these expressions take on unique symptom patterns or characteristics not found at all in the diagnostic nosology as outlined by the *Diagnostic and Statistical Manual of Mental Disorders* (Fourth Edition, Text Revised) (DSM-IV-TR),[10] and are referred to as culture-bound syndromes. For example, many Caribbean-origin Latinos describe a constellation of depressive, anxiety, somatic, and dissociative symptoms known as *nervios* (nerves) illness, and can experience an acute syndrome termed *ataques de nervios*, which combines these symptoms as well as agitation, dissociation, and even brief psychosis. These culturally specific idioms of distress or syndromes are based on explanatory models that are founded on or invoke spiritual, supernatural, or unique interpersonal beliefs, Such explanatory models and expressions may lead families to seek help from a spiritual healer rather than a mental health professional, thus making diagnosis and treatment more challenging.[11–14]

Diagnosing culturally diverse minority children is also more challenging due to the frequent presence of comorbidities. For example, stresses associated with immigration, acculturation stress, discrimination, and community violence contribute not only to depression but also to comorbidities of anxiety, disruptive behavior, substance abuse, and/or posttraumatic stress disorders.[15–17] As with many people of lower socioeconomic status, people of immigrant and minority backgrounds tend to postpone seeking treatment until either the child's situation is fairly critical, or the family is under significant distress from his or her symptoms. This situation may be related to their socioeconomic background, lack of insurance, multiple economic and social demands, stigma of mental illness, perceived barriers to treatment, and cultural values that are more present-focused and not as future- or prevention-oriented (see the article by Alegria and colleagues elsewhere in this issue for further exploration of this topic).

Biological factors related to culture have risen in importance as we have come to rely more on pharmacological treatments. Various genes control the metabolism of drugs through their effects on metabolizing enzymes, receptor regulation, and transporters, and their polymorphisms are associated with different racial and ethnic populations. The article by Lawson and colleagues elsewhere in this issue review the importance of ethnopharmacology in the mental health of culturally diverse children and youth. The rapidly growing knowledge from this field and its related field of pharmacogenomics will need to be rapidly incorporated into the knowledge base and treatment armamentarium of clinicians serving diverse populations.

Culturally Informed Clinical Assessment

Language and communication are critical in obtaining accurate clinical information and establishing a therapeutic alliance, especially with family members. However, many immigrants (particularly recent immigrant youth and especially parents) may have limited English proficiency and may not be able to fully participate in the clinical process. In those situations, translation and interpretation are critical to effective care, and interpreters should be readily available and have proper training in both translation and psychiatric terminology and services. These professionals should not only serve as linguistic interpreters but also as cultural consultants, helping to decipher verbal and nonverbal communication. The lack of interpreter services leads to the use of untrained translators, including family members, siblings, or even the affected child, without regard to the adverse impact of these practices. The use of the affected child should be always forbidden, given its demonstrated deleterious effects on family function.[18] Similarly, any rating instruments used should not only be translated to the language of the family member or child but should also (if possible) be validated and normed for that given ethnic/racial population.[19,20]

At times, diverse families may seek treatment under external pressure from social agencies, such as school, child welfare, or juvenile justice officials, or during an emergent situation as a result of postponement of services. Treatment thus tends to start on an adversarial and more urgent basis, with higher rates of involuntary commitment and premature termination from treatment.[4] These trends have significant implications for treatment effectiveness, as symptomatic improvement without remission because of premature termination is often associated with poor prognosis, more recurrences, and poorer outcomes. Stigma is also a major culturally related barrier to seeking mental health services. Many cultures have major negative associations with mental illness, while the fear of double discrimination (being culturally different as well as "crazy") also presents diverse families and youth from accessing services.[21] Some of these attitudes may originate historically in negative experiences with the mental health system by minority populations in the United States and by immigrants in their home nations.[22] The patient and family should be explicitly reassured about patient confidentiality to the fullest extent possible, because some immigrant families are very concerned about people in their community having knowledge about what is revealed.

Clinicians' self-awareness about their attitudes and perceptions of diverse patients is a critical aspect of effective cross-cultural evaluation and treatment. The report by the Institute of Medicine[23] titled *Unequal Treatment* has outlined how racial/ethnic disparities are related to subtle factors at the level of clinicians affecting their ability to objectively evaluate diverse populations in the face of cultural difference. The report hypothesizes 3 main factors contributing to health disparities: health systems-level factors—financing, structure of care, cultural and linguistic barriers; patient-level factors—patient preferences, refusal of treatment, poor adherence, and biological differences; and disparities arising from the clinical encounter. The investigators found that the main clinician factors were related to clinicians' possible tendencies to engage in bias, uncertainty, and stereotyping when encountering diverse patients. No evidence suggests that providers are more likely than the general public to express racial/ethnic biases, but some evidence suggests that unconscious biases may exist. Uncertainty was found to be plausible, particularly when providers treat patients who are dissimilar in cultural or linguistic background and they are uncertain about how to approach their care. There is evidence that suggests that clinicians, like everyone else, use "cognitive shortcuts" that result from stereotyping.

Effectiveness in addressing cultural factors is related not only to knowledge about the family's cultural background but also to the clinician's ability to form a patient- and family-centered alliance in which he or she respect the family's knowledge and unique perspectives on the child, avoids stereotyping, and empowers them to make critical treatment decisions. Cooper and colleagues[24] demonstrated that the failure to form such alliances contributes to significant barriers in assessment and subsequent use of health services by minority patients, whereas race-concordant clinician-patient pairs tended to prevent such misalliance. The initial interview is a critical juncture to establish a strong therapeutic alliance. Factors such as the maintenance of appropriate distance, eye contact, use of appropriate gestures in greetings, and demonstrating genuine warmth can serve as grounds for establishing trust or developing mistrust of the clinician.[25]

It is also important to obtain critical contextual information during the initial evaluation about how culture influences the child's and family's understanding of the presenting problems and perceptions of needs. This interview includes asking about beliefs and attitudes about treatment, and inquiring after whether treatment was coerced in any way or whether there is conflict in the family around accessing services. The clinician should address these concerns as best possible, and empower the family and older child to make the most appropriate treatment choices available, addressing the perceptions of power differentials with the clinician. The clinician should inquire about barriers that may prevent the family from obtaining services for their child or adolescent, including bureaucratic barriers common in hospitals or clinics. Diverse children and their families are usually best served in community clinics located in familiar community locations where families feel comfortable, and should be affiliated with institutions that are favorably viewed by the community.[20]

The clinician should assess the strengths and needs of both the child or adolescent and of key family members, taking into account the danger of prematurely assigning diagnoses to the patient. The clinician should attend to variations in the expression of affect and behavior to prevent misdiagnosis, taking into account idioms of distress, differential expressions of normal emotions/affect and symptoms, and culture-bound syndromes.[13,14] The diagnosis and treatment of diverse children must be contextual, addressing psychosocial and cultural needs and being consonant within the values and beliefs of the minority family. The cultural and family context of symptomatology (eg, normative crises such as grief or mourning) must be considered in the assessment of a minority child. One must also assess the level of assimilation and acculturation of both the child and his or her parents and family, the presence of acculturation stress influencing symptoms, or whether cross-cultural dynamics may play a role in symptomatology (such as acculturative family distancing, discrimination, or marginalization from the majority culture or the youth's own culture).[26,27]

It is important to inquire about the family's cultural values, spiritual and religious beliefs and practices, family and gender roles, and language preference and fluency of key family members, the latter serving as a proxy for level of acculturation. The use of a cultural consultant, with the family's consent, can also be useful in dealing with issues related to traditional beliefs and values, as well as their potential distortion (for example, whether spiritual preoccupations are consistent with the family's cultural or religious practices or are a psychotic distortion).[20] The inclusion of extended family members and nonblood relatives who possess an equivalent emotional bond (ie, "fictive kin"[28]) have been shown to be essential in obtaining the necessary collateral input needed for appropriate diagnosis and subsequent treatment recommendations.

A history of the immigrant child's and family's migration experience and possible traumatic experiences should be an essential part of the diagnostic interview. The history should include traumas before immigration (such as natural disasters, terrorism, warfare, or famine), during their journey (such as arduous journeys or victimization), or subsequent to arrival (such as prolonged and traumatic separations and reunifications from family members, social uprooting, and abrupt geographical relocations). For inner city children, it is important to inquire about exposure to violence at home or in their community, including the death of peers, sequential losses of parenting figures, and abuse or punitive childrearing.[20,29]

Models of Cultural Formulation

The DSM-IV-TR Outline for Cultural Formulation[30] provides a systematic method of considering and incorporating sociocultural issues into the clinical formulation. The Outline for Cultural Formulation is incorporated in the American Psychiatric Association Practice Guideline for the Psychiatric Evaluation for Adults. Although it may not be possible to do a complete cultural formulation based on the findings of the initial interview, these issues may be explored further during subsequent sessions with the patient and family. The information contained within the cultural formulation may be integrated with the other aspects of the clinical formulation or recorded separately. The cultural formulation includes the following 5 sections:

1. *Cultural identity* includes not only the individual's race/ethnicity, acculturation/biculturality, and language but also age, gender, gender identity, socioeconomic status, sexual orientation, religious and spiritual beliefs, disabilities, political orientation, and health literacy, among other factors.
2. *Cultural expressions and explanations of the illness* includes symptom expression and dysfunction, the patient's explanatory models of illness, and idioms of distress through which symptoms or needs may be communicated. Treatment history and preferences (including complementary and alternative medicine and indigenous approaches) are also identified. Due to possibly varying cultural identities and values of the child/adolescent and their parents due to acculturation, there may be varying cultural expressions and explanations of illness resulting in different treatment preferences.
3. *Cultural factors related to development, psychosocial environment, and level of functions* includes cultural factors related to psychosocial stressors, available social supports, and levels of function or disability, including the roles of family/kin and religion/spirituality in providing emotional and instrumental support. For children, one should also consider the impact of normal developmental expectations. All of these factors should be evaluated within the context of the youth's cultural reference group. As with the previous section, varying cultural identities may lead to value differences, which can cause intergenerational stress among family members.
4. *Cultural elements influencing the relationship between the individual and the clinician.* Differences in the cultural identities between the clinician and the child/adolescent and parents including race/ethnicity, language, and socioeconomic

status, among other factors, may add to the complexities of the clinical encounter. Transference and countertransference may be influenced by these cultural identity differences, interfering with or facilitating the treatment relationship. The impact of the clinician's sociocultural identity on the patient should be taken into account in the subsequent formulation of a diagnostic opinion. It is important for clinicians to know their limits of knowledge and skills rather than to reinforce damaging stereotypes and overgeneralizations.

5. *Overall cultural assessment* of the ways in which these cultural considerations will specifically apply to differential diagnosis and treatment planning.[30,31] As to differential diagnosis, the clinician must distinguish at the phenomenological level what is culturally congruent and what is psychopathological based on the information gathered in the previous sections. For example, hearing the voice of a deceased relative especially during bereavement may be culturally congruent for the cultural identity of the patient and family, and should not be misdiagnosed as an auditory hallucination. Second, the clinician must understand the possible misdiagnoses at the categorical level for a child or adolescent from a particular cultural background. For example, the DSM-IV-TR section on Specific Culture, Age, Gender Features for the diagnosis of schizophrenia notes that schizophrenia may be diagnosed more often in individuals who are African American and Asian American than in other racial groups.

Tseng[32] proposed the Cultural Analysis as a framework to understand patients' world views, with an emphasis on the importance of self and its relationships with others and with the world. The Cultural Analysis includes 3 broad domains: self, relations, and treatment. Within these domains basic elements are identified, with culture affecting the way in which each element is conceptualized, its relative importance, and its ideal or desired state. The *self domain* focuses on how the individual's overall self-concept is intrinsically tied to one's culture. Culture may affect the very building blocks of internal psychological experiences and observable actions, including affect, cognition, and behavior. Individual aims, goals, and motivating forces in life also depend on culture. Culture also influences the conceptualization of mind-body (dualistic vs more integrated), self-constructs, or theory of mind (individualistic or collectivistic); and the interpretation, antecedents, and acceptability (per cultural standards) of specific personal emotions. The *relations domain* addresses the cultural influence over the patients' world views regarding their relationships. This domain includes the patients' relationships with family and significant people in their life (hierarchical vs collateral vs exclusive nature of relationships); their relationship with nature and their environment (subservience, harmonious, or dominant); their relationship with and importance of material possessions; and their relationship with time orientation (the relative importance allocated to the past, present, or future) and how this affects such issues as spirituality and existential issues. The *treatment domain* highlights elements of therapy that may be especially influenced by culture. These elements include communication patterns, both verbal and nonverbal; problem-solution models (how patients conceptualize their difficulties); and the therapist-client relationship (including specified roles and transferences). Culture not only influences each element within the 3 domains individually but may also contribute to interactions within and across domains. In children and youth, the self domain will naturally be evolving developmentally and according to the youth's transition through the acculturation process. The relationship domain, which is very culturally value based, may be blended in its various orientation but will be abutting against what is usually a more traditional family interpretation. The therapist will most likely be bridging traditional and Western elements in the treatment domain in the individual and family components of therapy and treatment, given the usual cultural differences across generations.

CULTURALLY INFORMED TREATMENT: GENERAL PRINCIPLES

Treatment of minority children must also be contextual and integrative, addressing psychosocial and cultural needs as well as psychological and biological ones. The clinician must evaluate and mobilize familial, neighborhood, and community resources, address contributing and sustaining environmental factors, and enhance strengths that the child and family bring to treatment. The clinician should support parents in the development of appropriate behavioral management skills consonant with their cultural values and beliefs. Parents must respect culturally established means of communication and family role functioning but also foster family flexibility in dealing with their bicultural offspring.[20] At the same time, the clinician should address internal acculturative conflict resulting from the clash between values/beliefs from the culture of origin versus mainstream culture.[17]

Psychological interventions should be congruent with the values and beliefs of culturally diverse children and their families. More traditionally acculturated children and families may be more accepting of and responsive to therapeutic approaches with a practical problem-focused, here-and-now orientation. Clinicians must be realistic about the acceptability of therapeutic interventions that may not be consonant with the family's cultural values. At the same time, clinicians must advise families about naturalistic parenting approaches that may be acceptable in their culture of origin but may be considered unacceptable or illegal in mainstream culture, such as the use of corporal punishment. Consultation from and collaboration with traditional healers (such as curanderos, santeros, shamans, and religious ministers or priests), including the use of rituals and ceremonies from the youth's culture, may be an important component of treatment of children from more traditional families. This component helps to prevent conflict between healing orientations that families may experience, and can help develop traditional healers as potential collaborators. Referral to same-culture clinicians or culturally specific programs (for example, community-based clinics oriented to specific cultural groups) has been associated with improved attendance and adherence.[20]

A value-neutral approach, whereby the clinician models openness to the diverse cultural influences on the child and judicious self-disclosure of similar experiences, is a helpful technique. Confidentiality in psychotherapy must be addressed so that the clinician is not perceived as "driving a wedge" between the child and his or her family, nor used by the patient to resist dealing with family issues. Home-based or community-based alternatives to hospitalization usually result in better outcomes for diverse children and youth, whereas involuntary hospitalization tends to recreate past traumas of oppression. If at all possible, out-of-home placement should be accomplished with the cooperation of the family and youth. An interagency system of care approach is consistent with cultural competence, because it uses community resources and empowers the child and family to a maximum extent.[20]

In addition to being mindful and addressing ethnopharmacological issues, there are numerous interpersonal aspects of pharmacotherapy with minority children that require attention. These aspects include proper informed consent and family collaboration, particularly with traditional cultural family decision-makers (typically outside of the nuclear family); demystification of medications (not only education on their mechanisms of action but also addressing suspicions and myths); and empowerment of children and families to make medication choices and address power differentials with clinicians.[20]

There are several evidence-based interventions that are gaining considerable research support for use with minority and immigrant children and youth. Kataoka and colleagues elsewhere in this issue outline the current state of the evidence around psychological and community-based interventions for culturally diverse populations. It behooves child mental health clinicians to use psychological interventions with evidence specific to the population of origin to which that the child or youth being treated belongs. In the absence of such evidence, it may be indicated to make adaptations to broadly evidence-based interventions that enhance their acceptability and applicability without altering essential elements.

There is little psychopharmacological research on minority and immigrant children. The Treatment of Adolescent Depression Study (TADS[33]) had a 26% minority representation among its participants, and minority status was found not to be significant moderator of acute outcome. However, no separate data analyses on the effectiveness of the treatments examined has been published. For attention-deficit hyperactivity disorder, atemoxetine appears to have equal efficacy for Latinos and African Americans in open-label trials,[34,35] while stimulants have demonstrated effectiveness, but there is some question as to whether behavioral interventions are needed in addition to reach equal effectiveness.[36] There are significant problems concerning minority inclusion in research trials, and one of the unfortunate results of such lack of evidence may be the significantly lower numbers of minority children and youth who receive pharmacotherapy.[37–39]

Culturally Informed Psychotherapy

There are several evidence-based psychotherapy interventions that are gaining considerable research support for use with minority and immigrant children and youth. Some research evidence exists on cognitive-behavioral and interpersonal psychotherapies with Latino and African American youth.[40,41] Some therapists have developed interventions that are specific for particular ethnic and racial groups, which have been evaluated for efficacy, such as storytelling through pictures,[42] the use of Magical Realism for traumatized Hispanic children,[43] and the use of classroom drama therapy for immigrant and refugee children.[44] Family therapy interventions have been used successfully to address at-risk minority and immigrant youth, and have focused on issues of acculturative family distancing, family-related separations, intrafamilial conflicts, and the effects of discrimination.[45,46] Group psychotherapy, particularly approaches that integrate cultural and ethnic identity themes, psychoeducation, and culturally consonant coping approaches, have been reported as both well accepted and successful.[47,48]

Psychodynamic psychotherapy, which had been discarded by many for lacking an empirical base, has been reevaluated through the rigorous lens of meta-analysis and effect size. Psychodynamic psychotherapy has been found to be as effective as cognitive-behavioral therapy (CBT) and pharmacotherapy for the treatment of depression and generalized anxiety.[49] In addition, recent empirical analysis of psychodynamic psychotherapy reveals that it also works by helping develop the person's inner capacities and strengths, and that the improvement continues after the therapy has ended. Rothe[29] has outlined a model for treating immigrant Hispanic adolescents and their families with psychodynamic therapy that has utility with other immigrant and minority groups. The model includes: (1) providing a holding environment and a safe place for the adolescent to express affects and experience containment and tolerance; (2) facilitating the mourning process associated with the losses of immigration, including the expression of sorrow, which may not be permitted by adult family members who may perceive it as the child's "ingratitude" for the parent's sacrifices;

(3) becoming an object of identification for the immigrant adolescent, so he can rehearse the newly acquired parts of his identity that belong to the new culture and delete the parts of his identity that are no longer useful in the receiving country; (4) allowing transferences to develop and analyzing them, using the therapy as a new, reconstructive emotional experience; (5) serving as a mediator of affects between the adolescent and his family, allowing for both to complete their process of adaptation to the new culture; and (6) serving as a mediator between the adolescent's family and the new culture, empowering the family, promoting their autonomy, and enabling them to create a new "American Milieu" in which to thrive.

In some cultures, psychotherapy is uncommon or stigmatizing. Testimonial therapy has proven to be successful with traumatized refugees whose culture has an oral tradition of storytelling. Narrating and reframing the story allows the person to translate pain into political and spiritual dignity and can serve to highlight resiliency factors, such as the courage and intelligence that it took to survive.[50] Rothe[51] has developed a psychotherapy model for treating child and adolescent refugees living inside refugee camps, to minimize psychological trauma and to prevent dissociative memories that result from these experiences.

Despite the recent progress in the development of culturally sensitive and evidence-based treatments, dropping out from psychotherapy among children and adolescents remains a significant problem, affecting 40% to 60% of the cases that receive outpatient treatment.[52] Of note, interpersonal psychotherapy was initially evaluated with a very large Hispanic sample[53] and was later shown to be more effective than CBT in a head-to-head trial,[54] lending support to the congruence between cultural values (*personalismo*, or interpersonal skills among Hispanics) and the effectiveness of psychotherapeutic interventions. Establishing a strong therapeutic alliance in the earliest points of contact with the family and the child and identifying factors that weigh on the burden of treatment continue to be important future challenges to clinicians who provide treatment to these culturally diverse populations.[29]

Cultural Transference and Countertransference

Cultural transference refers to a patient developing a certain relationship, feeling, or attitude toward the therapist because of the therapist's perceived cultural background; cultural countertransference implies the reverse phenomenon, namely, a therapist developing a certain relationship with the patient mainly because of the patient's perceived cultural background. Transference or countertransference is primarily based on the previous knowledge, impression, bias, or experience of a therapist or a patient, which has its own cultural influences in relation to a particular cultural group, but is also affected by the nature of the differences or similarities in the patient's and therapist's cultural background, race, gender, sexual orientation, socioeconomic background, and other identifying characteristics. Cultural transference or countertransference can be positive or negative, and can significantly influence the process of therapy, requiring timely attention and management. Cultural transference may express itself in various ways: mistrust, suspicion, and hostility; denial of therapist cultural differences; idealization and overcompliance; friendliness and overfamiliarity; or ambivalence toward the therapist. Countertransference can express itself as denial of patient's cultural differences, excessive curiosity about the patient's cultural background (often referred to as "cultural tourism"), or excessive feelings of anger, guilt, or ambivalence toward the patient.[32,55] It is important to remember that in work with children and youth, transference and countertransference principles apply to the therapeutic relationships with families, which in culturally diverse youth is perhaps more central to treatment than with mainstream culture youth.

CULTURAL CONSIDERATIONS IN CHILD SERVICES SETTINGS
School Settings

Schools are influential institutions for culturally diverse children and their families, given the frequent imperatives for achievement in school by families, and the child's exposure to peers as well as the mainstream culture primarily in that setting. However, they often face challenges in adapting to the increasing cultural/ethnic/racial diversity they face in the classroom, particularly around behavioral management. Weinstein and colleagues[56] proposed the model of culturally responsive classroom management (CRCM) to address the importance of culture in sociobehavioral management. Their conception of CRCM includes 5 essential components: (a) recognition of one's own ethnocentrism; (b) knowledge of students' cultural backgrounds; (c) understanding of the broader social, economic, and political context; (d) ability and willingness to use culturally appropriate management strategies; and (e) commitment to building caring classrooms. Another challenge faced by schools concerns bilingual education and teaching students with limited English proficiency. Elsewhere in this issue Toppleberg and Collins discuss the significance of language adaptation for culturally diverse students, including for their emotional and behavioral adjustment.

School-based services are generally well accepted and highly effective for diverse children. Cardemil and colleagues[57] demonstrated the effectiveness of a school-based cognitive intervention for depression as far out as 2 years. Kataoka and colleagues[58] demonstrated the effectiveness of school-based CBT for trauma-related depression or posttraumatic stress with Hispanic children and youth. Morsette and colleagues[59] have demonstrated effectiveness using CBT in schools with traumatized American Indian children and adolescents living on a reservation.

Child Welfare

The US Department of Health and Human Services[60] found that 22.5% of 3.5 million children who underwent an investigation for abuse or neglect were found to have been maltreated. The child welfare and juvenile justice systems are diverse culturally and ethnically. African American, American Indian, or Alaska Native children, as well as children of multiple races, had the highest rates of maltreatment (16.7, 14.2, and 14.0 per 1000 children, respectively). Hispanic and white children had lower rates (10.3 and 9.1 per 1000 children, respectively), and Asian children the lowest rate of 2.4 per 1,000 children of the same race or ethnicity. Black and Hispanic children are overrepresented in child welfare, with black children more likely to be referred and 3 times more likely than white children to be placed out of home, and Hispanic children more likely to be permanently placed out of home.[61,62] American Indian children had a historically high rate of referral to Caucasian foster homes and residential group homes and boarding schools, with the overt intent of protection from abusive families but with a hidden agenda of forced assimilation. The American Indian Child Welfare Act of 1978 was specifically passed to reverse such practices.[63]

Children in foster care are at high risk for having been abused, severely neglected, or neglected, and are at high risk for mental health problems.[64] Studies have shown that 50% to 80% of children in foster care suffer from mental health disorders.[65] Children in foster care have high use rates of mental health services,[66] and higher expenditures for mental health services and psychiatric drugs as well as for nonpsychiatric conditions than other low-income children.[65,67] However, McMillen and colleagues,[68] in a study of mental health services use by older youth in foster care, found that minority youth were less likely to receive outpatient therapy, psychotherapeutic medications, and inpatient services, and they were more likely to receive residential services.

There are many mental health issues to consider for children who are in sustained out-of-home placements, including the effects of multiple placements, changes of school, friends, family, and supports on a child's emotional state; the emotional and behavioral stressors that can result from a foster care system; and the emotional state of other children in the home as well as of the caregivers. For this reason, multiple sequential assessments are needed to evaluate changes in children's mental health as they adjust to new surroundings.[67] Older children, such as transition-age youth who are leaving child systems of care for the adult system, will need special services to ensure assistance in occupational, educational, and mental health needs.[69]

Clinicians should work through a culturally sensitive lens to be comprehensive. One particularly important issue is that of the racial/ethnic match between foster or adopted children and foster or adoptive families. Although many critics have asserted the "color blindness" of adoptions and the primacy of good intentions and affection, the importance of supporting the development of a strong ethnic/racial identity has been emphasized by researchers and policy-makers alike. The adoption of a child needs to be accompanied by the adoption of a child's culture of origin by the foster or adopted family, with that family having a responsibility for supporting the maintenance of meaningful connections between the child and his or her group of origin.[70] In the case of therapeutic foster care, foster parents from a similar racial/ethnic background can even serve as mentors and surrogate kin to the family of origin and facilitate family reunification. Kinship care has been a recommended method of foster care for minority families that strives to preserve the child's bond with his or her extended family.[71] In terms of clinical interventions, culturally diverse children in foster care have been reported to have a favorable response to a program combining wrap-around services with psychotherapy, trauma-focused CBT, and structured psychotherapy for adolescents, but have encountered difficulties with the implementation of such comprehensive interventions.[72]

Juvenile Justice

Juvenile justice involvement disproportionately involves minorities—the minority youth population in America is 34%, but more than 65% of the nation's detained youth are minorities.[73] African American youth are reported to engage in more aggressive behaviors compared with European American or Hispanic youth,[74] and are more likely to be referred to the juvenile justice system than the mental health treatment system, with Latino youth recently experiencing a similar pattern. Youth involved in the juvenile justice system have high levels of mental health needs. Incarcerated youth have been found to have similar prevalence rates of mental health disorders as hospitalized and community-treated youth in the mental health system. The majority of youth in the juvenile justice system meet criteria for at least one mental health disorder and also have high rates of comorbid mental disorders, with most having 3 or more mental health disorders.[75–77] There is a gender difference as well, with girls showing more internalizing disorders and being at higher risk (80%) than boys (67%) for having a mental health disorder.[78]

Referral to mental health services is variable, and is often based on sociodemographic variables: Caucasians, females, or African Americans[78] are more likely to be referred for mental health services. Rogers and colleagues[78] found that Latino youth specifically were under-referred, which may be due to cultural differences at an individual and systems level. Moreover, criminal history such as being a repeat[79] or violent offender[78] is related to referral, and the attitude or perception of need leads to referrals, because routine screening is often unavailable.

Child and adolescent psychiatrists have an important role in consultation with the juvenile justice system for evaluation, short-term treatment, and the development of aftercare plans for youth.[80] Effective programs are highly structured, intensive, use empirical treatments, use mental health professionals (not correctional staff) as treatment providers, collaborate, and deliver enough treatment.[81,82] Racial/ethnic representation among staff that reflects the population make-up of the youth allows for more positive identification and attachments by youth and more sensitive management and referral by staff.[78]

There are multiple therapeutic approaches that have been shown to be helpful in working with culturally diverse youth in the juvenile justice system. Multisystemic therapy is an intensive, multimodal, family-based treatment, with the goal of empowering families to cope with youth in the juvenile justice system, and to empower youth to cope with their surroundings. Wrap-around services integrate the child, family, school, and community to develop an individualized treatment plan.[82] Functional family therapy is a brief, family-centered approach for youth ages 11 to 18 and takes a culturally sensitive approach to motivate families.[83] Multidimensional treatment foster care (MTFC) is an alternative to residential treatment or incarceration for youths with severe delinquent behavior and emotional disturbance. Adolescents are placed into a structured living environment with local families who are trained and supervised.[71] Placing juveniles in adult prisons, youth curfew laws, and juvenile boot camps have been shown to be ineffective in decreasing recidivism or addressing the causes of youth crime.

Longitudinal studies looking at clinical factors that predict future involvement in the juvenile system is important. Further research on the influences of ethnicity as a risk indicator versus the confounded influence of poverty is needed, as well as identifying problems in the referral process that may overidentify minority youth in the juvenile justice system. The field also needs studies that look at how the referral source can influence a youth's access to mental health services. More broadly, long-term studies are needed to determine the factors regarding why some delinquent youths develop new psychopathology and others do not, protective factors, and how risk and resilience, along with vulnerable periods, differ by gender, race and ethnicity, and age.

CULTURALLY COMPETENT SYSTEMS OF CARE

As outlined by Cross and colleagues,[3] there are several main qualities to be demonstrated by culturally competent agencies or institutions: valuing and adapting to cultural diversity; ongoing organizational self-assessment; understanding and managing the dynamics of cultural difference; the institutionalization of cultural knowledge and skills through training, experience, and literature; and instituting service adaptations to better serve culturally diverse clients and their families.

Mental health services for minority and culturally diverse populations should be located in community settings where diverse populations feel comfortable accessing services. Services associated with institutions that are viewed favorably in the community, such as religious institutions, primary care settings, and nonmedical settings such as schools, are often less threatening and more easily accessed than a traditional mental health clinic. Tertiary medical centers are venues of last resort for diverse populations, being associated with death or involuntary long-term institutionalization. Reduced bureaucratic barriers and a personalized but respectful approach are important to facilitate access to services.[19]

Culturally competent practice can occur only within a system of care that has internalized and integrated cultural competence principles into every aspect of its organization and functioning. This integration requires an operationalization of how cultural competence is applied within these systems. Further impetus has been provided by the advent of managed care. Diverse and minority children are widely covered under Medicaid, which is largely under state-sponsored managed care programs. Public managed behavioral health, combined with privatization, has adopted approaches that fail to address the multiple stressors faced by diverse children and families. It has also relocated many mental health services away from minority community settings, and selected against minority practitioners in provider panels due to their fewer "formal" credentials and serving "higher-risk" inner-city or rural clients. In recent years, however, there has been greater recognition of the value of community-based services for diverse and mainstream populations with multiple needs, though the quality and cultural orientation of such services varies greatly by state and community.

The response to these challenges has been to further operationalize the definition of culturally competent mental health services at both the provider and the systems level, which has led to the development of standards for culturally competent mental health services for mental health practitioners, provider organizations, health plans, and organized systems of care. Examples of such standards include the Center for Mental Health Services cultural competence standards.[19] These guidelines outline specific system standards (including governance, benefit design, quality assurance/improvement, information systems, and staff training and support) and clinical standards (access portals, triage and assessment, care planning, case management, treatment services, case management, and linguistic support). Moreover, they outline cultural competence planning processes for systems of care based on needs assessments of diverse populations being served involving the leadership and front-line providers.

SUMMARY

Work in the area of cultural competence in children's mental health continues to evolve and develop in parallel with other fields (such as education, health care, human services, and even business) as our society becomes aware of its importance to our multicultural society. The US Surgeon General's supplement on mental health, culture, race, and ethnicity[84] has further outlined significant issues in ethnic/racial mental health disparities and the need for expanding research in this important area. This report has complemented the Federal initiative on health disparities, which involves the identification inequalities not only in mental health status but also in physical health. Research in epidemiology and treatment outcome, and services research examining mental health disparities are pointing the way toward the best practices and reforms in system of care needed to improve the cultural competence of child mental health services.[20,84]

However, as Cross and colleagues[3] clearly asserted, the advancement of knowledge and skills needs to be matched with similar progress in attitudes in order for true progress to be made toward a culturally pluralistic and proficient system of care. It will be up to us as front-line practitioners in community systems of care to use the new knowledge about the influence of culture, race, and ethnicity in mental health but also to face the old ugly specters of prejudice and discrimination that still affect all of us.

REFERENCES

1. U.S. Census. Population reports. Available at: http://www.census.gov/population/index.htlm; 2000. Accessed May 14, 2010.

2. Eaton D, Kann L, Kinchen S, et al. Youth risk behavior surveillance—United States, 2007. MMWR Surveill Summ 2008;57(S S04):1–130.
3. Cross T, Bazron B, Dennis K, et al. Towards a culturally competent system of care. Washington, DC: CASSP Technical Assistance Center, Georgetown University Child Development Center; 1989.
4. Kilgus M, Pumariega A, Cuffe S. Race and diagnosis in adolescent psychiatric inpatients. J Am Acad Child Adolesc Psychiatry 1995;34:67–72.
5. Hong V, Pumariega A, Licata C. Race, minority status, cultural isolation, and psychiatric diagnosis in children in public mental health. Proceedings of the 14th annual conference proceedings- A system of care for children's mental health: expanding the research base. Tampa (FL): University of South Florida, Research and Training Institute for Children's Mental Health; 2002. p. 313–7.
6. Malgady R, Rogler L, Dharma E. Cultural expression of psychiatric symptoms: idioms of anger amongst Puerto Ricans. Psychol Assmt 1996;8:265–8.
7. Glover S, Pumariega A, Holzer C, et al. Anxiety symptomatology in Mexican-American adolescents. J Child Fam Stud 1999;8:47–57.
8. Kataoka S, Zhang L, Wells K. Unmet need for mental health care among U.S. children: variation by ethnicity and insurance status. Am J Psychiatry 2002;159: 1548–55.
9. Chentsova-Dutton Y, Tsai J, Chu J, et al. Depression and emotional reactivity: variation among Asian Americans of East Asian descent and European-Americans. J Abnorm Psychol 2007;116:776–85.
10. American Psychiatric Association. Diagnostic and statistical manual of mental disorders, Version IV—text revision. Arlington (VA): American Psychiatric Press; 2000.
11. Kleinman A. Rethinking psychiatry. New York: Free Press; 1988.
12. Simons R, Hughes C. Culture bound syndromes. In: Gaw A, editor. Culture ethnicity and mental illness. Washington, DC: American Psychiatric Press; 1993.
13. Rogler L, Cortes D, Malgady R. The mental health relevance of idioms of distress. Anger and perceptions of injustice among New York Puerto Ricans. J Nerv Ment Dis 1994;182:327–30.
14. Lewis-Fernandez R, Das A, Alfonso C, et al. Depression in US Hispanics: diagnostic and management considerations in family practice. J Am Board Fam Pract 2005;18:282–96.
15. Jaycox L, Stein B, Kataoka S, et al. Violence exposure, posttraumatic stress disorder, and depressive symptoms among recent immigrant schoolchildren. J Am Acad Child Adolesc Psychiatry 2002;41:1104–10.
16. McFarlane J, Groff J, O'Brien J, et al. Behaviors of children who are exposed and not exposed to intimate partner violence: an analysis of 330 Black, white and Hispanic children. Pediatrics 2003;112:e202–7.
17. Romero J, Carvajal S, Valle F, et al. Adolescent bicultural stress and its impact on mental well-being among Latinos, Asian-Americans, and European-Americans. J Comp Psychol 2007;35:519–34.
18. Martinez C, McClure H, Eddy J. Language brokering contexts and behavioral and emotional adjustment among Latino parents and adolescents. J Early Adolesc 2009;29:71–98.
19. Four Racial Ethnic Panels. Cultural competence standards for managed care mental health for four racial/ethnic underserved/ underrepresented populations. Rockville (IN): Center for Mental Health Services, Substance Abuse and Mental Health Administration, U.S. Department of Health and Human Services; 1999.

20. Pumariega A, Rogers K, Rothe E. Culturally competent systems of care for children's mental health: advances and challenges. Community Ment Health J 2005;41:539–56.
21. Freedenthan S, Stiffman A. "They might think I was crazy": young American Indian's reasons for not seeking help when suicidal. J Adol Research 2007;22:58–77.
22. Suite D, LaBril R, Primm A, et al. Beyond misdiagnosis, misunderstanding, and mistrust: Relevance of the historical perspective in the medical and mental health treatment of people of color. J Natl Med Assoc 2007;99:879–85.
23. Institute of Medicine Unequal treatment. Confronting racial and ethnic disparities in health care. Washington, DC: National Academies Press; 2002.
24. Cooper L, Roter D, Johnson R, et al. Patient-centered communication, ratings of care, and concordance of patient and physician race. Ann Intern Med 2003; 139(11):907–15.
25. Napoles-Springer A, Santavo J, Houston K, et al. Patients' perceptions of cultural factors affecting the quality of their medical encounters. Health Expect 2005;8:4–17.
26. Szapocznik J, Kurtines W. Breakthroughs in family therapy with drug abusing and problem youth. New York: Springer; 1989.
27. Pumariega A, Rothe E. Leaving no children or families behind: the challenges of immigration. Am J Orthopsychiatry 2010;80(4), in press.
28. Chatters L, Taylor R, Jayakody R. Fictive kinship relations in black extended families. J Comp Fam Stud 1994;25:297–313.
29. Rothe E. Hispanic adolescents in the United States: psychosocial issues and treatment considerations. Adolesc Psychiatry 2004;28:251–78.
30. American Psychiatric Association. Diagnostic and statistical manual of mental disorders. text revision. 4th edition. Washington, DC: American Psychiatric Association; 2000. p. 897–904.
31. Lu F, Lim R, Mezzich J. In: Oldham J, Riba M, editors. Review of psychiatry, Issues in the assessment and diagnosis of culturally diverse individuals, vol. 14. Washington, DC: American Psychiatric Press; 1995. p. 477–510.
32. Tseng W. Culture and psychotherapy: review and practical guidelines. Transcult Psychiatry 1999;36:131–79.
33. Curry J, Rohe P, Simons A, et al. Predictors and modifiers of acute outcome in the Treatment for Adolescents with Depression Study (TADS). J Am Acad Child Adolesc Psychiatry 2006;45:1427–39.
34. Tamayo J, Pumariega A, Rothe E, et al. A comparison of Latino versus Caucasian pediatric outpatients with ADHD in a combined analysis of two acute open-label studies with atomoxetine. J Child Adol Psychopharm 2008;18:44–53.
35. Durell T, Pumariega A, Rothe, et al. Effects of open-label Atomoxetine on African-American and Caucasian pediatric outpatients with attention-deficit/ hyperactivity disorder. Ann Clin Psychiatry 2009;21:26–37.
36. Arnold E, Elloitt M, Sachs L, et al. Effects of ethnicity on treatment attendance, stimulant response/ dose, and 14-month outcome in ADHD. J Consult Clin Psychol 2003;71(4):713–27.
37. Zito J, Safer D, Dosreis S, et al. Racial disparity in psychotropic medications prescribed for youths with Medicaid insurance in Maryland. J Am Acad Child Adolesc Psychiatry 1998;32:179–84.
38. Snowden L, Evans-Cuellar A, Libby A. Minority youth in foster care: managed care and access to mental health treatment. Med Care 2003;41:264–74.
39. Leslie L, Weckerly J, Landsverk J, et al. Racial/ethnic differences in the use of psychotropic medication in high-risk children and adolescents. J Am Acad Child Adolesc Psychiatry 2003;42:1433–42.

40. Brown C, Schulberg H, Sacco D, et al. Effectiveness of treatments for major depression in primary care practice: a post-hoc analysis of outcomes for African-American and white patients. J Affect Disord 1999;53:185–92.
41. Rosello J, Jimenez-Chafey M. Cognitive-behavioral therapy for depression in adolescents with diabetes: a pilot study. Interam J Psychol 2006;40:219–26.
42. Constantino G, Malgady R, Rogler L. Storytelling through pictures: culturally sensitive psychotherapy for Hispanic children and adolescents. J Clin Child Psychol 1994;23:13–20.
43. De Rios M. Magical realism: a cultural intervention for traumatized Hispanic children. Cult Divers Ment Health 1997;3:159–70.
44. Rousseau C, Benoit M, Gauthier MF, et al. Classroom drama therapy program for immigrant and refugee adolescents: a pilot study. Clin Child Psychol Psychiatry 2007;12:451–65.
45. Mitrani M, Santiesteban D, Muir J. Addressing immigration related separations in Hispanic families with a problem-behavior adolescent. Am J Orthopsychiatry 2004;74:219–29.
46. Santisteban D, Mena M. Culturally informed and flexible family-based treatment for adolescents: a tailored and integrative treatment for Hispanic youth. Fam Process 2009;48:253–68.
47. Salvendy J. Ethnocultural considerations in group psychotherapy. Int J Group Psychother 1999;49:429–64.
48. Guerda L, Arntz D, Hirsh D, et al. Cultural adaptation of a group treatment for Haitian American adolescents. Prof Psychol Res Pr 2009;40:378–84.
49. Shendler J. The efficacy of psychodynamic psychotherapy. Am Psychol 2010;98–109.
50. Lustig S, Weine S, Saxe G, et al. Testimonial psychotherapy for adolescent refugees: a case series. Transcult Psychiatry 2004;41:31–45.
51. Rothe E. A psychotherapy model for treating refugee children caught in the midst of catastrophic situations. J Am Acad Psychoanal Dyn Psychiatry 2008;36:625–42.
52. Kazdin A. Dropping out of psychotherapy: issues for research and implications for practice. Clin Child Psychol Psychiatry 1996;1:133–56.
53. Mufson L, Dorta K, Wickramaratne P. A randomized effectiveness trial of interpersonal psychotherapy for depressed adolescents. Arch Gen Psychiatry 2004;61:577–84.
54. Rosello J, Bernal G. The efficacy of cognitive-behavioral and interpersonal treatments for depression in Puerto Rican adolescents. J Consult Clin Psychol 1999;67:734–45.
55. Comas-Diaz L, Jacobsen F. Ethno cultural transference and countertransference in the therapeutic dyad. Am J Orthopsychiatry 1991;61:392–402.
56. Weinstein C, Tomlinson-Clarke S, Curran M. Toward a conception of culturally responsive classroom management. J Teacher Educ 2004;55:25–38.
57. Cardemil E, Reivich K, Beevers C, et al. The prevention of depressive symptoms in low-income minority children: two year follow-up. Behav Res Ther 2007;45:313–27.
58. Kataoka S, Stein B, Jaycox L, et al. A school-based mental health program for traumatized Latino immigrant children. J Am Acad Child Adolesc Psychiatry 2004;42:311–8.
59. Morsette A, Gyda S, Saxe G, et al. Cognitive Behavioral Intervention for Trauma in Schools (CBITS): School-based treatment on a rural American Indian reservation. Transcult Psychiatry 2004;41:31–45.
60. US Department of Health and Human Services. Administration for children and families, administration on children, youth and families, children's bureau. Child

Maltreat 2007. Available at: http://www.acf.hhs.gov/programs/cb/pubs/cm07/index.htm. Accessed May 14, 2010.

61. Blumberg E, Landsverk J, Ellis-MacLeod E, et al. Use of the public mental health system by children in foster care: client characteristics and service use patterns. J Ment Health Adm 1996;23:389–405.

62. McCarthy J, Van Buren E, Irvine M. Child and family services reviews 2001–2004: a mental health analysis. Washington, DC: Georgetown University Center for Child and Human Development, National Technical Assistance Center for Children's Mental Health and the Technical Assistance Partnership for Child and Family Mental Health, American Institutes for Research; 2007.

63. Cross T, Earle K, Simmons D. Child abuse and neglect in Indian country: policy issues. Fam Soc 2000;81:49–58.

64. Pires S, Lazear K, Conlan L. A primer for child welfare. Washington, DC: National Technical Assistance Center for Children's Mental Health; Georgetown University Center for Child and Human Development; 2008.

65. dosReis S, Zito J, Safer D, et al. Mental health services for youths in foster care and disabled youths. Am J Public Health 2001;91:1094–9.

66. Harman J, Childs G, Kelleher K. Mental health care utilization and expenditures by children in foster care. Arch Pediatr Adolesc Med 2000;154:1114–7.

67. Halfon N, Zapeda A, Inkelas M. Mental health services for children in foster care. UCLA Center Healthier Children Fam Comm 2002;4:1–13.

68. McMillen J, Scott L, Zima B, et al. Use of mental health services among older youths in foster care. Psychiatr Serv 2004;55:811–7.

69. Clark H, Davis M. Transition to adulthood: a resource for assisting young people with emotional or behavioral difficulties. Baltimore (MD): Paul H. Brookes; 2000.

70. Courtney M, Barth R, Berrick J. Race and child welfare services: past research and future directions. Child Welfare 1996;75:99–137.

71. Leve L, Fisher P, Chamberlain P. Multidimensional treatment foster care as a preventive intervention to promote resiliency among youth in the child welfare system. J Pers 2009;77:1869–902.

72. Weiner D, Schneider A, Lyons J. Evidence based treatments for trauma among culturally diverse foster youth: Treatment retention and outcomes. Child Youth Serv Rev 2009;31:1199–205.

73. Hsia H, Bridges G, McHale R. Disproportionate minority confinement: 2002 update. Washington, DC: Department of Justice, Office of Juvenile Justice and Delinquency Prevention; 2004.

74. Kashani J, Jones M, Bumby K, et al. Youth violence: psychosocial risk factors, treatment, prevention, and recommendations. J Emot Behav Disord 1999;7:200–10.

75. Atkins D, Pumariega A, Montgomery L, et al. Mental health and incarcerated youth. I: Prevalence and nature of psychopathology. J Child Fam Stud 1999;8:193–204.

76. Teplin L, Abran K, McClelland G, et al. Psychiatric disorders in youth in juvenile detention. Arch Gen Psychiatry 2002;59:1133–43.

77. Shufelt J, Cocozza J. Youth with mental health disorders in the juvenile justice system: results from a multi-state prevalence study. Delmar (NY): National Center for Mental Health and Juvenile Justice Research and Program Brief; 2006. Available at: http://www.ncmhjj.com/pdfs/publications/PrevalenceRPB.pdf. Accessed August 14, 2010.

78. Rogers K, Zima B, Powell E, et al. Who is referred to mental health services in the juvenile justice system? J Child Fam Stud 2002;10(4):485–94.

79. Vander-Stoep A, Evens C, Taub J. Risk of juvenile justice system referral among children in a public mental health system. J Ment Health Adm 1997;24:428–42.

80. Zachik A, Naylor M, Klaehn R. Child and adolescent psychiatry leadership in public mental health, child welfare, and developmental disabilities agencies. Child Adolesc Psychiatr Clin N Am 2010;19:47–61.
81. Altschuler D. Intermediate sanctions and community treatment for serious and violent juvenile offenders. In: Loeber R, Farrington D, editors. Serious and violent juvenile offenders. Thousand Oaks (CA): Sage; 1998. p. 367–88.
82. Lipsey M, Wilson D, Cothern L. Effective intervention for serious juvenile offenders OJJDP Bull. Washington, DC: U.S. Department of Justice: Office of Juvenile Justice and Delinquency Prevention; 2000. Available at: http://www.ncjrs.gov/pdffiles1/ojjdp/181201.pdf. Accessed August 14, 2010.
83. Sexton T, Alexander J. Functional family therapy for at-risk adolescents and their families. In: Kaslow F, Patterson T, editors. Comprehensive handbook of psychotherapy: cognitive-behavioral approaches. New York: Wiley; 2002. p. 117–66.
84. U.S. Office of the Surgeon General. Mental health: race, ethnicity, and culture: a supplement to the surgeon general's report on mental health. Washington, DC: Substance Abuse and Mental Health Administration, U.S. Department of Health and Human Services; 2001.

Racial and Ethnic Disparities in Pediatric Mental Health

Margarita Alegria, PhD[a,b,]*, Melissa Vallas, MD[c],
Andres J. Pumariega, MD[d]

KEYWORDS

• Ethnic • Racial • Disparities • Youth • Mental health
• Minorities • Health care

Despite the enormous toll that mental health problems take on the well-being of youth and families ($247 billion annually)[1] disparities in access to and intensity of quality mental health services appear to persist for racial/ethnic minority children, who are more likely to receive fewer and inferior health services than their non-Latino white peers.[2] This fact has raised serious questions about the progress made in reducing disparities, even though it has been an explicit focus of public health surveillance since 2000, and continues to be monitored as part of the National Healthcare Disparities Report.[3] This article discusses the current state of disparities in pediatric mental health care, underlining the challenges and potential obstacles to successfully addressing these disparities. The authors first make explicit their definition of "disparity," then proceed to describe disparities as they exist in diagnostic assessment, prevention of mental health problems, need for mental health care, access to services, psychotherapy, pharmacologic treatments, and outcomes of care. The article concludes with necessary approaches and specific recommendations.

This work was supported by Grant MH073469-05 from the National Institute of Mental Health, Grant MD002261-03 from the National Center on Minority Health and Health Disparities, and Grant 62609 from the Robert Wood Johnson Foundation.
Disclosure: The authors have nothing to disclose.
[a] Department of Psychiatry, Harvard Medical School, MA, USA
[b] Center for Multicultural Mental Health Research, Cambridge Health Alliance, 120 Beacon Street, Fourth Floor, Somerville, MA 02143, USA
[c] Division of Child & Adolescent Psychiatry, Lucile Packard Children's Hospital at Stanford, 401 Quarry Road, Stanford, CA 94305-5719, USA
[d] Section of Child and Adolescent Psychiatry, The Reading Hospital and Medical Center, Temple University School of Medicine, Sixth Avenue and Spruce Street, Reading, PA 19612, USA
* Corresponding author. Center for Multicultural Research, Cambridge Health Alliance, 120 Beacon Street, Fourth Floor, Somerville, MA 02143, USA
E-mail address: malegria@charesearch.org

Child Adolesc Psychiatric Clin N Am 19 (2010) 759–774
doi:10.1016/j.chc.2010.07.001
1056-4993/10/$ – see front matter © 2010 Elsevier Inc. All rights reserved.

DEFINING DISPARITIES

In the face of the health disparities debate, several definitions have been used for the term "disparity." The definition provided by the National Institute of Medicine[2] describes a health service disparity as "differences in treatment or access not justified by the differences in health status or preferences of the groups." This statement implies that although differences between racial/ethnic groups in service use might be explained by several factors related to need for health care services (eg, differences in parental recognition of a child's need or divergent pathways into care between groups), only the remainder of the identified difference *after* adjusting for the mental health profile is defined as the *disparity*. The Institute of Medicine definition also posits that racial/ethnic disparities are unfair and worthy of remediation, even if they arise through racial/ethnic differences in socioeconomic status, insurance, or other mechanisms outside of need and preferences.[4] With that definition of disparity in mind, there has been not only a distinct body of literature that describes disparities in mental health care in racial and ethnic minority children, and in families of lower socioeconomic status, but it has also become increasingly apparent that ethnic/racial minority children are underserved relative to their non-Latino white counterparts in the areas of prevention, access, quality treatments, and outcomes of care. In this article, the authors summarize these important findings and provide recommendations for promising targets to reduce disparities.

PREVENTION OF MENTAL HEALTH PROBLEMS

The presence of psychiatric disorders in childhood has been linked to negative outcomes, including poor social mobility and reduced social capital. For example, childhood depression has been associated with increased welfare dependence and unemployment.[5] Many of these identifiable risk factors for mental illness disproportionately affect minority children, such as poverty, food insecurity, and exposure to violence, increasing the likelihood that ethnic/racial minority children are actually included in many preventive interventions. According to the United States Census, in 2007 approximately 18.0% of children were poor, and among these, black and Latino children were disproportionately affected.[6] Beiser[7] has shown how economic difficulties seriously affect the likelihood of psychiatric disorders in youth.

High rates of isolation and socioeconomic disadvantage of minority children can have significant adverse effects on children's mental health, including depression and behavior problems,[8] anxiety disorders such as posttraumatic stress disorder,[9] and a range of other adjustment difficulties. Food insecurity, or uncertain availability of food because of inadequate resources, is one of the many difficulties associated with poverty. Like poverty, risk of food insecurity is also patterned by race/ethnicity.[10] Many ethnic and racial minority children and adolescents also experience "compounded community trauma," which has been defined as the experience of children when they witness violence in *both* their homes and their neighborhoods.[11] Compounded community trauma has been linked to high rates of mental illness, including posttraumatic stress disorder, depression, and externalizing behaviors.[11,12] Additional factors that increase the risk for mental illness for minority youth are neighborhood exposure to violence,[13] neighborhood social disorganization,[14] repeated experiences of discrimination, and chronic exposure to racism.[15] As a result, early interventions in the lives of ethnic and racial minority children, intended to maximize their effective coping in these disadvantaged and at-risk environments, can be advantageous in terms of future outcomes.[1] Thus, effective service delivery systems that engage in early prevention and intervention are essential to reduce the burden of mental disorders for ethnic and racial minorities.[16]

Bayer and colleagues[17] have examined about 50 preventive interventions that have been evaluated in randomized controlled trials, most of which targeted children's behavioral problems. These investigators cite several United States programs for their robust evidence of efficacious outcomes. In infancy, the individual Nurse Home Visitation Program,[18] which provided individual home visits for mostly ethnic and racial minority, first-time mothers who screened as single or low income, showed efficacy in decreasing child abuse and adolescent delinquency at a 15-year follow up. During preschool age, Triple P[19] and Incredible Years[20] are the most widely known and respected preventive interventions for child behavior problems. Both programs are geared toward parents with children identified as already having behavior problems. Both indicated efficacy in decreasing behavior problems, and in improving parenting practices and mental health. The individual Family Check-Up Program[21] also provided brief family support offered to at-risk families in the home or in community centers, and was shown to be effective in promoting proactive and positive parenting skills that correlated with changes in children's disruptive behavior. For school-age children, the John Hopkins Prevention program,[22] a 1-year program for first graders in high-risk school settings, showed a decrease in teacher reports of problem behaviors, conduct disorder diagnosis at sixth grade, school suspension, special classroom placement, and medication. Lastly, the Good Behavior Game class program[23] was a 2-year whole school social skills curriculum that showed efficacy in improved attention and concentration, and less oppositional and conduct behavior problems, predominantly in children with moderate levels of initial inattention.[17] Most of these preventive measures in very young children have focused on parenting interventions, and have targeted children who have been identified either as being at risk or as already having behavior problems. These programs all show promise of minimizing the negative effects of at-risk environments and appear to effectively work for ethnic and racial minority youth.

In older children, prevention programs have focused directly on those children identified as having behavior problems, and have also included interventions with parents. One large study done in the United States was instrumental in providing evidence for the importance of available funding for preschools in urban areas. In 2001, Reynolds and colleagues.[24] found that in a large group of predominantly black urban children, preschool participation was associated with a notably higher rate of school completion, significantly lower rates of juvenile arrest, and lower rates of special education and grade retention by late adolescence.[24]

Although there are several well-researched early prevention interventions that have proved to be effective in reducing behavior problems in ethnic and racial minority children, most interventions target externalizing behavior (such as attention-deficit disorder or oppositional defiant disorder), with limited research geared toward interventions that tackle internalizing disorders (such as depression or some anxiety disorders). Exceptions are Kataoka's Cognitive-Behavioral Intervention for Trauma in Schools (CBITS), which effectively addresses traumatic stress in diverse communities,[25] and the study by Weisz and colleagues[26] in 2005. Kataoka and colleagues tested an intervention with third through eighth grade students with trauma-related depression and/or posttraumatic stress disorder symptoms, in which group cognitive-behavioral therapy was delivered in Spanish by bilingual, bicultural school social workers, with additional psychoeducation and support services available for parents and teachers. Students in the intervention groups showed significantly greater improvement than those placed on a waitlist for the program. Other community-based interventions that show promise include school-based services, mentoring programs, family support and education programs, and wilderness programs. Many of these have demonstrated effectiveness with African American, Latino, and American Indian children and families.[27] School-based prevention efforts such as those already mentioned have demonstrated positive outcomes when adaptations are done with a specific cultural context in mind, such as The Circles of Care, which are specially focused on the needs of American Indian children and youth.[28]

NEED FOR MENTAL HEALTH SERVICES

Mental health need is significantly higher amongst at-risk groups of children and youth, a group that is overwhelmingly of ethnic and racial minority background. Several studies have documented high rates of serious emotional disturbance amongst youth in the juvenile justice system[29] and in the child welfare system (rates of 50%). These systems also comprise high percentages (50%–70%) of underserved minority youth, principally African Americans, Latinos, and American Indians.[30] Many youth with mental disorders are typically referred to juvenile justice if they display aggressive or disruptive behaviors,[31] without consideration of whether these are untreated mental health problems.[32] There has also been increasing recognition that children in the child welfare system have extremely high mental health needs,[30] with prevalence rates estimated at close to 50%. However, they are significantly underserved with respect to mental health services, partly due to a shortage of mental health providers to address their needs. Minority children and youth experience higher rates of entry into juvenile justice and child welfare.[30,33]

Another less recognized, high-risk population is children of women who have experienced maternal depression. Longitudinal research has demonstrated the long-term impact on children of maternal depression, including estimated prevalence rates of emotional or behavioral disturbance of 50% to 80%, with increased risk for depression, separation anxiety, attention deficits, and conduct disturbances.[34] In addition, the rates of postpartum and maternal depression amongst underserved racial/ethnic minority groups are as high as 30% to 40%.[34]

Amongst minority populations, some studies have suggested higher population prevalence of psychiatric disorders such as depression, anxiety disorders, substance abuse, and even eating disorders.[35] For example, the Youth Risk Behavior Survey of the Centers for Disease Control found significant higher prevalence rates of sad mood, suicidal ideation, and suicidal attempts amongst Latino and African American youth as compared with non-Hispanic whites.[36] In terms of the abuse of illicit drugs, Latino youth have equal rates to whites, but higher rates than African Americans.[37]

DIAGNOSTIC ASSESSMENT

Significant diagnostic disparities have been documented in children's mental health, largely with African American and Latino children.[35,38,39] Similarly, the conceptual equivalence in the terminology of screening/diagnostic measures[40,41] may influence proper identification of minority cases in need for treatment. There is some evidence that the way in which questions are phrased may lead to response bias by minority youth, in that they may differentially endorse screener items compared with white youth with similar clinical profiles. Diagnostic disparities have also been associated with regional differences in the representation of minority populations.[42] In addition, significant delays have been identified in the diagnosis of autism in African American (7.9 years) versus white children (6.3 years).[43]

ACCESS TO FORMAL MENTAL HEALTH SERVICES

As evidence of racial and ethnic disparities in mental health care access continues to increase, efforts have been made to better understand gaps and limitations in the way that minority children's mental health services are provided. In the last 3 decades, there have been increased efforts to raise awareness of the need for comprehensive, community-based, child-centered, and culturally competent mental health care for children,[44] particularly ethnic and racial minority children. Developing appropriate health and mental health treatment services for ethnic minorities requires comprehensive and ongoing collaborative efforts that address issues of nonengagement in mental health treatments, such as cultural differences in the perception of illness and its causes, help-seeking behavior and attitude toward health care providers, and in how ethnic and racial minority families prioritize, respond to, and adhere to mental health treatments.[45] Caregivers of minority youth might have perceptions that can affect referral to professional treatment, leading to different help-seeking behaviors and underrecognition of mental health problems.[46–50] At the same time, a wide range of structural and sociopolitical constraints related to accessing services disproportionately affect minority youth, such as poverty, lack of insurance, and insufficient availability of behavioral health services in minority neighborhoods. Latino children, for example, have the lowest rate of public or private health insurance coverage of any ethnic group (37%), nearly half that of whites.[51] This factor is particularly critical when addressing the needs of minority children.

According to the Institute of Medicine Report,[1] minority youth are less likely to receive mental health care services than their non-Latino white counterparts. Kodjo and Auinger[52] analyzed the National Longitudinal Study of Adolescent Health (2003) and found that African American but not Latino youth were significantly less likely than non-Latino white youth to have received psychological counseling. Analyzing 3 nationally representative household surveys, Kataoka and colleagues[9] found that both African American and Latino youth had lower rates of mental health service use than their non-Latino white counterparts. Among regional studies, those by McCabe and colleagues,[53] Bui and Takeuchi,[54] and Sue and colleagues[55] found white and black youth to be overrepresented and Latino youth underrepresented across most treatment sectors, while Zahner and Daskalakis[56] found that black and Latino youth underuse services, after controlling for socioeconomic status. Cuffe and colleagues[31] found African American females much less likely to receive mental health services. Overall, the evidence seems to suggest that minority children have the highest rates of unmet need for mental health services.[57,58]

Even when they are able to access care, minorities are significantly undertreated compared with their white counterparts,[57,59] with linguistic minorities reporting worse care than English-speaking racial and ethnic minorities.[60] At the same time, there have been vast increases in the number of school-age children in the United States who do not speak English well, or who are from families in which the adults do not speak English proficiently. In the last projections of the Census, about 26.3% of children aged 5 to 17 years reported that they speak English worse than "very well,"[61] and about 19.7% of children live in linguistically isolated households where all household members older than 14 years have limited English proficiency.[62] This finding suggests that there might be great challenges in achieving equitable mental health care for ethnic and racial minority children in the United States, especially linguistic minorities.

Some studies have shown that most children with mental illnesses do not receive specialty mental health services, but that ethnic and racial minorities are at a more serious disadvantage.[9] Not surprisingly, poor and minority youth, despite equal if not higher need for services, often receive lower quantity and quality of mental health services. Indeed, one could infer a "greater burden of disease" in children, especially poor and minority children, if they are less likely to receive treatment for their illnesses, or receive poorer quality of treatment.[63]

PSYCHOTHERAPY AND ETHNIC AND RACIAL DISPARITIES

Psychotherapy is considered to be an evidence-based treatment for most major mental disorders. In fact, patients who receive both psychopharmacologic treatment and psychotherapy have better outcomes of treatment than do patients receiving only psychopharmacologic treatment, among those with numerous mental illnesses.[64] However, despite its importance as a treatment modality for mental illness, there remain disparities in psychotherapy's utility among ethnic minorities, and limited well-established, effective treatments for ethnic minority youth.[65] In a sample of children enrolled in the child welfare system, counseling access was found to be lower for African American children than for white children. The study also found that both private health insurance and a lack of insurance were negatively associated with counseling access, whereas a history of sexual abuse and greater caseworker efforts to secure services were positively associated with access.[66]

Despite the data suggesting that minorities are less likely to receive psychotherapy for mental illness, there are studies confirming that minority children can benefit from community-based psychotherapy. For example, one study demonstrated a successful implementation of a brief psychosocial intervention (individual psychotherapy) delivered by community-based clinicians in urban school-based health clinics serving minority students with depression.[67] Others have looked beyond the issue of disparity, and focused more on intervention efficacy by attempting to recognize evidence-based treatments geared specifically to minority youth. Community-based treatment of adolescents with substance abuse disorders is both accessible and efficacious, with considerable evidence for day treatment, night programs, and school-based programs. Few such community-based programs and treatment modalities are designed to treat the special needs of females, minority groups, and medically compromised individuals such as those with AIDS, but recent progress is being made in adopting the principles of cultural competence in the treatment of adolescent substance abuse disorders. Brief Strategic Family Therapy, an evidence-based family intervention, has been developed and tested with Latino and African American youth.[68] Ethnically specific programs for American Indian youth based on traditional values and rituals/ceremonies have also been developed and evaluated.[69,70]

Huey and Polo[65] reviewed research on evidence-based treatments for this population (ages 18 and younger), and found no well-established treatments defined as requiring at least 2 high-quality (eg, random assignment, adequate sample size) between-group trials by different investigative teams showing that treatment is superior to placebo or another treatment, or equivalent to an already established treatment. However, they were able to identify probably efficacious treatments for ethnic minority youth with anxiety-related problems, attention-deficit/hyperactivity disorder [ADHD], depression, conduct problems, substance use problems, trauma-related syndromes, and other clinical problems. Huey and Polo defined "probably efficacious treatments" as those that require only one high-quality trial comparing treatment to placebo (or alternative treatment) or 2 trials comparing treatment to no treatment.

PSYCHOPHARMACOLOGIC TREATMENTS

There is growing evidence that psychotropic prescribing frequency in child psychiatry continues to increase around the world, with stimulants, selective serotonin reuptake inhibitors (SSRIs), and antipsychotics being the most commonly prescribed.[71] The United States in particular is accountable for more than 80% of the world's use of stimulant medication. In addition, antidepressants and antipsychotics are much more frequently prescribed to children and adolescents in the United States than in most other industrialized countries.[72] However, despite the prevalent use of psychotropic prescription drugs in children and adolescents in this country, there continues to be concern that there are differences in prescription psychotropic drug use based on race and ethnicity. Treatment disparities include lower use of psychiatric pharmacotherapy, with significantly lower use amongst African Americans and Latinos,[73,74] higher rates of treatment noncompletion, and higher likelihood of receiving inadequate treatment.[75]

The adult literature has produced consistent findings suggesting that race is an independent predictor of mental health service use, and prescription drug use in particular, in a wide array of mental illnesses.[76] Race and ethnic disparities in psychotropic drug use in children has been studied in several samples: children enrolled in Medicaid, special education students, public school students, participants in the National Ambulatory Medical Survey (NAMCS), and high-risk children participating in the Patterns of Youth Mental Health Care in Public Service Systems (POC). In all studies, white children were at least 2 times more likely, if not more so, to receive psychotropic medication than nonwhite children. For example, Bussing and colleagues[77] found that in a special education population, minority children at risk for ADHD were twice as likely than nonwhite children to not receive stimulant medication. Also, Lasser and colleagues[78] found that in adolescents, visit rates per year to primary care providers or psychiatrists for mental health services were much lower for African Americans relative to whites for the same services, including psychotropic medication prescription. Similar findings have been seen in a sample of children aged 5 through 14 years enrolled in state Medicaid programs. African American children showed a distinctly lower rate of treatment with psychopharmacologic agents.[79] In the specific sample of high-risk youth who were participants in the Patterns of Care study[57] where the prevalence of psychotropic medication use was as high as 54%, minority race/ethnicity was associated with lower use of psychotropic medication, adjusting for factors such as age, gender, income, insurance status, need, or impairment. In this study, both African American and Latino youth had a reduced likelihood of using psychotropic medications after controlling for other factors.[73]

Several unanswered questions remain about the reasons for such disparity in the areas of both psychopharmacology treatment and use of psychotherapy as a treatment for mental illness in children. Many have postulated that there are several sociocultural issues that play a role in not only the initiation but also the continuation of mental health treatment.[72] Specifically, minority youth face several barriers to effective mental health care that have been defined in the literature; these include population barriers (socioeconomic disparities, stigma, poor health education, lack of activism), provider factors (deficits in cross-cultural knowledge, skills, patient orientation, and attitudinal sensitivity), and systemic factors (services location and organization, training, culturally competent services, and so forth).[35] There is a large body of literature recognizing the deficits in our mental health care system that negatively and disproportionately affect minority children.[80] Future research should lend itself to better understanding the barriers that perpetuate such dysfunction, as well as finding innovative and efficacious ways to combat them.

OUTCOMES OF TREATMENT

Few studies have compared racial/ethnic differences in the outcomes from mental health treatment. In studies of mainstream interventions, only 2 studies found ethnic minority children do not respond as well as white youth with similar characteristics. The Multi-site Treatment Study of Attention Deficit and Hyperactivity Disorders found that inner-city Latino and African American youth had higher levels of symptoms following pharmacotherapy, and required combination pharmacotherapy and behavioral therapy for equal response to whites.[81] However, these differences were not significant once socioeconomic disadvantage was taken into account. Another study found poorer outcomes in preventing depression in African American youth compared with white, Latino, and Asian youth in an intervention to increase optimism.[81]

Most studies find similar or improved outcomes of mental health treatment for ethnic and racial minority youth as for whites. One study examined cross-ethnic outcomes from public community mental health services in a California sample of youth. Asian American youth were found to improve significantly more on clinical and functional measures than youth of other ethnic/racial backgrounds, while parents reported them as having fewer problems at baseline.[82] In addition, there have been several community-based, evidence-based interventions that have demonstrated efficacy and effectiveness and are increasingly being implemented in child mental health programs. These interventions include intensive case management, therapeutic foster care, partial hospitalization, and intensive in-home wraparound interventions.

However, the literature in terms of differential outcomes of treatment remains sparse. Santisteban and colleagues[83] have outlined pressing issues in the transfer of empirically supported treatments in ethnic minority populations, specifically Latino youth. These issues include testing established treatments in specifically Latino samples both with and without elements of cultural competence in the treatment model. There may also be treatments that do not meet the stringent criteria of empirically supported treatment but that demonstrate an adequate balance of internal and external validity with ethnic and racial minority children, which should be evaluated for effectiveness and differential outcomes in comparison with those of their white counterparts.

APPROACHES TO ADDRESSING DISPARITIES

Several approaches are being used to improve the financing of children's mental health services at the Federal level, including the State Children's Health Insurance Program (SCHIP)[84] and Medicaid Expansion SCHIP (M-SCHIP) to expand children's health insurance coverage to uninsured children, and the Home and Community-Based Services (HCBS) waivers and the Tax Equity and Financial Responsibility Act (TEFRA) option under Medicaid. These expansions help prevent the entry of children into state custody as a result of lack of coverage for mental illness and emotional disturbances by funding children to be treated in the community, as long as the cost of that care does not exceed the estimated cost of institutional care. The Early Periodic Screening Detection and Treatment mandate also provides for states to deliver medically necessary mental health services for children covered by Medicaid who have a mental disorder identified as part of periodic screening, with some states using behavioral health screening tools.[84] In addition, the Affordable Care Act of 2010 (health care reform legislation) recently passed by Congress included sections addressing workforce shortages in child mental health disciplines through program grant support and payback for child mental health discipline graduates serving underserved communities. However, there is a great deal to be done in both increasing the diversity of the children's mental health workforce and the training of all children's mental health professionals on delivering culturally competent services.

Community-based systems of care for children's mental health has been a service philosophy that has been increasingly promoted and adopted nationally to better address both access to care and effectiveness of services, including endorsement by the US Surgeon General. The key principles of community systems of care include: access to a comprehensive array of services; treatment individualized to the child's needs; treatment in the least restrictive environment possible; full use of family and community resources; full participation of families as partners in services planning and delivery; interagency coordination; the use of case management for services coordination; no ejection or rejection from services due to lack of "treatability" or "cooperation"; early identification and intervention; smooth transition of youth into the adult service system; effective advocacy efforts; and nondiscriminating, culturally competent services. Community systems of care promote a flexible and individualized approach to service delivery for the child and family within the context of his or her home and community as an alternative to treatment in out-of-home settings, while attending to family and systems issues that affect such care. These factors include access, use, child and family empowerment, financing, and clinical- and cost-effectiveness of mental health services provided to children and adolescents, as well as the functioning and effectiveness of systems of care for child mental health.[27]

The Center for Mental Health Services (CMHS) Comprehensive Community Mental Health Services Program for Children and Their Families has funded more than 100 systems of care projects in diverse communities throughout the nation. The current phase of the grant program emphasizes culturally diverse populations and early childhood grants. The multisite national evaluation of the Comprehensive Mental Health Services Program for Children and Their Families has shown improved reduced out-of-home placements, improved school attendance, reduced service fragmentation, improved child and family functioning, reduced clinical symptoms, reduced family burdens, increased stability of living situation, and reduced cost of care when cost offsets in education, juvenile justice, child welfare, and general health are considered.[85] In addition, this program has demonstrated a significant reduction of racial/ethnic disparities in access to community mental health services, with 3 times the percentage of poor children, twice the percentage of African American children, and equal numbers of Latino children as in the populations of the targeted catchment areas.[86]

System of care integrated service strategies may include such activities as providing mental health consultation to Head Start, Early Intervention, primary care practitioners, community health nurses, and child care workers; and providing mental health services to adults whose children are at risk of out-of-home placement. States are also beginning to invest resources in training to improve the skills of early childhood clinicians.[34] Such approaches are even more critical for minority populations, which have a higher proportion of younger children and children at risk.

There are encouraging efforts toward enhancing and improving models of collaborative care between primary care and mental health providers. Some state Medicaid plans have adopted model or statewide programs to facilitate access to child mental health consultants by primary care practitioners, while others have invested in training for primary care practitioners on EPSDT (Early Periodic Screening, Diagnosis, and Treatment) tools, referral procedures, and consultative programs to enhance their function as mental health providers to high-risk populations.[84] Other more formal models of collaborative care, using such technologies as systematic screening tools and telemedicine, are being evaluated and found to be effective in improving access to community-based care. More formal evaluation is needed on the use of nurse practitioners and physician's assistants as extenders in the delivery of child psychiatric services, as well as the use of culturally competent models of community outreach, such as Promotoras de Salud in minority communities.[27]

An increasing consensus exists for delivering mental health services for ethnic/racial minority populations within the cultural awareness framework. This framework indicates the need to identify and address the special mental health needs of diverse populations through both clinician-related factors (such as acquiring knowledge, skills, and attitudes that enable them to serve populations different from their own) and system factors (such as reviewing and changing policies and practices that present barriers to diverse populations, staff training around cultural competence, and the recruitment of diverse staff and clinicians for planning service pathways and delivering care). It also calls for the use of natural strengths and resources in concert with professional services that are protective and support children and families in diverse communities and cultures dealing with emotional disturbance. Cultural awareness and competence also includes the adoption of culturally specific therapeutic modalities (such as use of native healers or cultural mediators), mainstream modalities evaluated with diverse populations, and the appropriate use of language interpreters.[35]

The cultural competence framework has been operationalized in consensus health and mental health cultural competence standards, such as the CMHS standards. These standards address cultural adaptations and modifications in clinical processes (such as assessment, treatment planning, case management, and linguistic support) and system processes (such as staff training and development, access protocols, governance of service systems, quality assurance and improvement, and information management). There is initial evidence that adopting such practices results in improved access to services and retention in treatment. The CMHS Comprehensive Community Mental Health Services Program for Children and Their Families has promoted the cultural competence model, with improved outcomes for children and youth of minority backgrounds correlating with the application of cultural competence principles.

RECOMMENDATIONS

1. The government should name a Task Force to address the enormous gaps in unmet need for care for youth in general, and ethnic/racial minority youth in particular. The task force should evaluate whether changes in the current approach to the provision of mental health services are needed, including major changes in health care policy.
2. Evaluating the role of different sources of care (eg, schools and/or community agencies) in service delivery may help minority families become more receptive to mental health treatments. Designing programs, including after-school preventive programs, that address ethnic and racial minority families' competing demands and linguistic capacity, may help surmount barriers to mental health services.
3. Providing decision rules that help parents identify the threshold for labeling a problem requiring professional mental health care is essential. Health literacy, to understand the trade-offs in postponing early intervention for minority youth, may also prove helpful.
4. There is almost no literature on treatment preferences among minority youth and their families, underscoring the importance of developing such a line of inquiry. Aligning treatment options with what families of color value is necessary. Ensuring

that minority parents collaborate with providers so that their cultural values are considered is central to parental satisfaction and youth entry into mental health care.

5. Assessment instruments must provide accurate identification of symptoms and screening processes across ethnic and racial minority youth. More emphasis on the validity of diagnostic and screening instruments for minority populations is required of both service systems and researchers.

6. Different patterns of social and mental health problems might be associated with diagnostic uncertainty in minority youth, resulting in differential needs for treatment such as combined treatments or more case management services; more attention should be paid to differential needs of ethnic and racial minority families in assessment and treatment design.

7. To reduce disparities in access, allocation of outpatient mental health treatment resources in foster care and juvenile justice settings should be investigated to determine proper allocation of providers and adequate treatment capacity.

8. Negative attitudes, lack of treatment information, and financial concerns about treatment should be minimized by social marketing campaigns (to address stigma) or by financial coverage and treatment availability through SCHIP.

9. Given significantly lower treatment completion rates among African Americans and Latinos, interventions such as enhanced access to medications and "virtual" interventions (telephone, computers) that provide anonymity and are less burdensome to complete should be explored.

10. Interventions to reduce negative provider attitudes toward minority youth and enhance adoption of evidence-based treatment should be incentivized and supported in community health care systems. Building coaching teams that facilitate supervision and monitoring to train providers in evidence-based and culturally specific therapeutic modality treatments should be encouraged with financial and institutional support.

REFERENCES

1. Institute of Medicine. Focusing on children's health: community approaches to addressing health disparities. Washington, DC: National Academy Press; 2009.
2. Institute of Medicine. Unequal treatment: confronting racial and ethnic disparities in health care. Washington, DC: The National Academies Press; 2002.
3. U.S. Department of Health and Human Services. National Healthcare Disparities Report. Washington, DC: Agency for Healthcare Research and Quality; 2006.
4. McGuire T, Alegría M, Cook B, et al. Implementing the Institute of Medicine definition of disparities: an application to mental health care. Health Serv Res 2006; 41(5):1979–2005.
5. Fergusson DM, Boden JM, Horwood L. Recurrence of major depression in adolescence and early adulthood, and later mental health, educational and economic outcomes. Br J Psychiatry 2007;191(4):335.
6. Bishaw A, Semega J. Income, earnings, and poverty data from the 2007 American community survey. Washington, DC: US Census Bureau; 2008.
7. Beiser M. The health of immigrants and refugees in Canada. Can J Public Health 2005;96(2):30.
8. Mollica RF, Poole C, Son L, et al. Effects of war trauma on Cambodian refugee adolescents' functional health and mental health status. J Am Acad Child Adolesc Psychiatry 1997;36(8):1098.

9. Kataoka SH, Zhang L, Wells KB. Unmet need for mental health care among US children: variation by ethnicity and insurance status. Am J Psychiatry 2002; 159(9):1548.

10. Slopen N, Fitzmaurice G, Williams DR, et al. Poverty, food insecurity, and the behavior for childhood internalizing and externalizing disorders. J Am Acad Child Adolesc Psychiatry 2010;49(5):444–52.

11. Horowitz K, Weine S, Jekel J. PTSD symptoms in urban adolescent girls: compounded community trauma. J Am Acad Child Adolesc Psychiatry 1995; 34(10):1353.

12. Flannery DJ, Wester KL, Singer MI. Impact of exposure to violence in school on child and adolescent mental health and behavior. J Community Psychol 2004;32(5):559–73.

13. Jaycox LH, Stein BD, Kataoka SH, et al. Violence exposure, posttraumatic stress disorder, and depressive symptoms among recent immigrant schoolchildren. J Am Acad Child Adolesc Psychiatry 2002;41(9):1104.

14. Sampson RJ, Morenoff JD, Earls F. Beyond social capital: spatial dynamics of collective efficacy for children. Am Sociol Rev 1999;64(5):633–60.

15. Gunew SM. Haunted nations: the colonial dimensions of multiculturalism. New York: Routledge; 2003.

16. Goenjian AK, Walling D, Steinberg AM, et al. A prospective study of posttraumatic stress and depressive reactions among treated and untreated adolescents 5 years after a catastrophic disaster. Am J Psychiatry 2005;162(12):2302.

17. Bayer J, Hiscock H, Scalzo K, et al. Systematic review of preventive interventions for children's mental health: what would work in Australian contexts? Aust N Z J Psychiatry 2009;43(8):695–710.

18. Olds D, Henderson CR Jr, Cole R, et al. Long-term effects of nurse home visitation on children's criminal and antisocial behavior: 15-year follow-up of a randomized controlled trial. JAMA 1998;280(14):1238.

19. Sanders MR, Markie-Dadds C, Tully LA, et al. The Triple P-Positive Parenting Program: a comparison of enhanced, standard, and self-directed behavioral family intervention for parents of children with early onset conduct problems. J Consult Clin Psychol 2000;68(4):624–40.

20. Gardner F, Burton J, Klimes I. Randomized controlled trial of a parenting intervention in the voluntary sector for reducing child conduct problems: outcomes and mechanisms of change. J Child Psychol Psychiatry 2006;47(11):1123–32.

21. Dishion TJ, Shaw D, Connell A, et al. The family check-up with high-risk indigent families: preventing problem behavior by increasing parents' positive behavior support in early childhood. Child Dev 2008;79(5):1395–414.

22. Ialongo N, Poduska J, Werthamer L, et al. The distal impact of two first-grade preventive interventions on conduct problems and disorder in early adolescence. J Emot Behav Disord 2001;9(3):146.

23. Hendricks Brown C, Kellman S, Ialongo N, et al. Prevention of aggressive behavior through middle school using a first-grade classroom-based intervention. In: Tsuang M, Lyons M, editors. Recognition and prevention of major mental and substance use disorders. Arlington (VA): American Psychiatric Publishing; 2007. p. 347–69.

24. Reynolds AJ, Temple JA, Robertson DL, et al. Long-term effects of an early childhood intervention on educational achievement and juvenile arrest: a 15-year follow-up of low-income children in public schools. JAMA 2001;285(18):2339.

25. Kataoka SH, Stein BD, Jaycox LH, et al. A school-based mental health program for traumatized Latino immigrant children. J Am Acad Child Adolesc Psychiatry 2003;42(3):311.

26. Weisz JR, Sandler IN, Durlak JA, et al. Promoting and protecting youth mental health through evidence-based prevention and treatment. Am Psychol 2005; 60(6):628.

27. Pumariega AJ, Winters NC, Huffine C. The evolution of systems of care for children's mental health: Forty years of community child and adolescent psychiatry. Community Ment Health J 2003;39(5):399–425.

28. Novins DK, Beals J, Roberts RE, et al. Factors associated with suicide ideation among American Indian adolescents: does culture matter? Suicide Life Threat Behav 1999;29(4):332–46.

29. Rogers KM, Pumariega AJ, Atkins DL, et al. Conditions associated with identification of mentally ill youths in juvenile detention. Community Ment Health J 2006; 42(1):25–40.

30. Garland AF, Hough RL, McCabe KM, et al. Prevalence of psychiatric disorders in youths across five sectors of care. J Am Acad Child Adolesc Psychiatry 2001; 40(4):409.

31. Cuffe SP, Waller JL, Cuccaro ML, et al. Race and gender differences in the treatment of psychiatric disorders in young adolescents. J Am Acad Child Adolesc Psychiatry 1995;34(11):1536–43.

32. Pescosolido BA, Gardner CB, Lubell KM. How people get into mental health services: stories of choice, coercion and "muddling through" from "first timers". Soc Sci Med 1998;46(2):275–86.

33. Farmer EMZ, Burns BJ, Chapman MV, et al. Use of mental health services by youth in contact with social services. Soc Serv Rev 2001;75(4):605–24.

34. Onunaku N. Improving maternal and infant mental health: focus on maternal depression. Los Angeles (CA): National Center for Infant and Early Childhood Health Policy at UCLA; 2005.

35. Pumariega AJ, Rogers K, Rothe E. Culturally competent systems of care for children's mental health: advances and challenges. Community Ment Health J 2005; 41(5):539–55.

36. Eaton DK, Kann L, Kinchen S, et al. Youth risk behavior surveillance—United States, 2007. MMWR Surveill Summ 2008;57(4):1–131.

37. Zambrana RE, Logie LA. Latino child health: need for inclusion in the US national discourse. Am J Public Health 2000;90(12):1827.

38. Stevens J, Harman JS, Kelleher KJ. Ethnic and regional differences in primary care visits for attention-deficit hyperactivity disorder. J Dev Behav Pediatr 2004; 25(5):318.

39. Disalver S. Unsuspected depressive mania in pre-pubertal Hispanic children referred for the treatment of 'depression' with history of social 'deviance'. J Affect Disord 2001;67(1–3):187–92.

40. Gelhorn H, Hartman C, Sakai J, et al. Toward DSM-V: an item response theory analysis of the diagnostic process for DSM-IV alcohol abuse and dependence in adolescents. J Am Acad Child Adolesc Psychiatry 2008;47(11):1329–39.

41. Wu LT, Ringwalt CL, Yang C, et al. Construct and differential item functioning in the assessment of prescription opioid use disorders among American adolescents. J Am Acad Child Adolesc Psychiatry 2009;48(5):563–72.

42. Hong V, Pumariega A, Licata C. Race, minority status, cultural isolation, and psychiatric diagnosis in children in Public Mental Health. Tampa (FL): University of South Florida, Research and Training Institute for Children's Mental Health; 2002.

43. Mandell DS, Listerud J, Levy SE, et al. Race differences in the age at diagnosis among Medicaid-eligible children with autism. J Am Acad Child Adolesc Psychiatry 2002;41(12):1447.

44. Walrath C, Garraza LG, Stephens R, et al. Trends in characteristics of children served by the children's mental health initiative: 1994-2007. Adm Policy Ment Health 2009;36(6):361–73.
45. Szczepura A. Access to health care for ethnic minority populations. Br Med J 2005;81(953):141–7.
46. Castaneda DM. A research agenda for Mexican-American adolescent mental health. Adolescence 1994;29(113):225–39.
47. Lieberman AF, Weston DR, Pawl JH. Preventive intervention and outcome with anxiously attached dyads. Child Dev 1991;62(1):199–209.
48. Constantino G, Malgady RG, Rogler LH, et al. Discriminant analysis of clinical outpatients and public school children by TEMAS: a thematic apperception test for Hispanics and Blacks. J Pers Assess 1988;52(4):670–8.
49. Malgady RG, Rogler LH, Costantino G. Culturally sensitive psychotherapy for Puerto Rican children and adolescents: a program of treatment outcome research. J Consult Clin Psychol 1990;58(6):704–12.
50. Szapocznik J, Santisteban D, Rio A, et al. Family effectiveness training: an intervention to prevent drug abuse and problem behaviors in Hispanic adolescents. Hisp J Behav Sci 1989;11(1):4.
51. Strug DL, Mason SE. Social service needs of Hispanic immigrants. J Ethn Cult Divers Soc Work 2001;10(3):69–88.
52. Kodjo CM, Auinger P. Predictors for emotionally distressed adolescents to receive mental health care. J Adolesc Health 2004;35(5):368–73.
53. McCabe K, Yeh M, Hough R, et al. Racial/ethnic representation across five public sectors of care for youth. J Emot Behav Disord 1999;7:72–82.
54. Bui KV, Takeuchi DT. Ethnic minority adolescents and the use of community mental health care services. Am J Community Psychol 1992;20(4):403–17.
55. Sue S, Fujino DC, Hu L, et al. Community mental health services for ethnic minority groups. A test of the cultural responsiveness hypothesis. J Consult Clin Psychol 1991;59(4):533–40.
56. Zahner G, Daskalakis C. Factors associated with mental health, general health, and school-based service use for child psychopathology. Am J Public Health 1997;87(9):1440–8.
57. Hough RL, Hazen AL, Soriano FI, et al. Mental health care for Latinos: mental health services for Latino adolescents with psychiatric disorders. Psychiatr Serv 2002;53(12):1556.
58. Yeh M, McCabe K, Hough RL, et al. Racial/ethnic differences in parental endorsement of barriers to mental health services for youth. Ment Health Serv Res 2003;5(2):65–77.
59. Pumariega AJ. Disparities among age groups. Treating child and adolescent depression. Philadelphia: Lippincott Williams & Wilkins; 2009; p. 117.
60. Flores G. Devising, implementing, and evaluating interventions to eliminate health care disparities in minority children. Pediatrics 2009;124(Suppl):S214.
61. US Census Bureau. Fact finder, S1601. Language spoken at home. American Community Survey. Available at: http://factfinder.census.gov/servlet/STTable?_bm=y&-geo_id=01000US&-qr_name=ACS_2008_3YR_G00_S1601&-ds_name=ACS_2008_3YR_G00_&-redoLog=false. Accessed July 7, 2010.
62. US Census Bureau. Fact Finder, S1603. Characteristics of People by Language Spoken at Home. American Community Survey. Available at: http://factfinder.census.gov/servlet/STTable?_bm=y&-geo_id=01000US&-qr_name=ACS_2008_3YR_G00_S1603&-ds_name=ACS_2008_3YR_G00_&-redoLog=false. Accessed July 7, 2010.

63. U.S. Department of Health and Human Services. Mental health: a report of the surgeon general. Rockville (MD): U.S. Department of Health and Human Services, Substance Abuse and Mental Health Services Administration, Center for Mental Health Services, National Institutes of Health, National Institute of Mental Health; 1999.

64. West JC, Wilk JE, Rae DS, et al. Economic grand rounds: financial disincentives for the provision of psychotherapy. Psychiatr Serv 2003;54(12):1582.

65. Huey SJ Jr, Polo AJ. Evidence-based psychosocial treatments for ethnic minority youth. J Clin Child Adolesc Psychol 2008;37(1):262–301.

66. Wells R, Hillemeier MM, Bai Y, et al. Health service access across racial/ethnic groups of children in the child welfare system. Child Abuse Negl 2009;33(5):282–92.

67. Mufson L, Dorta KP, Wickramaratne P, et al. A randomized effectiveness trial of interpersonal psychotherapy for depressed adolescents. Arch Gen Psychiatry 2004;61(6):577.

68. Szapocznik J, Williams RA. Brief strategic family therapy: Twenty-five years of interplay among theory, research and practice in adolescent behavior problems and drug abuse. Clin Child Fam Psychol Rev 2000;3(2):117–34.

69. Pumariega AJ, Rodriguez L, Kilgus MD. Substance abuse among adolescents: current perspectives. Addict Disord Their Treat 2004;3(4):145.

70. Novins DK, Beals J, Moore LA, et al. Use of biomedical services and traditional healing options among American Indians: sociodemographic correlates, spirituality, and ethnic identity. Med Care 2004;42(7):670.

71. Staller JA, Wade MJ, Baker M. Current prescribing patterns in outpatient child and adolescent psychiatric practice in central New York. J Child Adolesc Psychopharmacol 2005;15(1):57–61.

72. Rue DS, Xie Y. Disparities in treating culturally diverse children and adolescents. Psychiatr Clin North Am 2009;32(1):153.

73. Leslie LK, Weckerly J, Landsverk J, et al. Racial/ethnic differences in the use of psychotropic medication in high-risk children and adolescents. J Am Acad Child Adolesc Psychiatry 2003;42(12):1433.

74. Snowden LR, Evans Cuellar A, Libby AM. Minority youth in foster care: managed care and access to mental health treatment. Med Care 2003;41(2):264.

75. Chow JCC, Jaffee K, Snowden L. Racial/ethnic disparities in the use of mental health services in poverty areas. Am J Public Health 2003;93(5):792.

76. Han E, Liu GG. Racial disparities in prescription drug use for mental illness among population in US. J Ment Health Policy Econ 2005;8(3):131.

77. Bussing R, Zima BT, Belin TR. Differential access to care for children with ADHD in special education programs. Psychiatr Serv 1998;49(9):1226.

78. Lasser KE, Himmelstein DU, Woolhandler SJ, et al. Do minorities in the United States receive fewer mental health services than whites? Int J Health Serv 2002;32(3):567–78.

79. Zito J, Safer DJ, Dosreis S, et al. Racial disparity in psychotropic medications prescribed for youths with Medicaid insurance in Maryland. J Am Acad Child Adolesc Psychiatry 1998;37(2):179.

80. Alegria M, Atkins M, Farmer E, et al. One size does not fit all: taking diversity, culture and context seriously. Adm Policy Ment Health 2010;37(1):48–60.

81. Miranda J, Bernal G, Lau A, et al. State of the science on psychosocial interventions for ethnic minorities. Annu Rev Clin Psychol 2005;1:113–42.

82. Baker M. Youth clinical outcomes: does race/ethnicity matter? vol. 17. Portland (OR): Regional Research Institute for Human Services, Portland State University; 2003.

83. Santisteban D, Vega RR, Suarez-Morales L. Utilizing dissemination findings to help understand and bridge the research and practice gap in the treatment of substance abuse disorders in Hispanic populations. Drug Alcohol Depend 2006;84(S1):S94–101.
84. Beal AC. Policies to reduce racial and ethnic disparities in child health and health care. Health Aff 2004;23(5):171.
85. Foster EM, Connor T. Public costs of better mental health services for children and adolescents. Psychiatr Serv 2005;56(1):50.
86. Miech R, Azur M, Dusablon T, et al. The potential to reduce mental health disparities through the comprehensive community mental health services for children and their families program. J Behav Health Serv Res 2008;35(3):253–64.

The Practice of Evidence-Based Treatments in Ethnic Minority Youth

Sheryl Kataoka, MD, MSHS[a],*, Douglas K. Novins, MD[b], Catherine DeCarlo Santiago, PhD[a]

KEYWORDS

- Evidence-based treatment • Evidence-based practice
- Children • Minority

GENERAL OVERVIEW

The increasing diversity of the American society and the recognition of widening health disparities have resulted in the need to improve how issues of culture and context are addressed in mental health services and research.[1,2] Ethnic minority children continue to have substantial unmet mental health needs, and evidence-based treatments (EBTs) have proved challenging to disseminate widely among ethnic minority communities.[3] Indeed, policy makers have made an important distinction between EBTs, interventions that have proven efficacy in clinical trials, and evidence-based practice, which involves "the integration of the best available research with clinical expertise in the context of patient characteristics, culture, and preferences,"[4] and this is illustrated in **Fig. 1**. However, despite the publication of multiple cultural competence guidelines, researchers, policy makers, and service providers continue to debate over the

This work was supported by Grant No. R21MH082712 and P30MH082760 (Kataoka), R34MH077872 and R01DA022238 (Novins), T32MH073517 (Santiago) from the National Institutes of Health and SM59285 (Kataoka) from the Substance Abuse and Mental Health Services Administration.

The authors have nothing to disclose.

[a] University of California Los Angeles, Jane and Terry Semel Institute for Neuroscience and Human Behavior, Center for Health Services and Society and David Geffen School of Medicine, Department of Psychiatry and Biobehavioral Sciences, 760 Westwood Plaza, Los Angeles, CA 90095, USA

[b] Centers for American Indian and Alaska Native Health Research, Departments of Psychiatry, and Community and Behavioral Health, University of Colorado Anschutz Medical Campus, Mail Stop F800, PO Box 6508, Aurora, CO 80045, USA

* Corresponding author. UCLA Semel Institute, Center for Health Services and Society, 10920 Wilshire Boulevard, Suite 300, Los Angeles, CA 90024.

E-mail address: Skataoka@ucla.edu

Child Adolesc Psychiatric Clin N Am 19 (2010) 775–789

doi:10.1016/j.chc.2010.07.008

childpsych.theclinics.com

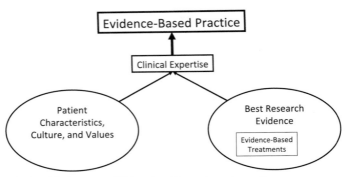

Fig. 1. The relationship between EBT and evidence-based practice.

conceptualization and implementation of cultural competence and key components of true evidence-based practice.[5] Moreover, the number of treatments that have a solid evidence base for use with ethnic minorities continues to lag behind that for the majority population.[6,7] This combination of very few EBTs for ethnic minorities and the continuing controversies around the operationalization of cultural competence in real-world settings has resulted in a paucity of robust models for the implementation of evidence-based practices as envisioned by the Institute of Medicine and other professional societies.[4,8]

Although the value of diversity and the importance of recognizing the effect of culture and context on treatment and treatment outcomes have been well established, research on cultural adaptation of treatments for specific ethnic groups is equivocal. Some works suggest that tailoring interventions for specific populations can increase its effectiveness,[9–12] whereas others argue that there is little support for ethnic-specific interventions.[13] In fact, some research also points to deleterious effects when core components of clinical treatments are diluted during the process of culturally adapting an intervention,[14] suggesting that fidelity to EBTs is important for improving outcomes for all communities. At the same time, culturally sensitive adaptations (eg, use of cultural concepts, addressing issues of migration, family values, language) and implementation (eg, client ethnic match, availability of materials in specific languages, working with cultural brokers) of services do relate to community and client engagement as well as retention in mental health treatment.[15–17] What seems to be important is to strike a balance between treatment fidelity to the original EBT and the incorporation of culturally informed care, resulting in the notion of evidence-based practice.

This article describes the historical context of culture-specific adaptations of EBTs for children and adolescents and recent frameworks for determining when adaptations are needed. It also addresses how to integrate culturally sensitive care while maintaining fidelity to an intervention and the broad public health perspective of engaging with ethnic minority communities and delivering these interventions in settings and ways that are accessible and acceptable to diverse children and their families. The authors then summarize the state of the literature of EBTs for several common psychiatric disorders of children as it pertains to ethnic minority populations and discuss recommendations for future research.

HISTORY/BACKGROUND

In 2001, the Surgeon General's Report on Mental Health—Race, Culture, and Ethnicity documented the paucity of studies demonstrating efficacious treatments for ethnic minorities of all ages.[2] Despite the growing awareness of disparities in care in the mental health field and the identification of key characteristics of cultural competence, few interventions had been designed to study efficacy in ethnic minority populations. To address this issue, some investigators have focused efforts on adapting EBTs for specific populations, although few have been rigorously studied. For example, one parenting program, adapted for Mexican American families,[18] identifies specific beliefs and attitudes about the intervention before implementation and then incorporates and tailors the intervention to address beliefs that may be counter to participating in the intervention. However, another adaptation for Cuban Americans participating in a family therapy intervention[19] did not demonstrate improvement over the standard intervention. Researchers are beginning to call into question whether or not adaptations are necessary for all interventions and are proposing that if adaptations are made, they be "selective and directed" and based on empirical evidence that suggests that without adaptations to address specific issues, there would be a high likelihood that the intervention would be less effective for the target population.[20]

Another approach to delivering interventions for ethnic minority youth has been in the actual implementation and tailoring of EBTs, while maintaining fidelity to the core components of the effective intervention and thereby not making significant adaptations to the original treatment.[21] An example of this is a community-partnered approach in which multiple stakeholders from a given community collaborate with clinicians and researchers in all aspects of the delivery of a program, including during the preplanning of an intervention, identifying ways to build on the strength of a given community in the implementation of a program, and addressing key concerns and needs within the community that should be addressed in delivering services.[22] Finally, providing access to EBTs that are delivered in a culturally sensitive manner in settings that are more acceptable and convenient for diverse youth and their families than hospitals and clinics (eg, schools, churches), may ultimately be an important way in which disparities are minimized.

Previous research has described important cultural issues to integrate into any treatment for ethnic minority children and families, such as help-seeking preferences, expressions of distress, communication styles, migration experiences, family values, and sociopolitical history.[9] These concepts are often central to understanding the experience of specific ethnic minority populations and are elaborated in other articles in this issue. Providing EBTs that incorporate these important and culturally relevant components to care, yet maintain fidelity to known effective treatments, is an important balance in delivering services to some of the most vulnerable populations and is at the heart of the concept of evidence-based practice but remains challenging to achieve.

Another challenge in implementing many EBTs is whether the human services institutions serving a particular minority community have the necessary financial, infrastructural, and human resources to implement a specific treatment.[23] For example, interventions that are designed for delivery by master's level professionals may be difficult to implement in service systems that are heavily reliant on bachelor's level providers and paraprofessionals.[24] EBTs that are highly complex require substantial training and supervision to implement, involve significant up-front costs to incorporate into a system, and are much less likely to be used by programs serving minority communities because they often lack the additional resources necessary to incorporate new treatments into the programs serving minority communities and maintain them over time.[8,23] Because many EBTs were first developed and implemented in well-resourced university-supported settings, they often have basic structural requirements that are beyond the reach of many programs serving minority communities.

DEVELOPMENTAL CONSIDERATIONS

Similar to cultural considerations, the importance of developmental factors has been historically important in child and adolescent psychiatry. Many EBTs were first developed for adult populations with little regard for important sociocultural factors affecting children, such as local beliefs regarding appropriate child rearing practices and the cultural norms for child behavior that are essential in treating children and adolescents. For example, many American Indian cultures emphasize the development of autonomy and independence at very young ages and reinforce learning skills that rely on observation and experience rather than on direct instruction.[25] In the review of EBTs in the following section, particular attention is paid to characteristics of the populations studied in terms of both age and culture.

MAJOR EMPIRICAL FINDINGS

Although not meant to be an exhaustive description of the child and adolescent psychotherapy treatment literature in the United States, this section highlights examples of EBTs. These psychotherapy interventions have been rigorously studied in at least 1 randomized controlled trial and also include most ethnic minority youth in the sample or have specific treatment analyses of ethnic minorities. For this discussion, the authors focus on interventions targeting the following conditions: depressive disorders, anxiety disorders, posttraumatic stress disorder (PTSD), conduct disorder, and substance use disorders. Given the limited scope of this discussion, preventive interventions have been excluded in this summary, although it is recognized that the prevention field has numerous examples of effective interventions that have included ethnic minority children and adolescents in evaluations. Illustrations of specific considerations for particular populations when applicable and ways in which the study captured the concept of evidence-based practice are presented.

Depressive Disorders

Treatment for child and adolescent depression has been widely studied with good evidence for the effectiveness of *cognitive-behavioral therapy* (CBT).[26,27] The American Academy of Child and Adolescent Psychiatry (AACAP) practice parameters (2007) on assessment and treatment of children and adolescents with depressive disorders included various studies on psychosocial interventions and recommendations for treatment.[28] Few of the studies discussed were conducted primarily with ethnic minority populations. Likewise, in the meta-analysis of 35 studies on psychotherapy for child and adolescent depression by Weisz and colleagues,[27] few studies were conducted with samples in which most children were of an ethnic minority. Exceptions with positive effect sizes include 2 studies examining Interpersonal Therapy for Adolescents (IPT-A),[29,30] 1 study comparing Interpersonal Psychotherapy (IPT) and CBT to wait-listed control,[31] 1 quality improvement intervention including CBT, and 1 study examining attachment-based family therapy.[32]

IPT-A has been evaluated in Hispanic adolescent females with low income. IPT-A has been successfully implemented in urban school-based health clinics serving minority students and has been shown to significantly reduce depressive symptoms and improve social and general functioning.[29] Rosselló and Bernal[31] evaluated IPT and CBT in comparison to a wait-listed control among Puerto Rican adolescents. Both IPT and CBT were more effective than the wait-listed control group in reducing depressive symptoms. In addition, both interventions were adapted to include the interpersonal aspects of the Puerto Rican. For example, the cultural values of familism and respeto (respect) were incorporated into both IPT and CBT interventions. IPT had positive outcomes on self-concept and social adaptation over the wait-listed control. No such changes were evident for CBT. The investigators suggest that IPT may be more compatible with Puerto Rican cultural values of personalismo (personalism, the preference for personal contacts in social situations) and familismo (familism, the tendency to place the interest of the family over the interests of the individual) shared by most Latino groups.[33–35]

A follow-up study in Puerto Rican adolescents compared individual and group formats of both IPT and CBT and found that both the CBT arms were superior to IPT, and no differences were found between individual and group modality for either intervention.[36] Although both IPT and CBT can be effective in this population, CBT resulted in a greater reduction in depressive symptoms. The investigators suggest that CBT may offer faster symptom relief than IPT owing to its structured, concrete, and directive approach, which may be consonant with the cultural value of respeto (eg, looking up to authoritative figures for guidance).

The Youth Partners in Care (YPIC) quality improvement intervention also included a CBT component (in addition to medications), which was delivered in a primary care setting to a large sample of ethnic minority youth.[37] The YPIC training included a focus on cultural sensitivity and tailoring of examples to fit within the cultural context of each youth and family. For example, the concept of simpatico (warm and caring interactions and concern for the whole family) was integrated into the care of Hispanic/Latino clients. While examining the differential effects of the YPIC intervention in Latino, African American, and white youth, African Americans in YPIC were found to have significantly greater improvement in depressive symptoms than those in usual care and YPIC Latino adolescents reported significantly greater treatment satisfaction than those in usual care. No intervention effects were found for white youth.[38]

Although CBT and IPT have the greatest evidence base, Diamond and colleagues[32] developed and evaluated attachment-based family therapy among a sample of 32 adolescents (78% girls, 69% African American). The treatment showed a greater reduction in depression symptoms when compared with a wait-listed control group. The investigators noted that the sample was composed mostly of inner-city African American women with low income, who were family oriented and had experienced high rates of trauma and loss. Thus, the investigators believed that the goals of improving communication, repairing trust, and resource building were engaging, important, and relevant for this population.

Anxiety Disorders

Similar to the literature on depression interventions, studies have also supported the use of CBT as probably efficacious in treating anxiety symptoms in youth for separation anxiety, generalized anxiety, social phobias,[39–41] and specific phobias,[42] with benefits extending up to 5 years posttreatment.[40] However, few studies have examined CBT for childhood anxiety in ethnic minority youth. Silverman and colleagues[43] found that group CBT compared with wait-listed control improved anxiety symptoms, with no differences found in treatment effect between white and Hispanic youth. Ginsburg and Drake[44] adapted this group CBT for African American adolescents from low-income families. These adaptations included shortening the number and length of sessions for easier delivery within the school setting that was specifically selected to improve access for these African American students. Treatment adaptations included modifications of specific examples used throughout treatment, which allowed for more relevant situations to be discussed within the context of learning new coping skills. Finally, the parent component was excluded from this adaptation owing to the parents' work schedules and transportation barriers in attending the sessions. In a small pilot study, this adapted group CBT intervention was found to be more effective than an attention-support control condition for African American adolescents.

Aside from CBT, anxiety management training, study skills training, and a combination of both were found to improve test anxiety in African American youth compared with either an attention control condition or no treatment.[45]

PTSD

Trauma specific therapies have been shown to be more effective than nonspecific therapies in decreasing symptoms of PTSD in preschoolers, school-aged children, and adolescents.[46] In addition, there is growing evidence that these trauma treatments are effective in ethnic minority youth with PTSD symptoms, without major adaptations to the original interventions needed for effectiveness. The most well-studied intervention for traumatized children is trauma focused-cognitive behavioral therapy (TF-CBT), a 12-session individual CBT that also involves parent-child dyadic sessions. In a multisite randomized controlled trial for sexually abused children, Cohen and colleagues[46] found that TF-CBT resulted in greater improvement in PTSD and other symptoms when compared with those who received child centered therapy. Although most children studied were white, 28% were African American children, and no differences in effectiveness by ethnicity were found.

A 10-session group trauma intervention, the cognitive behavioral intervention for trauma in schools (CBITS), was originally developed within a community-partnered framework to serve a multiethnic inner-city population and was designed to be implemented within the school settings to enhance the access to trauma services for underserved ethnic minority youth.[47] In a randomized controlled study of 126 primarily Latino sixth-grade students, CBITS significantly improved symptoms of both PTSD and depression in traumatized students receiving the intervention when compared with those in a wait-listed control group.[48] This intervention has also been found to be effective in a study of Latino immigrant students (majority of Mexican origin), delivered in Spanish by bilingual, bicultural, school-based clinicians.[49]

Another approach that has been found to be effective in treating childhood trauma is a long-term treatment (50 weeks) that alleviates trauma symptoms in preschool children by improving the child-mother relationship and the support for the child in coping with trauma. Child-parent psychotherapy (CPP), an intervention based on attachment theory, has been studied in a sample of ethnically diverse preschoolers exposed to marital violence.[50] The strategies used in CPP are also influenced by an ecological and theoretic framework that builds the strengths of traditional cultural practices and takes into account the effects of discrimination, poverty, and social inequities. Results of this study indicate that children who received CPP had greater improvement in traumatic stress symptoms and overall behavior problems compared with those randomized to case management.

Conduct Disorder

There is now strong evidence for the effectiveness of several treatments, most of which take a multimodal family-centered approach to address the problems associated with conduct disorder.[51,52] Conduct disorder is also an area of child psychotherapy research in which several studies have been conducted with ethnic minority youth, especially African American and Latino youth.

Multisystemic therapy (MST) has been studied in several randomized controlled studies of multiethnic, mainly African American, populations with delinquency and conduct symptoms and has been found to be effective in reducing outcomes such as rearrest rates, incarcerated period, and self-reported offenses.[53–56] Using a social-ecological framework, MST intervenes with multiple systems by individualizing the treatment with the family, peers, and school and takes into account the sociocultural context of each youth and family.[56] MST emphasizes the multidetermined nature of antisocial behavior and strives to deliver services to adolescents and their families in naturalistic settings. Studies of MST have demonstrated its positive effect on family correlates of antisocial behavior as well as adjustment in family members. Moreover, after a 4-year follow-up, MST was shown to significantly reduce future criminal behavior.[54]

The coping power intervention has also been shown to improve disruptive and delinquent behaviors in preadolescent aggressive white and African American boys.[57,58] The coping power intervention includes a cognitive behavioral school-based group component for children and this group teaches skills such as use of self-statements, distraction, relaxation, and social problem solving. A group parent training component is also included in this intervention. These studies have been conducted assessing the overall effectiveness of the intervention, and no moderation effect due to ethnicity has been found.[58]

Substance Use Disorders

The AACAPs practice parameters for substance use disorders identified CBT with or without motivational enhancement therapy[59,60] and family therapy approaches[61,62] as having the strongest evidence base for use with adolescents, but few of the studies have focused on the efficacy of substance abuse interventions for minority youth. In 2 randomized clinical trials that examined substance use problems, participants (53%–69% from ethnic minority groups) who received MST had reduced use of alcohol and marijuana in comparison to youths who received usual community services. Multidimensional family therapy (MDFT) focuses on developing better problem-solving, coping, and interpersonal skills.[62] Three clinical trials of MDFT[60,62–64] have included 49% to 96% of ethnic minority adolescent population in the sample and have consistently demonstrated the superiority of MDFT for reducing substance use in comparison with other treatments including adolescent/peer group therapy, CBT, and a multifamily educational intervention. The Adolescent Community Reinforcement Approach (ACRA) focuses on building communication and problem-solving skills in both individual and family sessions with the goal of reducing substance use and related problems.[65] One of the clinical trials of ACRA focused on a sample of homeless adolescents (59% from ethnic minority groups) and found that adolescents who received this intervention had significantly reduced substance use when compared with usual care.[65]

GUIDELINES FOR PRESENT PRACTICE

As these examples from the literature suggest, the present evidence base is far from optimal in guiding the selection, tailoring, and implementation of specific EBTs in minority communities. Although the authors are acutely aware of these scientific limitations, multiple studies have now clearly documented that ethnic minority youth have a greater unmet need for mental health services than the general population. Minority communities are in great need for access to interventions that are effective, feasible, and acceptable, while researchers continue to build this evidence base. From the brief summary of some of the EBTs that have been studied in ethnic minority populations, there seems to be growing empirical support that EBTs can be implemented effectively in ethnic minority communities. The following suggested guidelines support such efforts, while also being mindful of the significant limitations of the scientific literature.

Partnerships First

Collaboration with community stakeholders who have cultural knowledge and clinical expertise is critical to selecting interventions that are consistent with community priorities and needs and implementing them in ways that are congruent with and respectful of a community's cultural context. Local community partners can also help identify ways to increase access, engagement, and retention in treatment. **Fig. 2** illustrates the broad extent to which community partnerships can improve each stage of delivering EBTs.

Delivering EBTs in community settings and with local providers may also help address barriers to care, including those that accompany poverty. Ethnic minority children are disproportionately poor, with an estimated 35% of African American children, 31% Latino/Hispanic children, 31% American Indian children, and 15% Asian children living in poverty compared with 11% of white children.[66] Parents of poor and ethnic minority children often report cost, language, distance, transportation, time, belief that treatments may not help, and possible stigma as barriers to seeking services for their children. By partnering with communities and addressing identified needs, parents may feel more positive about the treatment helping them and their children and this may reduce stigma. In addition, partnerships within communities can work with parents to minimize barriers such as time, transportation, and distance, which may also increase acceptability of these treatments among community members.

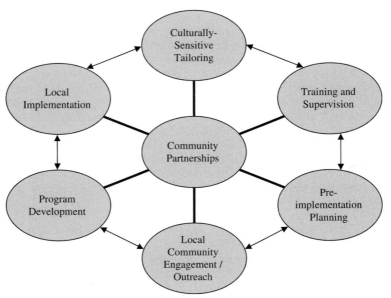

Fig. 2. A model for using community partnerships to provide culturally sensitive EBT. (*From* Ngo V, Langley AK, Kataoka SH, et al. Providing evidence-based practice to ethnically diverse youths: examples from the Cognitive Behavioral Intervention for Trauma in Schools (CBITS) program. J Am Acad Child Adolesc Psychiatry 2008;47:859; with permission.)

Choosing What to Implement

Specific EBTs should be assessed for their ability to address the specific priorities and needs that are identified through the community collaborative process mentioned earlier. This assessment of EBTs should also determine whether or not the intervention relies on techniques or materials that might violate local norms and beliefs or require human, infrastructural, and fiscal resources necessary to implement the EBT. From the summary of interventions presented in this article, there is evidence to suggest that EBTs are effective for ethnic minority populations and in some cases, more effective than in the majority group.[38] Thus, it is prudent for clinicians to choose EBTs over other less well-studied interventions, even if data are not available for the specific population to be treated, unless there is evidence that an EBT is ineffective in that population.[20] After choosing an EBT, there needs to be a balance between maintaining fidelity to the original treatment model while practicing the EBT in a culturally sensitive manner, what the authors refer to as evidence-based practice (see **Fig. 1**).

Considering Systems Issues When Choosing and Implementing EBTs

Delivering EBTs in community settings and non–mental health specialty sectors such as schools, primary care settings, and perhaps even community organizations, such as churches, can be especially important in ethnic minority communities. The summary of the empirical literature also points to several EBTs that have been effectively implemented in such settings with ethnic minority youth. This point is exemplified in a recent study of ethnic minority youth who were in need of treatment for trauma-related mental health symptoms after the Hurricane Katrina.[67] When youth were randomized to receive EBTs either in a school or clinic setting, striking differences in uptake of EBTs emerged. In the school-based setting, 98% of youth began treatment and 91% completed treatment. In contrast, 37% of youth assigned to receive treatment in the clinic came to their first appointment and only 15% completed treatment. It cannot be emphasized enough not only how important providing EBTs can be for improving the quality of care for ethnic minority youth but also how vital it is for providing these services in places where youth can readily receive them.

Monitoring the Implementation of EBTs and Remaining Open to Further Tailoring of these Treatments as Needed

It is impossible to fully anticipate the way a particular EBT performs in a given clinical setting, even if it is selected carefully. Incorporating a continuous quality improvement framework that seeks to systematically assess how clients are responding to a particular EBT is particularly important if an EBT has not been well studied in a community. Collaborating with indigenous community partners to identify the key outcomes to be monitored and to adjust the implementation strategy as necessary can be invaluable, especially in delivering EBTs to ethnic minority communities.

RESEARCH PRIORITIES

Finally, the summary of the present state of the science of EBTs for ethnic minority youth presents a compelling argument for the need for researchers to address several highly salient questions for the implementation of true evidence-based practice in minority communities.

How can Community Partnership and Engagement in Research Facilitate the Development and Implementation of EBTs and Practice

Just as service providers should partner with the community in selecting and implementing interventions, researchers should also develop such partnerships to guide their development and evaluation of the evidence base.[68] A method of balancing treatment fidelity and adhering to culturally informed care is through a process of community-based participatory research (CBPR), in which there is equal partnership between community members and researchers from the inception of the intervention, through all stages of development, implementation, and evaluation of a treatment program.[22,69] Present efforts to study the effect of CBPR on disseminating EBTs for adult depression is underway[70]; however, rigorous evaluations of a similar approach in a child's mental health are lacking. Studies that determine the effect of CBPR on development and implementation of EBTs and dissemination of evidence-based practices could provide new innovations to further decrease the disparities in mental health services for ethnic minority youth populations.

Priority of Dissemination and Implementation be as EBTs are Designed and Evaluated

It is critical that new interventions be designed at their outset to be culturally appropriate, acceptable, feasible, and sustainable. A CBPR process can be extremely helpful in this regard. The present evidence base largely consists of studies of efficacy conducted with carefully selected participants and highly trained, closely supervised clinicians. Although efficacy studies can demonstrate that a given intervention works in optimal conditions, the programs serving minority communities are rarely able to deliver care in such an exacting way. Thus, there is a substantial need for effectiveness research that is conducted in real-world clinical settings serving minority communities, uses less-stringent selection criteria, addresses barriers when possible, and supports clinicians in ways that are consistent with community practice. Frameworks such as reach, efficacy or effectiveness, adoption, implementation, and maintenance and cost (RE-AIM) contrasts efficacy and effectiveness research on several domains: RE-AIM[71] can be a useful rubric for balancing research efforts across all aspects of supporting evidence-based practice rather than focusing specifically on demonstrating efficacy.

One way to address the lack of available clinicians in ethnic minority communities with low income is to focus research efforts on developing treatments delivered by lay health workers and the existing nonclinical workforce in community settings to expand the access of EBTs. For example (1) research that explores the roles of non–mental health providers in either supporting the delivery of EBTs or actually implementing the intervention altogether is an important next step in increasing care to the broad number of children and families not receiving needed care at present and (2) similar to the role of teachers in school-based prevention efforts, studies of EBTs that target psychiatric symptoms in youth, which are designed for teachers and other school staff to deliver, are underway.[72]

How can the Understanding of Factors Relevant to the Effect of EBTs Be Increased with Ethnic Minority Youth and Families

One continued recommendation that has been sounded by several others in the past is the need to increase the inclusion of ethnic minority populations in treatment research studies.[73] There is a particular paucity of studies that include Asian and American Indian youth in psychosocial intervention research across psychiatric conditions. Immigrant populations, especially the growing immigrant Latino populations and other non-English speakers, have frequently been excluded from participation in research and are significantly underrepresented in treatment studies despite having unique risks for poor access to mental health treatments. There is a need not only for more funding agencies to support these efforts but also for researchers to develop new ways of creatively expanding participation of communities in research. Creating an infrastructure within underrepresented communities of color to better support community participatory research may be one strategy to expand the diversity of research samples that presently exist in research studies.

SUMMARY

The dissemination of EBTs to ethnic minority children, adolescents, and families can be challenging. The present research evidence suggests that several interventions have been found to be effective in ethnic minority populations without a need for major adaptations of the original interventions. However, in this article the authors have highlighted the need to deliver evidence-based practice, which is defined as the implementation of EBTs delivered with fidelity and with the integration of important cultural systems and community factors.

REFERENCES

1. Smedley BD, Stith AY, Nelson A, editors. Committee on Understanding and Eliminating Racial and Ethnic Disparities in Health Care. Unequal treatment: confronting racial and ethnic disparities in health care. Washington, DC: National Academies Press; 2003.
2. US Department of Health and Human Services. Mental health: culture, race, and ethnicity- a supplement to mental health: a report of the surgeon general. Rockville (MD): U.S. Department of Health and Human Services, Public Health Service, Office of the Surgeon General; 2001.
3. Kataoka SH, Zhang L, Wells KB. Unmet need for mental health care among U.S. children: variation by ethnicity and insurance status. Am J Psychiatry 2002;159: 1548–55.
4. American Psychological Association Presidential Task Force on evidence-based treatment. Evidence-based practice in psychology. Am Psychol 2006;61:271–85.
5. Stork E, Scholle S, Greeno C, et al. Monitoring and enforcing cultural competence in Medicaid managed behavioral health care. Ment Health Serv Res 2001;3:169.
6. Hall G. Psychotherapy research with ethnic minorities: empirical, ethical, and conceptual issues. J Consult Clin Psychol 2001;69:502–10.
7. Miranda J, Bernal G, Lau AS, et al. State of the science on psychosocial interventions for ethnic minorities. Annu Rev Clin Psychol 2005;1:113–42.
8. Committee on Crossing the Quality Chasm. Adaptation to mental health and addictive disorders: improving the quality of health care for mental and substance-use conditions: quality chasm series. Washington, DC: The National Academies Press; 2006.
9. Bernal G. Intervention development and cultural adaptation research with diverse families. Fam Process 2006;45:143–51.
10. Botvin GJ, Baker E, Dusenbury L, et al. Long-term follow-up results of a randomized drug abuse prevention trial in a white middle-class population. JAMA 1995; 273:1106–12.
11. Harachi T, Catalano R, Hawkins J. Effective recruitment for parenting programs within ethnic minority communities. Child Adolesc Social Work J 1997;14:23–39.

12. Szapocznik J, Santisteban D, Rio A, et al. Family effectiveness training: an intervention to prevent drug abuse and problem behaviors in Hispanic adolescents. Hisp J Behav Sci 1989;11:4–27.
13. Kazdin A. Adolescent mental health: prevention and treatment programs. Am Psychol 1993;48:127–40.
14. Kumpfer K, Alvarado R, Smith P, et al. Cultural sensitivity and adaptation in family-based prevention interventions. Prev Sci 2002;3:241–6.
15. Flaskerud JH, Liu PY. Effects of an Asian client-therapist language, ethnicity and gender match on utilization and outcome of therapy. Community Ment Health J 1991;27:31–42.
16. Sue S, Fujino DC, Hu L, et al. Community mental health services for ethnic minority groups: a test of the cultural responsiveness hypothesis. J Consult Clin Psychol 1991;59:533–40.
17. Takeuchi DT, Sue S, Yeh M. Return rates and outcomes from ethnicity-specific mental health programs in Los Angeles. Am J Public Health 1995;85:638–43.
18. McCabe KM, Yeh M, Garland AF, et al. The GANA program: a tailoring approach to adapting parent-child interaction therapy for Mexican Americans. Educ Treat Children 2005;28:111–29.
19. Szapocznik J, Rio A, Perez-Vidal A, et al. Bicultural effectiveness training (BET): an experimental test of an intervention modality for families experiencing intergenerational/intercultural conflict. Hisp J Behav Sci 1986;8:303–30.
20. Lau AS. Making the case of selective and directed cultural adaptations of evidence-based treatments: examples from parent training. Clin Psychol Sci Pract 2006;13:295–310.
21. Ngo V, Langley AK, Kataoka SH, et al. Providing evidence-based practice to ethnically diverse youths: examples from the Cognitive Behavioral Intervention for Trauma in Schools (CBITS) program. J Am Acad Child Adolesc Psychiatry 2008;47:858–62.
22. Kataoka SH, Fuentes S, O'Donoghue VP, et al. A community participatory research partnership: the development of a faith-based intervention for children exposed to violence. Ethn Dis 2006;16:S89–97.
23. Greenhalgh T, Robert G, Macfarlane F, et al. Diffusion of innovations in service organizations: systematic review and recommendations. Milbank Q 2004;82:581–629.
24. Barlow A, Varipatis-Baker E, Speakman K, et al. Home-visiting intervention to improve child care among American Indian adolescent mothers: a randomized trial. Arch Pediatr Adolesc Med 2006;160:1101–7.
25. Sarche M, Spicer P. Poverty and health disparities for American Indian and Alaska Native children: current knowledge and future prospects. Ann N Y Acad Sci 2008;1136:126–36.
26. Kennard BD, Silva SG, Tonev S, et al. Remission and recovery in the Treatment for Adolescents with Depression Study (TADS): acute and long-term outcomes. J Am Acad Child Adolesc Psychiatry 2009;48:186–95.
27. Weisz JR, McCarty CA, Valeri SM. Effects of psychotherapy for depression in children and adolescents: a meta-analysis. Psychol Bull 2006;132:132–49.
28. Birmaher B, Brent D, AACAP Work Group on Quality Issues, et al. Practice parameter for the assessment and treatment of children and adolescents with depressive disorders. J Am Acad Child Adolesc Psychiatry 2007;46:1503–26.
29. Mufson L, Dorta KP, Wickramaratne P, et al. A randomized effectiveness trial of interpersonal psychotherapy for depressed adolescents. Arch Gen Psychiatry 2004;61:577–84.

30. Mufson L, Weissman MM, Moreau D, et al. Efficacy of interpersonal psychotherapy for depressed adolescents. Arch Gen Psychiatry 1999;56:573–9.
31. Rosselló J, Bernal G. The efficacy of cognitive-behavioral and interpersonal treatments for depression in Puerto Rican adolescents. J Consult Clin Psychol 1999;67:734–45.
32. Diamond G, Brendali R, Diamond GM, et al. Attachment-based family therapy for depressed adolescents: a treatment development study. J Am Acad Child Adolesc Psychiatry 2002;41:1190–6.
33. Bernal G, Shapiro E. Cuban families. In: McGoldrick M, Giordano J, Pearce JK, editors. Ethnicity and family therapy. 2nd edition. New York: Guilford Press; 1996. p. 155–68.
34. Falicov C. Mexican families. In: McGoldrick M, Giordano J, Pearce JK, editors. Ethnicity and family therapy. 2nd edition. New York: Guilford Press; 1996. p. 229–41.
35. Garcia-Preto N. Puerto Rican families. In: McGoldrick M, Giordano J, Pearce JK, editors. Ethnicity and family therapy. 2nd edition. New York: Guilford Press; 1996. p. 242–55.
36. Rossello J, Bernal G, Rivera-Medina C. Individual and group CBT and IPT for Puerto Rican adolescents with depressive symptoms. Cultur Divers Ethnic Minor Psychol 2008;14:234–45.
37. Asarnow JR, Jaycox LH, Duan N, et al. Effectiveness of a quality improvement intervention for adolescent depression in primary care clinics: a randomized controlled trial. JAMA 2005;293:311–9.
38. Ngo VK, Asarnow JR, Lange J, et al. Outcomes for youths from racial-ethnic minority groups in a quality improvement intervention for depression treatment. Psychiatr Serv 2009;60:1357–64.
39. Kendall P. Treating anxiety disorders in children: results of a randomized clinical trial. J Consult Clin Psychol 1994;62:100–10.
40. Kendall P, Southam-Gerow M. Long term follow-up of a cognitive-behavioral therapy for anxiety disordered youth. J Consult Clin Psychol 1996;64:724–30.
41. Kendall PC, Flannery-Schroeder E, Panichelli-Mindel SM, et al. Therapy for youths with anxiety disorders: a second randomized clincal trial. J Consult Clin Psychol 1997;65:366–80.
42. Spence S, Donovan C, Brechman-Toussaint M. The treatment of childhood social phobia: the effectiveness of a social skills training-based, cognitive-behavioural intervention, with and without parental involvement. J Child Psychol Psychiatry 2000;41:713–26.
43. Silverman W, Kurtines W, Ginsburg G, et al. Treating anxiety disorders in children with group cognitive-behavioral therapy: a randomized clinical trial. J Consult Clin Psychol 1999;67:995–1003.
44. Ginsburg G, Drake K. School-based treatment for anxious African-American adolescents: a controlled pilot study. J Am Acad Child Adolesc Psychiatry 2002;41:768–75.
45. Wilson N, Rotter J. Anxiety management training and study skills counseling for students on self-esteem and test anxiety and performance. Sch Couns 1986;34:18–31.
46. Cohen JA, Bukstein O, Walter H. Practice parameter for the assessment and treatment of children and adolescents with posttraumatic stress disorder. J Am Acad Child Adolesc Psychiatry 2010;49:414–30.
47. Stein BD, Kataoka S, Jaycox LH, et al. Theoretical basis and program design of a school-based mental health intervention for traumatized immigrant children: a collaborative research partnership. J Behav Health Serv Res 2002;29:318–26.

48. Stein BD, Jaycox LH, Kataoka SH, et al. A mental health intervention for schoolchildren exposed to violence: a randomized controlled trial. JAMA 2003;290:603–11.

49. Kataoka SH, Stein BD, Jaycox LH, et al. A school-based mental health program for traumatized Latino immigrant children. J Am Acad Child Adolesc Psychiatry 2003;42:311–8.

50. Lieberman AF, Van Horn P, Ippen CG. Toward evidence-based treatment: child-parent psychotherapy with preschoolers exposed to marital violence. J Am Acad Child Adolesc Psychiatry 2005;44:1241–8.

51. Steiner H, Dunne JE. Summary of the practice parameters for the assessment and treatment of children and adolescents with conduct disorder. J Am Acad Child Adolesc Psychiatry 1997;36:1482–5.

52. Eyberg SM, Nelson MM, Boggs SR. Evidence-based psychosocial treatments for children and adolescents with disruptive behavior. J Clin Child Adolesc Psychol 2008;37:215–37.

53. Borduin CM, Mann BJ, Cone LT, et al. Multisystemic treatment of serious juvenile offenders: long-term prevention of criminality and violence. J Consult Clin Psychol 1995;63:569–78.

54. Henggeler SW, Clingempeel WG, Brondino MJ, et al. Four-year follow-up of multisystemic therapy with substance-abusing and substance dependent juvenile offenders. J Am Acad Child Adolesc Psychiatry 2002;41:868–74.

55. Henggeler SW, Melton GB, Brondino MJ, et al. Multisystemic therapy with violence and chronic juvenile offenders and their families: the role of treatment fidelity in successful dissemination. J Consult Clin Psychol 1997;65:821–33.

56. Henggeler SW, Melton GB, Smith LA. Family preservation using multisystemic therapy: an effective alternative to incarcerating serious juvenile offenders. J Consult Clin Psychol 1992;60:953–61.

57. Lochman JE, Wells KC. Effectiveness of the coping power program and of classroom intervention with aggressive children. Behav Ther 2003;34:493–515.

58. Lochman JE, Wells KC. The Coping Power Program for preadolescent aggressive boys and their parents: outcomes effects at the 1-year follow-up. J Consult Clin Psychol 2004;72:571–8.

59. Azrin NH, Donohue B, Teichner GA, et al. A controlled evaluation and description of individual-cognitive problem solving and family-behavior therapies in dually-diagnosed conduct-disordered and substance-dependent youth. J Child Adolesc Subst Abuse 2001;11:1–43.

60. Dennis M, Godley SH, Diamond G, et al. The Cannabis Youth Treatment (CYT) study: main findings from two randomized trials. J Subst Abuse Treat 2004;27:197–213.

61. Henggeler SW, Pickrel SG, Brondino MJ. Multisystemic treatment of substance abusing and dependent deliquents: outcomes, treatment fidelity, and transportability. Ment Health Serv Res 1999;1:171–84.

62. Liddle H, Dakof G, Parker K, et al. Multidimensional family therapy for adolescent drug abuse: results of a randomized clinical trial. Am J Drug Alcohol Abuse 2001;27:651–87.

63. Liddle H, Rowe C, Dakof G, et al. Early intervention for adolescent substance abuse: pretreatment to posttreatment outcomes of a randomized clinical trial comparing multidimensional family therapy and peer group treatment. J Psychoactive Drugs 2004;36:49–63.

64. Liddle HA, Dakof GA, Turner RM, et al. Treating adolescent drug abuse: a randomized trial comparing multidimensional family therapy and cognitive behavior therapy. Addiction 2008;103:1660–70.

65. Slesnick N, Prestopnik JL, Meyers RJ, et al. Treatment outcome for street-living, homeless youth. Addict Behav 2007;32:1237–51.
66. Wight VR, Chau M, Aratani Y. Who are America's poor children? The Official Story. National Center for Children in Poverty. 2010. Available at: http://www.nccp.org/publications/pub_912.html. Accessed July 29, 2010.
67. Jaycox LH, Cohen J, Mannarino A, et al. Children's mental health care following Hurricane Katrina: a field trial of trauma-focused psychotherapies. J Trauma Stress 2010;23:223–31.
68. Kataoka SH, Nadeem E, Wong M, et al. Improving disaster mental health care in schools: a community-partnered approach. Am J Prev Med 2009;37:S225–9.
69. Wells KB, Jones L. "Research" in community-partnered, participatory research [commentary]. JAMA 2009;302:320–1.
70. Chung B, Jones L, Dixon EL, et al. Using a community partnered participatory research approach to implement a randomized controlled trial: planning the design of Community Partners in Care to improve the fit with the community. J Health Care Poor Underserved 2010;21:780–95.
71. Glasgow RE, Vogt TM, Boles SM. Evaluating the public health impact of health promotion interventions: the RE-AIM framework. Am J Public Health 1999;89: 1322–7.
72. Jaycox LH, Langley AK, Stein BD, et al. Support for students exposed to trauma: a pilot study. School Ment Health 2009;1:49–60.
73. Huey SJ, Polo AJ. Evidence–based psychosocial treatments for ethnic minority youth. J Clin Child Adolesc Psychol 2008;37:262–301.

Culturally Adapted Pharmacotherapy and the Integrative Formulation

Mansoor Malik, MD[a],*, James Lake, MD[b,c],
William B. Lawson, MD, PhD[a], Shashank V. Joshi, MD[d]

KEYWORDS

- Culture • Ethnopharmacology
- Cytochrome P450 enzyme system • Pharmacotherapy
- Ethnopsychopharmacology • Integrative formulation
- Integrative medicine
- Complementary and alternative medicine

Ethnicity is reported to be an important, but often ignored factor in psychopharmacology.[1] Clinical observations and survey findings have repeatedly suggested the existence of dramatic cross-ethnic and cross-national differences in the dose requirement and side-effect profiles of various psychotropic and nonpsychotropic medications.[2] The United States is becoming more diverse, ethnically and culturally. This process is happening primarily through immigration and also to some extent from differential birth rates of various ethnic groups. More than one-third of today's Americans are ethnic minorities. Currently, Hispanics and African Americans each make up about 15% of the population. It is anticipated that individuals of Western European ancestry will become less than a majority in 2050.[3,4] Thus, clinicians increasingly need to understand the role of ethnicity, culture, and spirituality when diagnosing and providing psychiatric care to diverse populations. Cross-cultural psychopharmacology represents an

Dr William Lawson disclosed he has grant/research support from Pfizer and AstraZeneca and he is a consultant for Reckitt Benckiser.
Drs Lake, Malik, and Joshi have nothing to disclose.
[a] Department of Psychiatry and Behavioral Sciences, Howard University, 2041 Georgia Avenue Northwest, Washington, DC 20060, USA
[b] Department of Psychiatry and Behavioral Sciences, Stanford University, Stanford, CA, USA
[c] Department of Medicine, Arizona Center for Integrative Medicine, University of Arizona College of Medicine, Tucson, AZ, USA
[d] Division of Child & Adolescent Psychiatry, Lucile Packard Children's Hospital, 401 Quarry Road MC 5719, Stanford, CA 94305, USA
* Corresponding author.
E-mail address: mamalik@howard.edu

Child Adolesc Psychiatric Clin N Am 19 (2010) 791–814
doi:10.1016/j.chc.2010.08.003
1056-4993/10/$ – see front matter © 2010 Elsevier Inc. All rights reserved.

childpsych.theclinics.com

approach that "seeks to determine whether differences exist between ethnic groups in their response to psychotropic medications, as well as the reasons for such variations, including genetic, biologic, environmental, and psychosocial factors. ... However, research studies [examining, for example, CYP450 effects] have often yielded conflicting findings, and many questions remain unanswered, [particularly in pediatrics]." [p31]

The authors wish to be clear that when we write about diverse populations, we most definitely include the Caucasian diaspora among them. As stated in the preface of this issue, we and others[5] are striving to change the "misguided perspective that the close relationship between culture and illness occurs strictly in the lives of ethnocultural minorities only." This relationship and these connections are human ones, and they occur in persons of all races and ethnicities.

For the purposes of this article, we use the term 'race' to refer to the grouping of persons based on physical traits, and the term 'ethnicity' to include not only aspects of race but also "belonging to a group of people with a common origin and with shared social and cultural beliefs and practices. It entails the notion of identity and ... an individual's self-image and intrapsychic life."[6–8] Furthermore, we are in strong agreement with Dell and colleagues,[6] who have described how cross-racial variations occur both in the pharmacokinetics (absorption, distribution, metabolism, and excretion) of medications and their pharmacodynamics (how medicines act on target organ receptors to produce their effects). Genetic variation, especially polymorphisms of important enzymes in drug metabolism processes, and nongenetic biologic factors such as diet, smoking, and complementary and alternative medicine (CAM) treatments, are all crucial factors to consider in clinical work with patients from all ethnic backgrounds. Psychosocial and spiritual aspects of culture potentially important to the psychotropic prescription process include patient and family understandings of disease and mental illness, attitudes toward physicians, beliefs about traditional healing processes, illness behaviors, and meanings attributed to the medication color, form, and route of administration **Box 1**.[9–16]

Differences in the clinical presentation of mental illnesses notwithstanding, there are also significant differences in psychotropic drug treatment and clinical response across ethnicities. Several of these variations have been found in the genetic and nongenetic mechanisms affecting pharmacokinetics and dynamics of psychotropic drugs, which might underlie the differences in drug use and response across ethnic minorities.[17]

However, these variations are not well reflected in clinical trials of drugs in different ethnic populations. Instead, research conducted in the West has tended to be extrapolated to other parts of the world. The resultant use of medications without adequate clinical trials focused on specific ethnic and minority populations leaves them at risk for possible idiosyncratic side effects or inappropriate dosing.[18]

These issues spotlight the importance of the disparity in participation of ethnic minorities in clinical trials. The Surgeon General's Supplemental Report on Mental Health reviewed minority participation in clinical trials and noted that participation was small compared with whites of Western European ancestry.[4] In the trials surveyed, no single nonwhite ethnic group exceeded 10%. Such small numbers meant that there was insufficient statistical power in most studies to analyze treatment efficacy for any 1 particular ethnic minority group. One of the authors of this article (WL) surveyed all biologic psychiatry studies carried out during the 1980s and found similar results. Ethnicity was rarely identified and when it was, no more than 6% of the subjects were African Americans.[19]

In general, the issue of ethnicity effects on outcome has gained attention only during the latter part of the past decade, and most of the published literature or the papers

---

Box 1
Children, medication, and meaning

Physical properties of the medication itself:

- Name of the medicine: may help to enhance or decrease adherence, depending on association

- Form: liquid, tablet, capsule, or injectable form may each carry specific and different meanings

- Size: the bigger the pill, the bigger the problem (and vice versa)

- Labeling and printing: personalized associations tend to be made with imprinted numbers or letters

The need to take medicine:

- Only kids who are "sick" or "bad" have to take medicine

Timing of the dose:

- Frequency: greater frequency may be seen as more trouble, or perhaps, more help

- AM or PM: AM is for school, and may be neglected (with or without MD agreement) on weekends; PM is for sleeping and/or dreaming troubles.

- During school: concern about stigma

Who administers: self-administration is good, mature; teacher/parent administration is the doctor's agent

Adapted from Pruett K, Joshi SV, Martin A. Thinking about prescribing: the psychology of psychopharmacology. In: Martin A, Scahill L, Kratochvil CJ, editors. Pediatric psychopharmacology, principles and practice. New York: Oxford University Press; in press; with permission.

---

presented at national meetings have dealt with the adult population.[20] There is even less awareness of ethnic and cultural variation of the effects of psychotropic medications in children and adolescents. The situation is even more complicated, given that evidence-based practice in pediatric psychopharmacology, with the exception of attention-deficit/hyperactivity disorder (ADHD), is still early in development. Practitioners have generally tried to extrapolate the findings of adult psychopharmacology to children, and researchers have attempted to catch up with the off-label use in the community by conducting studies of already widely used medications. Recent surveys have reported a sizable increase in the use of psychotropic medications such as stimulants, antidepressants, and clonidine in children, including preschoolers aged 2 to 5 years.[21] Most of the medications identified in these surveys have not been adequately tested for efficacy or safety in this age group. Among all treatment approaches in psychiatry, children are more likely to receive pharmacotherapy, especially if they are suffering from ADHD, obsessive-compulsive disorder, or a mood disorder.[22] Although there may be limited research data exploring psychopharmacologic decision making among black and other minority children, there are several cultural considerations that clinicians assessing or treating these youngsters must be aware of for optimal effectiveness. These considerations were first introduced to the general medical audience in 1977 by Kleinman,[23] and are still relevant today:

Here the clinician mediates between different cognitive and value orientations. (S)he actively negotiates with the patient [or parent], as a therapeutic ally, about treatment and expected outcomes. No simple outline suffices at this stage, because negotiation between explanatory models depends on where discrepancies lie and whether they affect care. For example, if the patient [or parent] accepts the use of antibiotics but believes that the burning of incense or the wearing of an amulet or a consultation with a fortune-teller is also needed, the physician must understand this belief but need not attempt to change it. If, however, the patient regards penicillin as a "hot" remedy inappropriate for a "hot" disease[24] and is therefore unwilling to take it, one can negotiate ways to "neutralize" penicillin or one must attempt to persuade the patient of the incorrectness of his belief, a most difficult task.

Negotiation may require mediation between patient and family explanations, when they are discrepant. Indeed, the family model should be routinely elicited to check for such problems. This process of negotiation may well be the single most important step in engaging the patient's [and family's] trust, preventing major discrepancies in the evaluation of therapeutic outcome, promoting compliance, and reducing patient dissatisfaction.(p257)

INTEGRATIVE FORMULATION AND TREATMENT PLANNING IN PEDIATRIC PSYCHIATRY

The integrative formulation is a variation on case[25] or biopsychosocial[26] formulation. It is constructed from all pertinent social, cultural, psychological, and medical factors that are causing or exacerbating symptoms. In patients whose history is not clearly established or whose symptoms are vague, formal neuropsychological assessment may provide additional information on which to base the formulation. In patients who are reliable historians (or whose parents are reliable historians), whose symptoms are clearly defined, and who have no active medical problems, a comprehensive history (across settings, especially school) and examination are often all that is needed to develop an accurate formulation and treatment plan. The integrative treatment plan naturally flows from an assessment of the patient's unique medical, psychiatric, family, social and cultural history, symptom type and severity, a review of previously tried (conventional and alternative) treatments, along with cultural preferences and financial constraints (if any) affecting realistic treatment options. This plan includes adapting treatments based on knowledge of ethnic variations in pharmacokinetics or pharmacodynamics. One can infer in hindsight that the formulation was correct and that the treatment plan adequately addressed underlying factors when there is sustained clinical improvement. When the initial treatment plan is not successful, future sessions are used to gather additional pertinent information until underlying factors causing or exacerbating symptoms are correctly identified. On this basis a more accurate formulation is derived, resulting in a more appropriate and more effective integrative treatment plan. Previous work in this area has highlighted the importance of formulation, particularly as it relates to pharmacotherapy[9,27]:

The formulation should always precede the prescription, and not vice versa.[9] [As an integrative process], case formulation synthesizes how one understands the complex, interacting factors implicated in the development of a patient's presenting problems. It is explicitly comprehensive and takes into account the child and family's strengths and capacities that may help to identify potentially effective treatment approaches.

...Described most succinctly by Nurcombe and colleagues,[28] the formulation asks what is wrong, how it got that way, and what can be done about it. The case formulation is not static. Just as a child's "story" continues to unfold throughout the clinical process with added information, the case formulation evolves and is continually modified. It may start as rudimentary and become more elaborate over time.(p112)

In terms of culturally adapted pharmacotherapy, the following descriptions, adapted from Winters and colleagues,[25] may be helpful.

The information gathered in the assessment is put into a biopsychosocial framework with regard to 5 important domains, referred to in previous work as the *4 Ps*,[27,29] herein expanded to *5 Ps*[25]:

1. *Predisposing* factors are areas of vulnerability that increase the risk for the presenting problem. Examples of biologic predisposing factors include genetic loading for affective illness, ADHD, or prenatal exposure to alcohol, or possessing a PM (poor metabolizer) allele at CYP4502D6*4, as in some patients with European Caucasian ancestry,[30] which could lead to abnormal metabolism of many psychiatric drugs.
2. *Precipitating* factors are typically thought of as stressors or other events (they could be positive or negative) that have a temporal relationship with the onset of the symptoms and may serve as precipitants. Examples of psychological precipitating factors include conflicts about identity or separation-individuation that arise at culturally relevant developmental transitions, such as puberty onset or graduation from high school. Biologic precipitants can include relapse of substance use leading to reemergence of psychotic symptoms. Inquiry regarding CAM treatments is relevant here, as some have important drug interactions.
3. *Perpetuating* factors include any conditions in the patient, family, community, or larger systems that serve to maintain rather than ameliorate the problem. Examples include unaddressed parental conflict, unsafe neighborhood, poor teacher-child fit, or inadequate educational services to meet the child's learning needs.
4. *Protective* factors (strengths) include the patient's own areas of competency, talents, and interests as well as supportive elements in the family and the child's extrafamilial relationships. Examples in the sociocultural domain could include the child having a good relationship with a mentor from the local Boys & Girls Club or with a favorite uncle. In the biologic domain, the child might have a talent in sports, music, or video gaming that can be helpful in engaging them in treatment and enhancing self-esteem or self-efficacy.
5. *Prognosis* and *potential for change* is an additional P that should be included in the case formulation. This P includes identification of areas most amenable to change and potential obstacles to successful treatment, such as when a youngster with school avoidance is rewarded by being allowed to stay home for long periods.

For further description on how to use these descriptors in developing a treatment plan, please see the article by Winters and colleagues, from a previous edition of the *Clinics*.[25]

In the next sections we attempt to bridge what is known thus far about allopathic psychiatric approaches with what has been formally studied in CAM treatments. We also review what appears to be effective in pharmacotherapeutic engagement and alliance formation, and present examples of a culturally adapted approach to the needs of our increasingly diverse patients and families.

HISTORY/BACKGROUND

Early clinical trials with antipsychotics and antidepressants showed that ethnic minorities may respond faster at the same doses as European whites, and may have more side effects.[19,31] Moreover, ethnic minority patients are often prescribed lower doses.[32] In an early study, Lin and Finder[33] found that adult Asian patients required lower doses of chlorpromazine equivalents than white patients to show clinical improvement. However, dosing alone cannot be used as a measure of appropriate pharmacotherapy because an extensive literature has shown that African Americans, for example, often receive higher doses of antipsychotics and these doses may be based more on the therapist's relationship with the patient rather than the patient's clinical condition.[31,32] Lawson and colleagues[34,35] reported that African American patients with schizophrenia were *perceived* as being more violent even when they were *actually* less violent than their European white counterparts in the same setting. Others have reported higher dosing related to the lack of willingness of the physician to become involved with the patient.[36] This excessive dosing may explain in part the doubling of the risk for the persistent movement disorder tardive dyskinesia in African Americans receiving first-generation antipsychotics.[37–40]

Biologic factors that may influence pharmacologic response and side effects include pharmacokinetics such as protein binding, distribution, metabolism, or excretion, and pharmacodynamics such as receptor or tissue sensitivity.[32] However, recent research has focused on the cytochrome p450 family of liver isoenzymes (CYP450).[41] More than 90% of drugs in clinical use are metabolized by this system. These drugs include the antipsychotics, mood stabilizers, and antidepressants in common use. This enzyme may show reduced, normal, or enhanced activity, leading to decreased or increased drug metabolism, and increased or lower plasma concentrations of a medication, and this may have clinical consequences.[42] Moreover, there is now a great deal of documentation about CYP2D6, which, although it accounts for less than 2% of total CYP450 liver content, accounts for 25% of the metabolism of drugs in common use.[41] Recent studies have shown that individuals with certain CYP2D6 alleles are more likely to have extrapyramidal side effects on antipsychotics and to discontinue treatment.[43,44]

Racial and ethnic differences in CYP2D6 have been more thoroughly documented than with the other isoenzymes. For instance, more than 70% of whites but only about 50% of Asians, Sub-Saharan Africans, and African Americans have functional CYP2D6 alleles that code for normal metabolic activity.[41] Approximately 50% of Asians and people of African ancestry have reduced function or nonfunctioning alleles. As a consequence, many older psychotropic medications are metabolized more slowly and plasma levels may be higher. Thus, individuals of African and Asian ancestry may have an increased risk of side effects and need lower doses for a therapeutic response to many medications when compared with European whites.[32,41,42,45]

In contrast, newer antipsychotic agents may not be so heavily metabolized through the CYP2D6 system. A multisite randomized control trial compared haloperidol (HAL), a first-generation antipsychotic agent metabolized through CYP2D6, with olanzapine (OZP), a second-generation agent metabolized through CYP1A2, with CYP2D6 as a minor pathway. More movement-disordered side effects were seen with HAL.[46] A postanalysis by race found fewer reports of extrapyramidal symptoms and dyskinesia (4%) in patients of African descent on OZP than on HAL (22%).[47] In addition, there was ethnic variation in the risk for movement disorders between those of African, Asian, and European white ancestry for HAL, but no such variation was seen for OZP. However, while newer antipsychotic agents may reduce the risk for movement-disordered side effects for ethnic minorities, it may come at the price of increased risk for obesity, diabetes, and the metabolic syndrome.[48,49]

Lithium presents another model of ethnic variation in side effects and response. It is well established that African Americans show a higher red blood cell (RBC)/plasma ratio of lithium concentration when compared with Asians and whites.[50–52] Presumably, this difference is a result of the tendency of African Americans to retain sodium. Sodium retention offered a selective survival advantage for slaves brought to America over the middle passage, because hyponatremia was believed the major cause of mortality.[53]

The clinical significance of this racial difference for psychiatry was not known. A study examining lithium tolerability found more side effects in African American patients with high RBC/plasma ratio even when the lithium levels were in the therapeutic range.[51] It is not known whether African Americans require lower doses and respond with lower plasma levels. African Americans with mood disorders are less likely to be prescribed lithium either as primary treatment or adjunctive therapy.[54,55] It is unknown whether the lack of tolerability at usual therapeutic doses is a factor.

A recent study showed yet another mechanism for ethnic differences in pharmacologic response. Patients in the T Sequenced Treatment Alternatives for Depression (STAR*D study), a prospective study of the effectiveness of the newest generation of antidepressants, were genotyped to find genetic predictors of treatment response to the specific serotonin reuptake inhibitor (SSRI), citalopram. A relationship was found between the HTR2A gene, which codes for the serotonin 2A receptor, and treatment response.[56] The allele is 6 times more frequent in whites than African Americans, and African Americans were less responsive to citalopram. The *A* allele had an 18% reduction in absolute risk of having no response to treatment. It is unknown whether these findings can be generalized to other SSRIs. It is significant that African Americans are less likely to be treated with SSRIs[57] compared with other medications used for similar conditions. For a more detailed discussion of CYP450 subtypes and pharmacogenetics among different ethnic groups, please see Lin and colleagues.[30]

EMPIRICAL FINDINGS IN CHILDREN

By far the most studied condition in pediatric pharmacogenetics is ADHD. Lower levels of medication treatment of ADHD have been documented in ethnic minorities and in developing countries despite similar prevalence of the disorder across different cultural backgrounds.[58] In a systematic review, Samuel and colleagues[59] found that of 16 articles that dealt with ADHD in African American youth, only a handful of these articles had ethnicity as the primary focus of research. In a meta-analysis performed by Miller and colleagues,[60] African Americans were treated only two-thirds as often as whites for ADHD. This pattern was not explained by teacher rating bias or by socioeconomic status, but may have been influenced by parent beliefs about ADHD, higher rates of risk, and lack of treatment access and use. Although increasing awareness of the different sociocultural factors contributing to these inequalities is fostering more culturally sensible approaches to diagnosis and treatment, the existence of specific response or tolerability patterns of ADHD medications across ethnic groups is unclear.

When African American children do receive ADHD medications, there may be significant differences of response, compared with white children. Some, but not all studies have found greater nonresponse to ADHD medication in African American children. For instance, in a study sample of African Americans with ADHD, Winsberg and Comings[61] reported that patients homozygous for the 10-repeat allele of the dopamine transporter gene were nonresponsive to methylphenidate. There was no white comparison group in this study to determine if this was an ethnic effect, but the proportion of nonresponders (14 of 30) was considerably higher than reported in samples with more diversity (a 66%–85% response rate is customarily quoted), raising a question of possible lower stimulant response rate in African Americans. However, Waldman and colleagues[62] did not find any ethnic differences in the dopamine transporter gene. Arnold and colleagues, in the multimodal treatment of ADHD (MTA) study, also found a tendency in the direction of more nonresponders among African Americans; however, this difference was not deemed statistically significant.[63]

Although few studies have evaluated the tolerability of ADHD medication in children who are members of minority groups, these studies point toward greater adverse effects of these medications in African American children. In a small study of 11 male African American adolescents with attention-deficit disorder, Brown and Sexson[64] found that methylphenidate exerted improvement in attention and impulsivity, with a linear dose effect. This study also found a trend for an increase in side effects with increasing methylphenidate dose, including a mean increase in diastolic blood pressure. Although it was noted to be within the normal pediatric blood pressure range, these findings point toward the need for more studies in African American and other ethnic minority populations.

In a subgroup analysis performed by Starr and Kemner[65] for the African American participants of The Formal Observation of Concerta versus Strattera (FOCUS) study, they found that both methylphenidate and atomoxetine showed improvement in baseline symptoms and similar incidences of adverse events in African American children. Although it was concluded that there was no ethnic difference in tolerability of these agents, the study was not powered prospectively to study the African American subgroup; therefore, these data should be considered exploratory in nature.

These findings emphasize the importance of including ethnic minorities in clinical trials in sufficient numbers and to perform intraethnic analysis. Failure to do so means that new pharmacologic products will be selected primarily based on research of European whites. Ethnic minorities are left at risk for possible idiosyncratic side effects, inappropriate dosing, or lack of efficacy. The argument is often made that ethnic minorities do not participate in clinical trials because they do not want to. African Americans specifically are often suspicious because of previous experiences of exploitation of vulnerable minority groups.[57,66] The Tuskegee syphilis study is often cited as a reason for mistrust.[67,68] This was a federally funded study of the long-term consequences of syphilis on African American men, initially begun before antibiotics were available. However, the participants were not given treatment when effective treatment did become available, and were not informed that optimal treatment was withheld in order to follow the natural course of the disease. African Americans aware of this study are less willing and less likely to participate in research.[68,69] Even African Americans unaware of the study often mistrust research that might involve physically intrusive methods.[69] This mistrust is present for psychiatric research participation as well, even if participants are unaware of the Tuskegee study.[70]

Recent findings have challenged the view that lack of participation is a result of ethnic minority attitudes about research. The consent rate by race and ethnicity was examined in all of the published health research studies performed in the United States, Western Europe, and Australia.[70–72] No significant racial or ethnic differences in consent rate were seen, even when the United States alone was studied. All groups had more than 80% consent rates. For clinical intervention studies, Hispanics had a significantly higher consent rate than non-Hispanic whites, and African Americans had a nonsignificantly higher rate.

In an increasingly multiethnic country such as the United States, Canada, or Great Britain in 2010, pharmacologic and genetic research is showing that race and ethnicity must be considered in the development of new treatments for psychiatric disorders. Small efficacy studies and large effectiveness studies are showing the value of addressing interethnic variation in pharmacotherapy. Participation by ethnic minorities in clinical trials seems to be low not because of participant attitudes, but because of an inadequate focus on minority recruitment for studies.

Overall it must be contended that there is a paucity of empirical evidence to guide ethnopharmacologic practices in children and adolescents. Much of the (limited) work conducted thus far has focused on African American youth, and more investigation is needed into ethnopharmacologic differences among other cultural groups.

The Sociocultural Context of Pediatric Pharmacotherapy

As Lin and colleagues[30] described, "pharmacotherapy is fundamentally a process of social transaction, and its outcome is determined by contextual factors impinging on the patient, [family], and the clinician by forces that powerfully shape their interactions." Furthermore, these investigators highlight the need for clinicians to acknowledge "that [they] are just as malleable, consciously and unconsciously, by their sociocultural environment and prevailing ideologies." They invite us to struggle against certain prevailing notions of modern pharmacotherapy, which can undermine effectiveness. These notions include that (1) the therapeutic effects of medications are determined exclusively by their biologic properties; (2) the patient is a passive recipient of the prescription, and will be fully adherent with instructions; and (3) psychiatric and medical treatment represents (or is supposed to be) the only source of care available and used by the patient.[30] Culture influences the same areas that are central to mental health, such as behavioral expectations and tolerance, language, emotion, attention, attachment, traumatic experiences, conduct, personality, motivation, limit setting, and other aspects of parenting in general. Cultural context plays an important role not only in structuring the environment in which children with emotional and behavioral disorders function but also in the way such children are understood and treated.

Shame can be another cultural paradigm that enters the clinical setting. For both parent and (especially teen-aged) patient, the stigma of mental illness may be further fed by being referred to the psychiatrist by the primary-care provider (PCP). From the family/patient perspective, the implication is that the problems are so serious, too threatening, or so time consuming as to require a specialist,[73] beyond what the PCP (who is often a trusted adult in the teen/child's life) can handle. Metzl[73] has described how clinicians should strive to promote an "open and honest exchange of affect," especially because patients and families are often "sent" to our offices "to relate deep and highly personal aspects of their lives to a total stranger."(p39)

Broucek and Ricci[74] encourage us to "reduce the patient [and family's] shame and anxiety to levels more conducive to self-revelation. Intense shame [particularly among parents of some cultures] can be so aversive, noxious, and self-fragmenting that the [pharmacotherapist] may have to assist [them] in modulating it."(p435)

Another influential piece of writing comes from Havens[75] (modified version for families in Ref.[76]) who describes the use of "psychological analgesics", which can be prescribed in much the same way as our medical predecessors may have told the patient to "take 2 aspirin and call me in the morning":

1. *Protect self-esteem*: the patient has been potentially affected by having to come to a psychiatrist, and the parent may feel guilty for having caused the illness through bad parenting, poor gene contribution, or both.
2. *Emote a measure of understanding and acceptance*: when this technique is successful, the patient's problem is grasped intellectually, and the patient's and family's predicament is understood from *their* point of view.
3. *Provide a sense of future*: many families have experienced frustration and failure in attempting to find solutions and may have lost hope. Discussion about

expectations for treatment that still acknowledges fears or even hopelessness may still preserve opportunities for change: "It seems hopeless to you *now*."

Sabo and Rand[77] emphasize the importance of spending adequate time with the patient (and family) in the initial evaluation. Patients too often feel as though they are merely "the next appointment" unless the doctor listens to the personal and unique elements of their story. Interpreters in the initial appointment can be crucial here. Active empathic listening is necessary to create a special, common language between the patient and therapist. If a full work-up cannot be completed in the first appointment, follow-up sessions (preferably within 1–2 weeks) may be necessary to sustain the developing alliance. This situation becomes especially true with those families sufficiently unfamiliar with mental health disorders and their treatment that they may be unsure of what to expect in terms of treatment planning and treatment response. In families from cultures in which somatization is a frequent way to present mental health symptoms, the attuned pharmacotherapist finds ways to selectively use the medical model or chemical imbalance explanation to gain buy-in, but may also use the opportunity to help families conceptualize how mental health problems can greatly impair daily function (eg, school performance, peer and family relationships, self-worth). Choi[5] writes how "becoming familiar with the language for emotional distress and understanding cultural beliefs embedded in [certain cultural or culture-bound] expressions are critical steps for culturally competent communication between [clinicians] and adolescents."[(p79)]

Pharmacotherapeutic Engagement

Despite perceptions by the general public—and sadly, even many clinicians—to the contrary, the act of prescribing psychotropic medications is one of tremendous [potential] psychodynamic significance to children, adolescents, families, and caregivers. Particularly in the cultural context of every patient, we must not only "uncover and appreciate the attributions given to medication," but we must also realize that without attention to this, we will have an incomplete picture of the underlying psychopathology, the real-life contexts that matter to the patient, and that affect and are affected by her neuropsychiatric issues, issues that influence adherence to all recommended treatments and treatment response. Furthermore, even the briefest of encounters with a prescribing physician [may] carry [significant meaning] and psychotherapeutic weight.[6(p95)]

Readers are referred to several articles in the literature devoted to this topic,[9,76,78] which have highlighted that a strong therapeutic alliance lays the foundation on which positive outcomes in mental health treatment generally, and psychopharmacology specifically, are built. Culturally attuned pharmacotherapists should be mindful of not only the target symptoms but also the context and settings in which they occur. In addition to the psychiatrist's office, these principles apply in other treatment settings such as that of the PCP, where psychotropic medicines are often prescribed for children and adolescents. In pediatric psychopharmacology specifically, there is always at least a *dual alliance* that must be acknowledged and nurtured. Prescribing clinicians should strive to include both patient and parent/guardian into the working alliance paradigms of goal identification, task consolidation, and therapeutic bond establishment.[76] Research reviews have shown that knowledge of the psychological factors and developmental implications present when medicines are prescribed improves therapeutic outcomes.[9,76] The following case vignette illustrates how cultural attunement by the pharmacotherapist helped a teenager and family in need of multimodal interventions (individual psychotherapy, pharmacotherapy, family therapy, school engagement) continue to participate in all forms of treatment, despite wishes to withdraw from care:

> Jodie was a 16-year-old second-generation Filipina-American girl who lived in a household with 4 younger siblings and both parents. Several youth from her high school had died by suicide in the previous year, and among the victims was Jodie's best friend. School staff members were concerned about Jodie's sensitive nature, and asked that the School Mental Health Team (SMHT) consult with her and the family to assess for depression and self-harm potential. After consent was obtained, the team was able to quickly gain the patient and family's trust by doing the following:

> Begin the consultation by calling the family and outlining the specific steps to SMHT consultation, assuring them that although the consult would start at school, it would continue in whatever context the family felt most comfortable. In their case, it was the home.

> A home visit was conducted after the leader of the team, a child & adolescent pharmacotherpaist met with the teen at school that afternoon for initial assessment. The pharmacotherapist met the teen and parents together briefly, and then asked to meet the parents alone for about 30 minutes, to gain their trust and engage them in a culturally focused way: being mindful of the potential for stigma, their potential fears about whether contact with the team might affect her chances to go to the best college, and employed the selective use of a medical model to allow the family to conceptualize her need for treatment using a more familiar paradigm.

> The pharmacotherapist highlighted the need for the school counselor and pharmacotherapist to work closely together, and recommended that family therapy be started to address dysfunctional patterns and to learn new parenting and coping strategies for the mood swings Jodie was experiencing.

> A diagnosis of major depressive disorder and posttraumatic stress traits was made, and after full discussion of possible medication interventions, the pharmacotherapist told the patient and family that he would start with a low dose of medicine, mindful of the potentially good response at lower doses in some Asian patients, and also that this patient had been tried on medicine in the past, with the teen and family stopping treatment because "she was so sleepy and couldn't do her school work." He also supported the teen and family request to continue the omega fatty acid (OFA) supplement, because they believed this was important to her overall functioning, and the pharmacotherapist believed it was at least doing no harm and may have carried some meaning effect. (The teen who had died had suffered from ADHD and depression, and was nonadherent with the prescribed OFAs, stimulant and SSRI. Jodie believed she should "honor the memory" of her friend by trying to take the medicine as prescribed.)

> The supporting alliance[79] among doctor, parent, family therapist, schoolteacher, and guidance counselor was facilitated by the pharmacotherapist actively endorsing the role of the school in supporting Jodie, and highlighting their role on the team as the "watchful clinical eyes" during the school day.

> Jodie responded well to low-dose SSRI and standard-dose OFA, in conjunction with interpersonal therapy (IPT), family therapy, and regular mental health checkups with the school counselor. The pharmacotherapist continued to see her monthly, and had brief phone meetings with the IPT therapist weekly for the first 6 weeks.

The parents, although tempted many times to withdraw from this intensity of treatment, kept encouraging Jodie and supporting her continued participation, "because the doctor (SMHT psychiatrist) asked us to make sure she attends (and we participate where needed) all these meetings, and also because he said the treatment may not last forever—it will depend on how she responds."

Pruett and colleagues[9] remind us that, particularly with teens, the attuned child & adolescent clinician needs to remain alert to changes in the *meaning* of the drugs to the patient as s/he navigates the new developmental terrain of adolescence. The dramatic changes in bodily preoccupation, impulsive discharge, and mood lability that occur with puberty may cast any agent that in the past may have affected weight (gain or loss), endocrine function (galactorrhea), skin appearance (acne), genital arousal or dysfunction, or mood itself into an entirely different light. What might have been acceptable effects before are now intolerable because they emerge during, or simply exacerbate, already exquisitely sensitive developmental tasks. This is made even more complex by the fact that nearly all "side" effects, from extrapyramidal symptoms to nausea, are generally less well tolerated in child and adolescent populations to begin with.

The next sections describe adapted approaches within pharmacotherapy and also nonpharmacologic CAM treatments that may be useful when working with families who may be hesitant to use an allopathic approach. (We find it interesting that in modern psychiatric vernacular, the phrase "traditional (or conventional) approaches" refers to allopathic ones, whereas CAM providers use "traditional approaches" to refer to herbal and folk remedies. Many of these herbal remedies have become the basis for allopathic medicines, and many herbal products have important biologic effects at CYP450, which must be accounted for in integrated treatment.)

INCREASING USE OF NONPHARMACOLOGIC THERAPIES

Kemper and colleagues[80] recently wrote a comprehensive review of CAM treatments in pediatric medicine, and found that use of CAM therapies seems to vary among different ethnic and cultural groups. Excluding prayer, CAM is used less commonly by Hispanic and black individuals than by white individuals, and its use by Hispanic and black people is less likely to be disclosed to clinicians.[81] Families of varying cultural backgrounds may use herbs, over-the-counter remedies, and other items traditionally used for cooking as home remedies.[82,83] Many ethnic and cultural groups also use traditional healing practices such as Traditional Chinese Medicine (TCM), ayurvedic medicine, and American Indian/Alaska Native healing practices, which can include a variety of diverse therapies and native healers within a coherent cultural belief system.[84,85] Use of these remedies is often integrated with conventional medicine, but may not be reported *unless the clinician specifically inquires about them.*[81]

Concerns about inappropriate or overprescribing by physicians of stimulant medications and poor understanding of long-term risks have led to increasing use of nonpharmacologic therapies for ADHD in particular.[86] It is estimated that more than 50% of parents of children diagnosed with ADHD rely on CAM therapies in addition to conventional pharmacologic treatment, including vitamins, dietary changes, and expressive therapies, but few disclose CAM use to their child's pediatrician.[87] Research findings suggest that select nonpharmacologic or integrative therapies ameliorate some symptoms of ADHD; in most cases the evidence is preliminary. The next section is a concise review of the evidence for nonpharmacologic and integrative treatments of childhood ADHD.

DIETARY MODIFICATION

Elimination diets refer to those that exclude food colorings and additives, dairy products, sugar, wheat, corn, citrus, eggs, soy, yeast, nuts, and chocolate, and are widely used by parents of children diagnosed with ADHD. However, an early review of controlled studies was inconclusive.[88] Another review of elimination diets in ADHD noted serious methodological flaws including heterogeneity of patient populations, absence of standardized outcome measures, high dropout rates, and nonblinded raters.[89] A more recent review of studies shows possible benefits in eliminating food additives and artificial colors for some children with ADHD.[90] Popular diets for children with ADHD eliminate refined sugar. However, research evidence supporting a relationship between a diet high in sugar or foods with a high glycemic index and hyperactivity is inconclusive.[91] Large prospective trials on dietary restrictions in ADHD are challenging because of difficulties controlling children's eating behaviors.[92]

NATURAL PRODUCTS

Essential fatty acids (EFAs) are frequently used adjunctively with stimulants in the treatment of childhood ADHD. However, research findings to date are inconsistent.[93,94] At the time of this writing, only one placebo-controlled trial on EFAs as a monotherapy for ADHD had been published.[95] The study reported positive outcomes. However, Weber and Newmark[91] noted that a high dropout rate biased findings in a positive direction. It has been suggested that future studies should be of longer duration and include higher doses of EFAs to adequately examine the hypothesis that particular fatty acids result in more permanent beneficial long-term changes in neuronal membrane structure required for sustained clinical improvement.[93] Research findings suggest that there is an inverse correlation between omega-3 fatty acid levels and the severity of ADHD symptoms. Children with the most severe ADHD symptoms tend to have the lowest serum and RBC membrane docosahexaenoic acid (DHA) levels.[94,96–98] However, findings of clinical trials show that combinations of omega-3 and omega-6 fatty acids are more efficacious than omega-3 acids alone. Two controlled trials on adjunctive omega-3 DHA in ADHD-diagnosed children showed no benefit.[93,97] Two subsequent placebo-controlled trials found that children with learning disorders and ADHD-type symptoms receiving a mixture of omega-3 and omega-6 fatty acids together with vitamin E experienced significant improvements over placebo in standardized ratings of attention and hyperactivity.[99,100] Preliminary findings of a small open trial on OFAs (up to 16 g/d of EFA-DHA preparations) as an adjunct to stimulants suggest that higher doses correlate with greater clinical improvement in ADHD symptoms[101]; however, large placebo-controlled studies are needed to replicate these findings. Findings on EFAs in ADHD require replication by large, well-designed prospective trials before they can be generalized to children diagnosed with ADHD.

Zinc may play a role in information processing and it has been reported that children with ADHD may have abnormally low plasma zinc levels.[102] Preliminary findings suggest that zinc (150 mg/d) improves response to stimulants in children diagnosed with ADHD; however, large placebo-controlled trials are needed to confirm these findings and determine optimum dosing strategies.[103]

Emerging findings suggest that low serum ferritin levels may play a causal role in hyperactivity in children with ADHD.[104] In a small 12-week placebo-controlled trial, nonanemic children with ADHD and abnormal low serum ferritin levels were randomized to oral iron in the form of ferrous sulfate 80 mg/d versus stimulants, and experienced comparable improvements.[105]

Acetyl-L-carnitine (ALC) is required for energy metabolism and synthesis of fatty acids. Preliminary findings suggest that L-carnitine (500–1500 mg twice a day) may reduce the severity of ADHD symptoms. However, design flaws limit the significance of these findings.[106] These preliminary findings need to be confirmed by large controlled trials.

Herbal Medicines

Findings of a small 4-week placebo-controlled study suggest that a compound herbal formula containing *Ginkgo biloba* and American ginseng (*Panax quinquefolium*) improves symptoms of ADHD.[107] Preliminary findings from open trials suggest that the extract of French maritime pine (*Pinus pinaster*) bark improve ADHD symptoms. In the only placebo-controlled study published to date, 61 children and adolescents randomized to a standardized bark extract (Pycnogenol) 1 mg/kg/d for 1 month experienced significant and sustained improvements in hyperactivity, inattention, and visual-motor coordination over placebo. ADHD symptoms returned to pretreatment baseline levels after 1-month washout.[108] Large prospective trials are needed to replicate these findings and determine optimal dosing before this botanic extract can be recommended as an evidence-based treatment of ADHD. Preliminary findings from case reports suggest that an ayurvedic herbal called brahmi (*Bacopa monnieri*) is beneficial for ADHD symptoms. However, studies have not been carried out with individuals formally diagnosed with ADHD, and the only placebo-controlled trial failed to show differential benefit over placebo in tests of short-term memory, working memory, executive processing, planning, problem solving, and information-processing speed.[109] A systematic review identified 34 controlled trials (published in Chinese or English language journals) comparing traditional Chinese herbal treatments (also known as TCM) and methylphenidate in children diagnosed with ADHD.[110] These specific reviewers concluded that Chinese medicinal herbals were at least as effective as stimulant medication for short-term symptom management in certain patients. Some studies reported improved response when Chinese medicinal herbals were combined with methylphenidate. These findings are limited by poor methodological quality of all studies included in the review, heterogeneity of study designs, the likelihood of publication bias, and few long-term trials. All studies reviewed were conducted in China and included only ethnically Chinese patients, thus positive group expectation effects cannot be ruled out. High-quality and larger prospective trials in China and Western countries (ideally in ethnically diverse populations) are needed to replicate these preliminary findings before Chinese herbals can be recommended as treatments for ADHD in children.

Case Vignette

Jeffrey was a bright 9-year-old Caucasian boy who was delivered at term following an uncomplicated pregnancy. Neonatal and developmental history was unremarkable, including a lack of in utero exposure to toxins. Jeffrey was diagnosed with ADHD, primarily hyperactive type, at age 5 years and had subsequently been maintained continuously on stimulants. Jeffrey's parents were young professionals in excellent mental and physical health. Medical review of systems was noncontributory, including no history of serious medical disorders or injuries. Psychological testing at age 7 years revealed normal intelligence and ruled out specific learning disorders, other psychiatric disorders, and auditory or visual processing deficits. Jeffrey had a "big sweet tooth" and sometimes skipped school lunches "because he can't sit still long enough to finish …" Jeffrey's parents and teachers reported moderate improvement with a slow release form of methylphenidate. However, they were concerned about

Jeffrey's loss of appetite, irritability, moodiness, insomnia, complaints of abdominal pain, and afternoon fatigue, all of which interfered with his general quality of life, playtime with peers, and his ability to pay attention in class and complete homework assignments. In addition to medication, Jeffrey and his parents had been working with a psychologist in behavioral therapy. Jeffrey's parents had become increasingly frustrated by his limited response to conventional forms of pharmacologic treatment and were also concerned about adverse effects. For these reasons, they decided to see an integrative psychiatrist who was knowledgeable about both pharmacologic and nonpharmacologic treatments for ADHD.

The initial treatment plan involved dietary modifications (including elimination of refined sugar, juices and fruits with a high glycemic index, food colorings, and additives), adding zinc (150 mg/d) and a chewable OFA supplement (eicosapentaenoic acid [EPA] 1 g twice a day with meals) to Jeffrey's current regimen of methylphenidate. Self-directed biofeedback training (reviewed later) was also recommended in the form of a children's computer game. At 1-month follow-up Jeffrey reported that playing the computer game "makes me feel quieter inside," and his teacher and parents observed some improvement in symptoms of impulsive behavior and hyperactivity. There were no apparent adverse effects to the OFAs and zinc. Jeffrey's eating habits remained unchanged and he continued to skip some lunches and eat highly refined sugar snacks during the day. In view of Jeffrey's improvement, the psychiatrist agreed with the parents that it was reasonable to reduce Jeffrey's daily methylphenidate regimen by one-half (to 10 mg/d). He encouraged the parents to be more consistent with Jeffrey's eating behavior and to reinforce healthy food choices with daily reward charting. One month later Jeffrey had made progress, adopting a more selective ("restrictive") diet, was functioning well at school and home, had slowed down noticeably at school, and was less moody and irritable at home. Since reducing the methylphenidate, Jeffrey had had no complaints of insomnia or abdominal pain, and his appetite had improved. His parents described him as "a happy camper," and agreed with recommendations to continue daily biofeedback training along with Jeffrey's current reduced regimen of methylphenidate, together with zinc and OFAs, and were rewarding Jeffrey for making healthy food choices.

This vignette illustrates how an integrative treatment plan that included a psychostimulant, select supplements, dietary changes, and biofeedback training resulted in significant and sustained clinical improvement in symptoms of hyperactivity and impulsivity. This strategy permitted reductions in stimulant dosing, with commensurate reductions in adverse effects. Adjunctive treatment with high-purity OFAs and zinc is a reasonable strategy in this case, and carries no known risks when used concurrently with stimulants. Self-directed biofeedback at home using a simple computer game reinforced Jeffrey's capacity to focus on tasks, and likely contributed to improved study skills. A restrictive diet that eliminates refined sugar, food additives, and colorings may also have contributed to symptomatic improvement.

Yoga and Massage

Small controlled trials suggest that adjunctive yoga and massage may reduce symptom severity in children with ADHD more than stimulants alone.[111,112]

ELECTROENCEPHALOGRAPHY BIOFEEDBACK

Research findings suggest that children diagnosed with ADHD have abnormal brain electrical activity.[113] Electroencephalography (EEG) biofeedback (also called neurofeedback) aims at normalizing electrical brain activity, thereby mitigating the cognitive and behavioral symptoms of ADHD.[114] Sensorimotor rhythm (SMR) training reinforces brain activity in the faster beta frequency range (16–20 Hz) and is used principally to reduce impulsivity and hyperactivity. In contrast, theta suppression is aimed at reducing activity in the slower theta frequency range (4–8 Hz) and targets symptoms of inattention. Controlled studies comparing EEG biofeedback with a stimulant medication versus a waitlist report positive clinical effects and EEG normalization. However, the significance of findings is limited by small study sizes, heterogeneous populations, absence of a control group in many studies, and inconsistent outcome measures.[115] Future studies should incorporate a sham EEG biofeedback arm to rule out group expectation effects.

Vignette

Christina, a second-generation daughter of Mexican immigrants, was diagnosed with ADHD, predominantly inattentive type, when she was 8 years old. At age 14 years, she had already had therapeutic trials on multiple stimulants and atomoxetine, with moderate improvement in symptoms of inattention and distractibility. There was no confounding social, psychiatric or medical history. However, her father had always had difficulty staying focused and believed he had undiagnosed ADHD. Christina had a healthy diet, was a good student, and enjoyed playing team soccer and spending time cooking with her *abuelita* (grandmother) on weekends. She was adherent with atomoxetine (60 mg/d) and there were no significant adverse effects. Her parents had recently heard a news report about a promising new therapy called EEG biofeedback and wished to explore this alternative approach with their daughter because "it would be nice if she didn't have to take drugs all her life." Through a national association of certified biofeedback therapists, they identified a local psychologist who had experience treating ADHD with different kinds of biofeedback.

After reviewing Christina's school and home history and conducting a clinical assessment, the psychologist confirmed a diagnosis of ADHD, predominantly inattentive type, and suggested a specific EEG biofeedback protocol called theta suppression. Christina had her first 30-minute biofeedback training during the intake and seemed to enjoy the experience. "It's like playing a computer game with my mind!" She reported feeling "calmer, quieter inside" immediately after the session. The therapist explained that the goal of biofeedback training was to help individuals learn how to achieve the same quiet mental state (ie, that takes place during biofeedback) at other times. Christina was excited by the prospect of learning "how to control my brain better," and her parents scheduled 8 consecutive biofeedback sessions at semi-weekly intervals. The psychologist encouraged Christina to use a simple handheld biofeedback device at home and during breaks in school. After 4 weeks of EEG biofeedback training Christina's teachers observed improvements in her attention span in class. Her parents reported fewer problems in her completing homework assignments on time, and she felt "more focused" overall. She was consistently using the handheld biofeedback device during breaks and when studying at home. Her *abuelita* had also noticed that Christina seemed more engaged with cooking activities and more confident in her social interactions. In view of these improvements, Christina's parents were considering reducing or discontinuing her medication, and they made an appointment with her family physician to discuss this option.

This vignette illustrates how sustained clinical improvement achieved through consistent EEG biofeedback training can permit dosage reduction (and in some cases discontinuation) of conventional pharmacologic treatment without symptomatic worsening. In this case there was no evidence that social, medical, or nutritional factors played a role in her presentation. Therefore, interventions addressing these issues were not indicated. EEG biofeedback training is a reasonable adjunct to conventional pharmacologic treatment, with the goal of further diminishing symptom severity in children who respond partially to medications. Research findings (see earlier discussion) suggest that regular sessions of a specific EEG biofeedback protocol using theta suppression may result in sustained improvement in symptoms of inattention and distractibility. EEG biofeedback poses no known safety issues and there are no contraindications to continuing conventional pharmacologic treatment.

Appropriate CAM and integrative treatment strategies for ADHD depend on the subtype of ADHD that is being addressed, symptom severity, previous treatment outcomes using conventional or nonpharmacologic modalities, adverse effect issues, psychiatric or medical comorbidities, patient or parental preferences, and the availability of qualified CAM practitioners or access to reputable brands of select supplements. Optimal integrative management of ADHD should be individualized, taking into account the unique history of each child, and starting with a careful assessment of any underlying genetic, physiologic, cultural, and biopsychosocial factors that may contribute to the syndrome. Conventional medications including stimulants and nonstimulants are often effective and well tolerated. However, when associated with significant adverse effects, dosage reductions or discontinuation are appropriate and often necessary. In such cases it is reasonable to consider the use of select natural products alone or adjunctively with conventional pharmacologic treatment. A careful review of dietary habits and food allergies suggests that a selective ("restrictive") diet, eliminating specific foods or additives, may be beneficial in some cases. Parents should consult with their child's PCP or nutritionist before initiating any kind of elimination or restrictive diet. Zinc supplementation at doses of 150 mg/d may be helpful when symptoms of hyperactivity and impulsivity do not improve with stimulants alone. Emerging findings suggest that supplementation with iron (ferrous sulfate up to 80 mg/d) or acetyl-L-carnitine (up to 1500 mg/d) may be especially helpful for symptoms of distractibility and inattention. High doses of omega-3, -6 or omega-3-6-9 EFAs including EPA and DHA (up to 16 g/d) may improve ADHD symptoms. Large well-designed studies are needed before any of these natural products can be generally recommended as first-line treatments of childhood ADHD. Preliminary findings suggest that standardized extracts of *Ginkgo biloba*, *Panax quinquefolium*, *Pinus pinaster,* and *Bacopa monnieri* may be safe and beneficial treatments of childhood ADHD symptoms. However, more conclusive findings from large well-designed placebo-controlled studies are needed to confirm efficacy, safety, tolerability, and optimal dosing strategies. More studies are also needed to evaluate use of select Chinese medicinal herbals before they can be recommended for ADHD. Provisional evidence suggests that regular yoga or massage may reduce the severity of ADHD symptoms. When conventional pharmacologic treatments are ineffective or poorly tolerated, select EEG biofeedback protocols including SMR training for primarily hyperactive type ADHD and theta suppression for primarily inattentive type ADHD should be considered. Research findings suggest that regular EEG biofeedback training may reduce ADHD symptom severity, permitting reduction in doses of conventional medications, resulting in fewer adverse effects and improved treatment adherence.

SUMMARY AND AREAS FOR FURTHER RESEARCH

Research has shown several ethnic differences in the clinical presentation, treatment, clinical response, and outcome of mental illnesses among children. Although there are more data on allopathic treatments compared with CAM interventions, ethnicity does seem to be an important influence on psychotropic drug response, and the role of culture, especially in the treatment of children and adolescents, cannot be ignored. Though there is a growing research literature in ethnopsychopharmacologic variations in drug responses in adults, much work remains to be done with pediatric populations.

Finally, attuned pharmacotherapists should never underestimate their role in helping families and patients *really learn* about mental health and illness. Perhaps a CAM treatment can be the beginning of a good alliance, which may allow for the prescription of a more conventional (allopathic) treatment in addition or as the next single therapeutic intervention. Culturally adapted pharmacotherapy includes being knowledgeable about dose modifications based on differential ethnic responses where appropriate, and attending to cultural beliefs about stigma, meaning effects, side effects, and benefits. If this is done successfully, the mind-brain dichotomy can be re-conceptualized as two sides of the same coin, and the integrative formulation will become common practice as we learn to culturally adapt to the needs of our diverse patients. Kandel[116] predicted the enlightened relationship that could develop between psychiatry and neurobiology, and how it applies to patient care:

As a result, when I speak to someone and he or she listens to me, we not only make eye contact and voice contact, but the action of the neuronal machinery in my brain is having a direct and, I hope, long-lasting effect on the neuronal machinery in his/her brain (and vice versa). Indeed, I would argue that it is only insofar as words produce changes in each others' brains that psychotherapeutic intervention produces changes in patients' minds. From this perspective, the biologic and psychological processes are joined.(p1036)

REFERENCES

1. Lin K, Anderson D, Poland R. Ethnicity and psychopharmacology: bridging the gap. Psychiatr Clin North Am 1995;18(3):635–47.
2. Chaudhry IB, Neelam K, Duddu V, et al. Ethnicity and psychopharmacology. J Psychopharmacol 2008;22:673.
3. US Census Figures. Available at: http://www.census.gov/. Accessed March 6, 2006.
4. US Department of Health and Human Services. Mental health: culture, race, and ethnicity - a supplement to mental health: a report of the Surgeon General. Rockville (MD): US Department of Health and Human Services, Substance Abuse and Mental Health Services Administration; 2001.
5. Choi H. Understanding adolescent depression in ethnocultural context. ANS Adv Nurs Sci 2002;25(2):71–85.
6. Dell ML, Vaughan BS, Kratochvil CJ. Ethics and the prescription pad. Child Adolesc Psychiatr Clin N Am 2008;17:93–111.
7. Mintz D. Meaning and medication in the care of treatment-resistant patients. Am J Psychother 2002;56(3):322–38.
8. Committee on Cultural Psychiatry of the Group for the Advancement of Psychiatry (GAP). Cultural assessment in clinical psychiatry. Washington, DC: American Psychiatric Press; 2002. p. 6–7.
9. Pruett K, Joshi SV, Martin A. Thinking about prescribing: the psychology of psychopharmacology. In: Martin A, Scahill L, Kratochvil CJ, editors. Pediatric psychopharmacology, principles and practice. 2nd edition. New York: Oxford University Press; in press.
10. Gaw AC. Cross-cultural psychopharmacology. In: Gaw AC, editor. Cross-cultural psychiatry. Washington, DC: American Psychiatric Press; 2001.

11. Gaw AC. Cultural context of nonadherence to psychotropic medications in psychiatry patients. In: Gaw AC, editor. Cross-cultural psychiatry. Washington, DC: American Psychiatric Press; 2001. p. 141–64.
12. Munoz R, Primm A, Ananth J, et al. Disparities. In: Life in color: culture in American psychiatry. Chicago: Hilton Publishing Company; 2007. p. 165–81.
13. Munoz R, Primm A, Ananth J, et al. Remedies in color. In: Life in color: culture in American psychiatry. Chicago: Hilton Publishing Company; 2007. p. 105–25.
14. Smith MW. Ethnopsychopharmacology. In: Lim RF, editor. Clinical manual of cultural psychiatry. Washington, DC: American Psychiatric Publishing; 2006. p. 207–35.
15. Tseng W-S. Culture, ethnicity, and drug therapy. In: Handbook of cultural psychiatry. San Diego (CA): Academic Press; 2001. p. 505–11.
16. Tseng W-S. Ethnicity, culture, and drug therapy. In: Clinician's guide to cultural psychiatry. Boston: Academic Press; 2003. p. 343–52.
17. Ng CH, Lin K-M, Singh BS, et al. Review of ethno-psychopharmacology: advances in current practice. New York: Cambridge University Press; 2008. p. 38–62.
18. Miskimen T, Marin H, Escobar J. Psychopharmacological research ethics: special issues affecting US ethnic minorities. Psychopharmacology (Berl) 2003;171:98–104.
19. Lawson WB. Biological markers in neuropsychiatric disorders: racial and ethnic factors. In: Sorel E, editor. Family, culture, and psychobiology. New York: Levas; 1990.
20. Vitiello B. Research in child and adolescent psychopharmacology: recent accomplishments and new challenges. Psychopharmacology (Berl) 2007; 191(1):5–13.
21. Olfson M, Marcus SC, Weissman MM, et al. National trends in the use of psychotropic medications by children. J Am Acad Child Adolesc Psychiatry 2002;41:514–21.
22. Timimi S, Taylor E. ADHD is best understood as a cultural construct. Br J Psychiatry 2004;184:8–9.
23. Kleinman A. Culture, illness, and care: clinical lessons from anthropologic and cross-cultural research. Ann Intern Med 1978;88:251–8.
24. Harwood A. The hot-cold theory of disease: implications for treatment of Puerto Rican patients. JAMA 1971;216:1153–60.
25. Winters NC, Hanson G, Stoyanova V. The case formulation in child and adolescent psychiatry. Child Adolesc Psychiatr Clin N Am 2007;16:111–32.
26. Engel GL. From biomedical to biopsychosocial: being scientific in the human domain. Psychosomatics 1997;38(6):521–8.
27. Barker P. The child and adolescent psychiatry evaluation: basic child psychiatry. Oxford (UK): Blackwell Scientific; 1995.
28. Nurcombe B, Drell M, Leonard H, et al. Clinical problem solving: the case of Matthew, part 1. J Am Acad Child Adolesc Psychiatry 2002;41(1):92–7.
29. Nurcombe B. Developmental psychopathology and the diagnostic formulation. Presented at the Annual Meeting of the American Academy of Child and Adolescent Psychiatry. Washington, DC, October 1992.
30. Lin K-M, Smith MW, Ortiz V. Culture and psychopharmacology. Psychiatr Clin N Am 2001;24(3):523–38.
31. Lawson WB. Clinical issues in the pharmacotherapy of African-Americans. Psychopharmacol Bull 1986;32:275–81.
32. Pi EH, Simpson GM. Cross-cultural psychopharmacology: a current clinical perspective. Psychiatr Serv 2005;56:31–3.
33. Lin K-M, Finder E. Neuroleptic dosage for Asians. Amer Jnl of Psychiatry 1983; 140:490–1.

34. Lawson WB. Racial and ethnic factors in psychiatric research. Hosp Community Psychiatry 1986;37:50–4.
35. Lawson WB, Yesavage JA, Werner RD. Race, violence, and psychopathology. J Clin Psychiatry 1984;45:294–7.
36. Segal SP, Bola JR, Watson MA. Race, quality of care, and antipsychotic prescribing practices in psychiatric emergency services. Psychiatr Serv 1996;47:282–6.
37. Morgenstern H, Glazer WM. Identifying risk factors for tardive dyskinesia among long-term outpatients maintained with neuroleptic medications: results of the Yale Tardive Dyskinesia Study. Arch Gen Psychiatry 1993;50:723–33.
38. Jeste DV, Caligiuri MP, Paulsen JS. Risk of tardive dyskinesia in older patients: a prospective longitudinal study of 266 patients. Arch Gen Psychiatry 1995;52:756–65.
39. Glazer WM, Morgenstern H, Doucette J. Race and tardive dyskinesia among outpatients at a CMHC. Hosp Community Psychiatry 1994;45:38–42.
40. Lindamer L, Lacro JP, Jeste DV. Relationship of ethnicity to the effects of anti-psychotic medication. In: Herrara JM, Lawson WB, Sramek JJ, editors. Cross cultural psychiatry. Chichester (West Sussex): John Wiley & Sons; 1999.
41. Bradford LD. CYP2D6 allele frequency in European Caucasians, Asians, Africans and their descendants. Pharmacogenomics 2002;3:229–43.
42. Lin KM. Biological differences in depression and anxiety across races and ethnic groups. J Clin Psychiatry 2001;62(Suppl 13):13–9.
43. Chillevoort I, de Boer A, van der Weide J, et al. Antipsychotic-induced extrapy-ramidal syndromes and cytochrome P450 2D6 genotype: a case-control study. Pharmacogenetics 2002;12:235–40.
44. de Leon J, Susce MT, Pan RM, et al. CYP2D6 poor metabolizer phenotype may be associated with risperidone adverse drug reactions and discontinuation. J Clin Psychiatry 2005;66:15–27.
45. Lawson WB. "Issues in the pharmacotherapy of African Americans". In: Ruiz P, editor. Review of psychiatry, vol. 19, no. 4. Washington, DC: American Association Press; 2000. p. 37–53.
46. Tollefson GD, Beasley CM, Tran VP, et al. Olanzapine versus haloperidol in the treatment of schizophrenia and schizoaffective and schizophreniform disorders: results of an international collaborative trial. Am J Psychiatry 1997;154:457–65.
47. Tran PT, Lawson WB, Andersen S, et al. Treatment of the African American patient with novel antipsychotic agents. In: Herrera J, Lawson WB, Sramek J, editors. Cross cultural psychiatry. Chichester (UK): John Wiley & Sons; 1999.
48. Bailey RK. Atypical psychotropic medications and their adverse effects: a review for the African-American primary care physician. J Natl Med Assoc 2003;95(2):137–44.
49. Fenton WS, Chavez MR. Medication-induced weight gain and dyslipidemia in patients with schizophrenia. Am J Psychiatry 2006;163:1697–704.
50. Okpaku S, Frazer A, Mendels J. A pilot study of racial differences in erythrocyte lithium transport. Am J Psychiatry 1980;137:120–1.
51. Strickland TL, Lin K-M, Fu P, et al. Comparison of lithium ratio between African-American and Caucasian bipolar patients. Biol Psychiatry 1995;37:325–30.
52. Strickland TL, Lawson WB, Lin K-M. Interethnic variation in response to lithium therapy among African-American and Asian-American populations. In: Lin K-M, Poland RE, Nakasaki G, editors. Psychopharmacology and psychobiology of ethnicity. Washington, DC: American Psychiatric Association; 1993. p. 107–23.

53. Hildreth C, Saunders O. Hypertension in blacks: clinical overview. Cardiovasc Clin 1991;21:85–96.
54. Valenstein M, McCarthy JF, Austin KL, et al. What happened to lithium? Antidepressant augmentation in clinical settings. Am J Psychiatry 2006;163:1219–25.
55. Kilbourne AM, Pincus HA. Patterns of psychotropic medication use by race among veterans with bipolar disorder. Psychiatr Serv 2006;57:123–6.
56. McMahon FJ, Buervenich S, Charney D, et al. Variation in the gene encoding the serotonin 2A receptor is associated with outcome of antidepressant treatment. Am J Hum Genet 2006;78:804–14.
57. Melfi CA, Croghan TW, Hanna MP, et al. Racial variation in antidepressant treatment in a Medicaid population. J Clin Psychiatry 2000;61:16–21.
58. Kuruppurachchi K, Wijeratne L. ADHD in developing countries. Br J Psychiatry 2004;185(5):439.
59. Samuel V, Curtis S, Thornell A, et al. The unexplored void of ADHD and African-American research: a review of the literature. J Atten Disord 1997;1(4):197–207.
60. Miller T, Nigg J, Miller R. Attention deficit hyperactivity disorder in African American children: what can be concluded from the past ten years? Clin Psychol Rev 2009;29(1):77–86.
61. Winsberg BG, Comings DE. Association of the dopamine transporter gene (DAT1) with poor methylphenidate response. J Am Acad Child Adolesc Psychiatry 1999;38:1474–7.
62. Waldman ID, Rowe DC, Abramowitz A, et al. Association and linkage of the dopamine transporter gene and attention-deficit/hyperactivity disorder in children: heterogeneity owing to diagnostic subtype and severity. Am J Hum Genet 1998;63:1767–76.
63. Arnold L, Elliott M, Sachs L, et al. Effects of ethnicity on treatment attendance, stimulant response/dose, and 14-month outcome in ADHD. J Consult Clin Psychol 2003;71(4):713–27.
64. Brown RT, Sexson SB. A controlled trial of methylphenidate in black adolescents. Attentional, behavioral and physiological effects. Clin Pediatr 1988;27:74–81.
65. Starr H, Kemner J. Multicenter, randomized, open-label study of OROS methylphenidate versus atomoxetine: treatment outcomes in African-American children with ADHD. J Natl Med Assoc 2005;97(Suppl 10):S11–6.
66. Corbie-Smith G, Thomas SB, Williams MV, et al. Attitudes and beliefs of African-American toward participation in medical research. J Gen Intern Med 1999;14:537–46.
67. Shavers VL, Lynch CF, Burmeister LF. Knowledge of the Tuskegee study and its impact on the willingness to participate in medical research studies. J Natl Med Assoc 2000;92:563–72.
68. Shavers VL, Lynch CF, Burmeister LF. Racial differences in factors that influence the willingness to participate in medical research studies. Ann Epidemiol 2002;12:248–56.
69. Hamilton LA, Aliyu MH, Lyons PD, et al. African-American community attitudes and perceptions toward schizophrenia and medical research: an exploratory study. J Natl Med Assoc 2006;98:18–27.
70. Wendler D, Kington R, Madans J, et al. Are racial and ethnic minorities less willing to participate in health research? PLoS Med 2006;3:e19.
71. Trivedi MH, Rush AJ, Wisniewski SR, et al. Evaluation of outcomes with citalopram for depression using measurement-based care in STAR*D: implications for clinical practice. Am J Psychiatry 2006;163:28–40.

72. Stroup TS, Lieberman JA, McEvoy JP, et al. Effectiveness of olanzapine, quetia-pine, risperidone, and ziprasidone in patients with chronic schizophrenia following discontinuation of a previous atypical antipsychotic. Am J Psychiatry 2006;163:611–22.

73. Metzl JA. Forming an effective therapeutic alliance. In: Tasman A, Riba MB, Silk KR, editors. The doctor-patient relationship in pharmacotherapy: improving treatment effectiveness. New York: Guilford Press; 2000. p. 25–47.

74. Broucek F, Ricci W. Self-disclosure of self-presence? Bull Menninger Clin 1998; 26(4):427–38.

75. Havens L. Forming effective relationships. In: Havens L, Sabo A, editors. The real world guide to psychotherapy practice. Cambridge (MA): Harvard University Press; 2000. p. 17–33.

76. Joshi SV. Teamwork: the therapeutic alliance in pediatric pharmacotherapy. Child Adolesc Psychiatr Clin N Am 2006;15:239–62.

77. Sabo A, Rand B. The relational aspects of psychopharmacology. In: Sabo A, Havens L, editors. The real world guide to psychotherapy practice. Cambridge (MA): Harvard University Press; 2000. p. 34–59.

78. O'Brien JD, Perlmutter I. The effect of medication on the process of psycho-therapy. Child Adolesc Psychiatr Clin N Am 1997;6(1):185–96.

79. Feinstein NR, Fielding K, Udvari-Solner A, et al. The supporting alliance in child and adolescent treatment: enhancing collaboration among therapists, parents, and teachers. Am J Psychother 2009;63(4):319–44.

80. Kemper KJ, Vohra S, Walls R, et al. The use of complementary and alternative medicine in pediatrics. Pediatrics 2008;122:1374–86.

81. Graham RE, Ahn AC, Davis RB, et al. Use of complementary and alternative medical therapies among racial and ethnic minority adults: results from the 2002 National Health Interview Survey. J Natl Med Assoc 2005;97(4):535–45.

82. Guenther E, Mendoza J, Crouch BI, et al. Differences in herbal and dietary supplement use in Hispanic and non-Hispanic pediatric populations. Pediatr Emerg Care 2005;21(8):507–14.

83. Smitherman LC, Janisse J, Mathur A. The use of folk remedies among children in an urban black community: remedies for fever, colic, and teething. Pediatrics 2005;115(3). Available at: http://www.pediatrics.org/cgi/content/full/115/3/e297. Accessed August 11, 2010.

84. Novins DK, Beals J, Moore LA, et al. Use of biomedical services and traditional healing options among American Indians: sociodemographic correlates, spiritu-ality, and ethnic identity. Med Care 2004;42(7):670–9.

85. Van Sickle D, Morgan F, Wright AL. Qualitative study of the use of traditional healing by asthmatic Navajo families. Am Indian Alsk Native Ment Health Res 2003;11(1):1–18.

86. Anderson SL, Navalta CP. Altering the course of neurodevelopment: a framework for understanding the enduring effects of psychotropic drugs. Int J Dev Neuro-sci 2004;22(5–6):423–40.

87. Chan E, Rappaport LA, Kemper KJ. Complementary and alternative therapies in childhood attention and hyperactivity problems. J Dev Behav Pediatr 2003; 24(1):4–8.

88. Wender EH. The food additive-free diet in the treatment of behavior disorders: a review. J Dev Behav Pediatr 1986;7(1):35–42.

89. Rojas NL, Chan E. Old and new controversies in the alternative treatment of attention-deficit hyperactivity disorder. Ment Retard Dev Disabil Res Rev 2005;11(2):116–30.

90. Diet and attention deficit hyperactivity disorder. The Harvard mental health letter [1057–5022] 2009;25(12):4–5.
91. Weber W, Newmark S. Complementary and alternative medical therapies for attention-deficit/hyperactivity disorder and autism. Pediatr Clin North Am 2007;54(6):983–1006.
92. Cormier E, Elder JH. Diet and child behavior problems: fact or fiction? Pediatr Nurs 2007;33(2):138–43.
93. Voigt RG, Llorente AM, Jensen CL, et al. A randomized, double-blind, placebo-controlled trial of docosahexaenoic acid supplementation in children with attention-deficit/hyperactivity disorder. J Pediatr 2001;139(2):189–96.
94. Stevens LJ, Zentall SS, Deck JL, et al. Essential fatty acid metabolism in boys with attention-deficit hyperactivity disorder. Am J Clin Nutr 1995;62(4):761–8.
95. Sinn N, Bryan J. Effect of supplementation with polyunsaturated fatty acids and micronutrients on learning and behavior problems associated with child ADHD. J Dev Behav Pediatr 2007;28(2):82–91.
96. Mitchell EA, Aman MG, Turbott SH, et al. Clinical characteristics and serum essential fatty acid levels in hyperactive children. Clin Pediatr (Phila) 1987;26(8):406–11.
97. Bekaroglu M, Aslan Y, Gedik Y, et al. Relationships between serum free fatty acids and zinc, and attention deficit hyperactivity disorder: a research note. J Child Psychol Psychiatry 1996;37:225–7.
98. Stevens LJ, Zentall SS, Abate ML, et al. Omega-3 fatty acids in boys with behavior, learning, and health problems. Physiol Behav 1996;59:915–20.
99. Richardson AJ, Puri BK. A randomized double-blind, placebo-controlled study of the effects of supplementation with highly unsaturated fatty acids on ADHD-related symptoms in children with specific learning difficulties. Prog Neuropsychopharmacol Biol Psychiatry 2002;26(2):233–9.
100. Stevens L, Zhang W, Peck L, et al. EFA supplementation in children with inattention, hyperactivity, and other disruptive behaviors. Lipids 2003;38(10):1007–21.
101. Sorgi PJ, Hallowell EM, Hutchins HL, et al. Effects of an open-label pilot study with high-dose EPA/DHA concentrates on plasma phospholipids and behavior in children with attention deficit hyperactivity disorder. Nutr J 2007;6:16.
102. Yorbik O, Ozdag MF, Olgun A, et al. Potential effects of zinc on information processing in boys with attention deficit hyperactivity disorder. Prog Neuropsychopharmacol Biol Psychiatry 2008;32(3):662–7.
103. Arnold LE, DiSilvestro RA. Zinc in attention-deficit/hyperactivity disorder. J Child Adolesc Psychopharmacol 2005;15(4):619–27.
104. Oner O, Alkar OY, Oner P. Relation of ferritin levels with symptom ratings and cognitive performance in children with attention deficit-hyperactivity disorder. Pediatr Int 2008;50(1):40–4.
105. Konofal E, Lecendreux M, Deron J, et al. Effects of iron supplementation on attention deficit hyperactivity disorder in children. Pediatr Neurol 2008;38(1):20–6.
106. Van Oudheusden LJ, Scholte HR. Efficacy of carnitine in the treatment of children with attention-deficit hyperactivity disorder. Prostaglandins Leukot Essent Fatty Acids 2002;67(1):33–8.
107. Lyon R, Cline JC, Totosy de Zepetnek J, et al. Effect of the herbal extract combination Panax quinquefolium and Ginkgo biloba on attention-deficit hyperactivity disorder: a pilot study. J Psychiatry Neurosci 2001;26(3):221–8.
108. Trebaticka J, Kopasova S, Hradecna Z, et al. Treatment of ADHD with French maritime pine bark extract, pycnogenol. Eur Child Adolesc Psychiatry 2006;15(6):329–35.

109. Nathan PJ, Tanner S, Lloyd J, et al. Effects of a combined extract of *Ginkgo biloba* and *Bacopa monnieri* on cognitive function in healthy humans. Hum Psychopharmacol 2004;19(2):91–6.
110. Lan Y, Zhang L-L, Luo R. Attention deficit hyperactivity disorder in children: comparative efficacy of traditional Chinese medicine and methylphenidate. J Int Med Res 2009;37(3):939–48.
111. Jensen PS, Kenny DT. The effects of yoga on the attention and behavior of boys with attention-deficit/hyperactivity disorder (ADHD). J Atten Disord 2004;7(4):205–16.
112. Khilnani S, Field T, Hernandez-Reif M, et al. Massage therapy improves mood and behavior of students with attention-deficit/hyperactivity disorder. Adolescence 2003;38(152):623–38.
113. Butnik SM. Neurofeedback in adolescents and adults with attention deficit hyperactivity disorder. J Clin Psychol 2005;61(5):621–5.
114. Monastra VJ. Quantitative electroencephalography and attention-deficit/hyperactivity disorder: implications for clinical practice. Curr Psychiatry Rep 2008; 10(5):432–8.
115. Gevensleben H, Holl B, Albrecht B, et al. Is neurofeedback an efficacious treatment for ADHD? A randomised controlled clinical trial. J Child Psychol Psychiatry 2009;50(7):780–9.
116. Kandel E. Psychotherapy and the single synapse: the impact of psychiatric thought on neurobiologic research. N Engl J Med 1979;301(19):1028–37.

Training Child and Adolescent Psychiatrists to Be Culturally Competent

Ayesha I. Mian, MD[a],*, Cheryl S. Al-Mateen, MD, DFAPA[b],
Gabrielle Cerda, MD[c]

KEYWORDS

- Child and adolescent psychiatry • Cultural competence
- Education • AACAP model curriculum

Cultural competence is the ability of health care professionals to communicate with and effectively provide high-quality care to patients from diverse sociocultural backgrounds. Aspects of diversity include—but go beyond—race, ethnicity, gender, sexual orientation, religion, and country of origin.[1] In response to the increasing diversity of many industrialized societies, educational efforts have been aimed at educating medical trainees to address the needs of a heterogeneous patient population. It is imperative that the child and adolescent psychiatric community prepare for the changing world to provide appropriate, accessible, and quality clinical care. The first step toward this goal is to understand the role of culture and cultural competence in clinical care. As the field of cultural competence has evolved, the goal has moved from educating clinicians in the categorical approach—that of becoming skilled at knowledge, attitudes, and practices of a particular cultural group of patients—to a focus on the development of a set of skills and framework. This culturally competent therapeutic stance is an orientation that places medicine and patients in a social, cultural, and historical context. The overall aim is the open acknowledgment of the dignity and autonomy of, and delivery of high-quality medical care to *all* members of society, regardless of gender, race, ethnicity, religion, sexual orientation, language, geographic origin, or socioeconomic background.[2]

[a] Menninger Department of Psychiatry and Behavior Sciences, Baylor College of Medicine, Houston, TX, USA
[b] Virginia Commonwealth University School of Medicine, Richmond, VA, USA
[c] Department of Psychiatry, University of California, San Diego, San Diego, CA, USA
* Corresponding author.
E-mail address: mian@bcm.tmc.edu

Child Adolesc Psychiatric Clin N Am 19 (2010) 815–831
doi:10.1016/j.chc.2010.08.004
1056-4993/10/$ – see front matter © 2010 Elsevier Inc. All rights reserved.

childpsych.theclinics.com

HISTORY

If one were to consider cultural psychiatry as the study of "unusual syndromes" by Western standards, then this field has existed for more than 100 years. It was Darwin who first talked about "primitive" people and described Westerners as possessing "advanced" evolutionary development. This fostered a predetermined value system of judging cultural groups and also influenced the medical assessment of seemingly culture-specific conditions.[3] For example, early colonial physicians condescendingly described unusual symptom patterns as "amok" among Malays as primitive expressions of stress.[4] Kraepelin observed that Western prototypes of mental disorders, although qualitatively variable in their presentations, were essentially culture-free constructs.[3] In 1977, Kleinman argued that these Western constructs of disorders could not be applied uniformly across different cultural contexts.[3] Furthermore, cultural contexts had an important shaping influence on disease categories. Cultural factors could not be subtracted from the disease without modifying its sufficient psychopathologic architecture, presentation, course, or outcome.[5] Also, in Rutter's textbook *Developmental Psychiatry*, he noted that creative capacities of adults and children reflected variations by gender and culture.[6]

Cultural evolutionism was also challenged in the early twentieth century by anthropologists who documented the great variability of social behaviors and stressed the importance of cultural factors in shaping the perceptions and hence the life of an individual.[7] Whiting and Child, in their book *Child Training and Personality,*[8] were the first to examine, in 6 cultural groups, how civilization affected the children in their later behavior. Indeed, cultural psychiatry involves much more than a focus on the "exotic." It embodies the concept that culture is relevant and important in *all* of our clinical interactions and that ongoing attention to cultural factors is *imperative* in the routine provision of clinical care.

Culture consists of the shared values, norms, traditions, customs, arts, history, folklore, and institutions of a group of people. It plays an important role in how people of different backgrounds express themselves, seek help, cope with stress, and develop social supports. Culture affects every aspect of an individual's life, including how we experience, understand, express, and address emotional and mental distress.

Cultural competence is defined as a set of knowledge-based and interpersonal skills that allow individuals to understand, appreciate, and work with individuals of cultures from other than their own. Five components comprise culturally competent care: (1) awareness and acceptance of cultural differences, (2) capacity for cultural self-awareness, (3) understanding the dynamics of difference, (4) developing basic knowledge about the patient's culture, and (5) adapting practice skills to fit the cultural context of the patient and family.[9] Failure to understand the cultural background of children and adolescents and their families can lead to the following problems: misdiagnosis, nonadherence, poor use of health services, and general alienation of the child/adolescent and family from the health care system.[10]

However, it was not until 1994, that a formal framework to assess the impact of culture on mental illness was included in the *Diagnostic and Statistical Manual of Mental Disorders*, 4th edition (DSM-IV).[11] This framework is the Outline for Cultural Formulation (OCF). It remains only in the Appendix along with a glossary of culture-bound syndromes in the current DSM-IV-TR (Text Revision), which was revised in 2000. The OCF includes the following 5 main areas: (1) cultural identity; (2) cultural explanation of the individual's illness; (3) cultural factors related to psychosocial, environmental, and functionality factors; (4) cultural elements of the relationship between the individual and the clinician; and (5) overall cultural assessment for diagnosis and care.

It is noteworthy that the OCF is primarily targeted toward the individual adult, not youth specifically and does not address the role of family, except in a general assessment of the cultural factors related to psychosocial, environmental, and functionality factors. Youth do not exist in a vacuum. The parent-child relationship is profoundly influenced by cultural forces. This relationship is often key to the child's clinical presentation. So, whereas the OCF is a significant contribution to the field of general psychiatry, when working with children and adolescents this framework must be expanded and modified. The cultural formulation must include some assessment of the child's family members and the impact of divergent (or similar) profiles on the child's life and clinical presentation. For optimal clinical care of the child, all 5 areas of the OCF should be touched on for at least the child's parents, and potentially other key individuals in the child's life.

The parents' cultural identity, cultural explanation of the child's illness, and cultural elements of the relationship between the parents and the clinician, are highly relevant to the overall cultural assessment for diagnosis and care of the child. The OCF is most clinically useful when considering all these variables in relation to the family as a whole, not just as they relate directly to the child or adolescent.

We must also assess issues such as the role of "differential" acculturation between family members. An acculturation differential exists when 2 individuals are not at the same level of acculturation. An example of this is a first-generation Mexican mother who speaks only Spanish, does not work outside the home, and adheres to traditional cultural values and gender roles (including the notion that a girl must remain a virgin until her wedding day), with a second-generation Mexican-American teenage daughter who prefers to speak English, identifies herself more with American pop culture than with her Mexican roots, has had several boyfriends, and is currently sexually active. This differential acculturation between parent and child can play a critical role in a youth's clinical presentation, and has even been suggested to be a risk factor for Latina teen suicide attempts and completions.[12]

As part of the OCF family assessment and in general, it is also important to recognize that the diversity that exists within an ethnic group is often overlooked. Even within a family, individuals may belong to or identify with different ethnic subgroups as well as groups. For example, the term Asian American includes people from a variety of nations, such as Afghanistan, China, India, Syria, and Japan. It includes both immigrants and those whose families have lived in the United States for generations. According to 2006 Census estimates, some 44.3 million Americans were identified as Hispanic. Within this group, 64.0% were Mexican, 9.0% Puerto Rican, 3.5% Cuban, 3.0% Salvadoran, and 2.7% Dominican. The remainders are of some other Central American, South American, or other Hispanic or Latino origin.

Until 1984, cultural competence was not stressed in the requirements for residency training in general or child psychiatry by the Accreditation Council for Graduate Medical Education (ACGME). The 1987 edition did not list any specific requirements for cultural training, but recommended broad clinical experience with families from "all social and economic levels." The 1991 revision was significant in that the ACGME required "didactic instruction about American culture and subculture" in addition to supervised clinical experiences with "patients of a variety of ethnic, racial, social and economic backgrounds." The 1995 revision stated that "Residents must receive training so that they have the opportunity to evaluate and to treat patients from various cultural backgrounds and socioeconomic levels." The 1999 revision added "sensitivity to a diverse patient population" as part of *Professionalism*, 1 of 6 core competencies that residents are expected to attain.[13]

Residency programs have responded to the ACGME's cultural competence standards. A 2004 article in the *Journal of the American Medical Association* found that among close to 8000 graduate medical educational programs surveyed in the United States, 50.7% offered cultural competence training in 2003–2004, up from 35.7% in 2000–2001. This was thought to be attributable to the recognition of the increasing diversity of the patient population, in response to pressure from ACGME.[14]

But there are still programs that do not offer formal cross-cultural training. There also seems to be a perception of lesser importance relative to other topics in the training curriculum.[15] Despite increasing requirements by the ACGME for training in cultural psychiatry, there has been little discussion of the content and method for teaching.[16] Some curriculum guidelines of cultural competence have been published.[15] Cultural curricula have been implemented in other disciplines besides psychiatry, including pediatrics and family medicine.[17–19]

MAJOR EMPIRICAL FINDINGS

As mentioned previously, psychiatrists entering medical practice are increasingly likely to provide services to culturally diverse patients. Data from the last census 2000–2050[20,21] show that the minority populations in the United States are increasing at a faster rate than the majority population. From the 2000 to 2050, the proportion of whites in the United States is projected to decrease while the proportion of other racial and ethnic groups (ie, black, Asian, Hispanic) is projected to increase. For child and adolescent psychiatrists, this trend toward diversity in patient population is already a reality. By 2020 the racial and ethnic distribution for school-age persons between 5 and 17 years old is projected to be 30 million white; 9 million African American; 13 million Latino/a; 3 million Asian/Pacific Islander; and 4 million other, which includes American Indians, Alaska Natives, and those of multiple race/ethnicities (U.S. Census Bureau, 2000; http://www.census.gov/census2000/demoprofiles.html). Because of the multifaceted, multicultural, and fluid nature of contemporary society, there are often significant challenges to providing culturally competent mental health services for culturally dissimilar as well as culturally similar therapeutic dyads.

A growing literature delineates the impact of sociocultural factors, race, and ethnicity on health and clinical care.[22,23] Patients present varied perspectives, values, beliefs, and behaviors regarding health and well-being. These include variations in patient recognition of symptoms, thresholds for seeking care, ability to communicate symptoms to a provider who understands their meaning, ability to understand the prescribed management strategy, expectations of care (including preferences for or against diagnostic and therapeutic procedures), and adherence to preventive measures and medications.[24,25] Considerable evidence supports the idea that sociocultural differences between patient and physician can influence communications and clinical decision making.[26] There is also literature that suggests that provider–patient communication is directly linked to patient satisfaction and adherence, and subsequently to health outcomes.[27] Thus, when sociocultural differences between patient and provider are not appreciated, explored, understood, or communicated in the medical encounter, patient dissatisfaction, poor adherence, and poorer health outcomes may result.[25] It is not only the patient's culture that matters; the provider's "culture" is equally important.[28] Historical factors for patient mistrust, provider bias, and their impact on physicians' decision making have also been documented.[25] Failure to take sociocultural factors into account may lead to stereotyping, and, in the worst cases, biased or discriminatory treatment of patients based on race, culture, language proficiency, or social status.[25]

HEALTH CARE DISPARITIES AND CULTURAL EDUCATION

In the United States, the results of these challenges can be seen in the existence of health care disparities.[29,30] The 2000 Institute of Medicine (IOM, 2001) Report, *Crossing the Quality Chasm,* listed patient-centered care and equity as 2 of 6 objectives that need to be met to improve quality of health care in the United States.[31] The 2002 IOM Report,[32] *Unequal Treatment: Confronting Racial and Ethnic Disparities in Healthcare,* was a landmark report that concluded that racial and ethnic disparities exist in health care and are unacceptable because they are associated with worse outcomes in many cases. The report defined "disparities" in health care as racial and ethnic differences in the quality of health care that are not attributable to access-related factors or clinical needs, preferences, and appropriateness of intervention. The 2002 report analyzed this evidence of disparities focusing on the operation of health care systems and the legal and regulatory climate and on discrimination at the individual patient provider level. Discrimination was defined in the report to refer to differences in care that result from biases, prejudices, stereotyping, and uncertainty in clinical communication and decision making. The report made 21 recommendations relating to education, which included increasing the proportion of underrepresented US racial and ethnic minorities among health professionals as well as integrating cross-cultural education into the training of all current and future health professionals. The 2004 Institute of Medicine report,[33] *In the Nation's Compelling Interest: Ensuring Diversity in the Healthcare Workforce,* summarized the evidence demonstrating that greater diversity among health professionals is associated with improved access to care for racial and ethnic minority patients, greater patient choice and satisfaction, better patient-provider communication, and better educational experiences for all students while in training. Many organizations, including the American Medical Association (AMA), have adopted recommendations made by these 3 IOM reports, of which training and education to increase physician cultural competency continues to be a strong focus. A year earlier in 2001, the Office of the Surgeon General had determined that in comparison with whites, ethnic minorities in the United States had less access to mental health care, were less likely to receive quality or expert care, were more likely to be misdiagnosed, and reported less effective mental health treatment.[30] The report cited considerable evidence that found that a disproportionate numbers of African Americans are represented in the most vulnerable segments of the population— people who are homeless, incarcerated, in the child welfare system, victims of trauma—all populations with increased risks for mental disorders. As many as 40% of Hispanic Americans report limited English-language proficiency. Because few mental health care providers identify themselves as Spanish speaking, most Hispanic Americans have limited access to ethnically or linguistically similar providers. The suicide rate among American Indians/Alaska Natives is 50% higher than the national rate; rates of co-occurring mental illness and substance abuse (especially alcohol) are also higher among Native youth and adults. Although some investigators have done important work (see the article by Kataoka and colleagues elsewhere in this issue for further exploration of this topic), even more data are needed with this population, so the full nature, extent, and sources of these disparities remain largely hypothetical. Both Asian Americans and Pacific Islanders who seek care for a mental illness often present with more severe illnesses than do other racial or ethnic groups. This, in part, suggests that stigma and shame are critical deterrents to service use. It is also possible that mental illnesses may be undiagnosed or treated later in their course because they are expressed in symptoms of a physical nature. The Youth Risk Behavior Survey of the Centers for Disease Control and Prevention[34] reports that

Latino and African American youths now have significantly higher rates of suicidal ideation and attempts compared with European Americans.

Based on the preceding information, many recommendations were made in the Surgeon General's report, out of which one was most relevant to education:

"*Minorities are underrepresented among mental health providers, researchers, administrators, policymakers, and consumer and family organizations. Furthermore, many providers and researchers of all backgrounds are not fully aware of the impact of culture on mental health, mental illness, and mental health services. All mental health professionals are encouraged to develop their understanding of the roles of age, gender, race, ethnicity, and culture in research and treatment. Therefore, mental health training programs and funding sources that work toward equitable representation and a culturally informed training curriculum will contribute to reducing disparities.*"[30]

It is evident from the previously cited empirical findings and the emphasis by medical education governing bodies that training our child and adolescent psychiatrists to be culturally attuned is not only imperative for optimal clinical care of our patients, but is the new frontier for competent training. Proper training in cultural psychiatry leads to increased awareness of social, cultural, and political issues that can enhance the effectiveness of clinical work. Attention to culture in psychiatric care also serves to articulate a vision of a pluralistic community that respects diversity. The effects of globalization on increased flows of knowledge and the confrontation of different value systems heighten the importance of cultural psychiatry both as an academic discipline and as a central pillar of clinical training.[3]

CULTURAL COMPETENCY CURRICULA IN CHILD AND ADOLESCENT PSYCHIATRY

Many organizations in American psychiatry recognize the need for formal training in cultural issues, and the development of cultural competency curricula in child and adolescent psychiatry training programs has been encouraged by many organizations, including the AMA, the American Psychiatric Association, American Academy of Child and Adolescent Psychiatry (AACAP), ACGME, American Association of Directors of Psychiatric Residency Training Programs (AADPRT), and the Residency Review Committee (RRC).[29] Several sample curriculum modules have been published.[35–39] Weissman and colleagues[40] found that there is a cohort of residents who feel unable to handle certain cross-cultural interactions at the time they finish training. This ranged from roughly 5% of study subjects not knowing how to address a patient in a culturally competent manner to 28% feeling very or somewhat unprepared to treat patients who had some distrust of the US Health system.[a]

The process of teaching about cultural competency has developed over the past 30 years, with the ideal course having evolved from a few didactic sessions focused on characteristics of minority group members, to a scaffolded multiyear curriculum encompassing an in-depth understanding of health care disparities, and exploring the knowledge, skills, and attitudes inherent in becoming a physician specialist able to provide culturally competent care in a multicultural society. There is wide recognition

---

[a] The first 3 organizations, the American Medical Association (AMA), American Psychiatric Association (APA), and the American Academy of Child and Adolescent Psychiatry (AACAP) are guild organizations that perform several functions, including representing the interests of practicing physicians and sponsoring education to physicians as well as the community-at-large. The latter 3, the Accreditation Council of Graduate Medical Education (ACGME), American Association of Directors of Psychiatric Residency Training Programs (AADPRT), and the Residency Review Committee (RRC) are responsible for oversight of graduate medical education programs.

throughout health care education that cultural competency concepts are integral to the care of patients. Anandaraja and colleagues[41] describe the development of a Global Health Residency Track that includes a core competency area "Health disparities, Human rights, and Cultural competency." This issue is equally relevant in dentistry, with recognition of the presence of dental disparities, a lack of diversity in the workforce, and dental schools continuing to integrate cultural competency concepts into their curricula.[42] Similarly, a variety of methods, including team-based learning, have been found useful in teaching cultural competency concepts to pharmacy students.[43] Although synonymous terms are "culturally effective health care" and "culturally effective pediatric care" (from the American Medical Association and from the American Academy of Pediatrics), the term "cultural competence" is more ubiquitous, and used throughout the various medical specialties. A newer, more process-oriented model, the "cultural sensibility" approach,[44] is described in detail elsewhere in this issue. Ideally, cultural competence related to the provision of health care will be couched in an understanding of health disparities, and the role of the health care provider in minimizing these disparities and ensuring the provision of care that is patient- and family-centered.[45] Such cultural education is no longer confined solely to the care of "minority patients," but is understood to extend to the more complete continuum of culture, including "the full spectrum of values, behaviors, customs, language, race, ethnicity, gender, sexual orientation, religious beliefs, socioeconomic status, and other distinct attributes of population groups."[46] Each of these is important, but may not receive needed attention in teaching. Of note, as of this writing, there are 381 languages spoken in the United States.[47] Although some studies have indicated the reverse, Boudreau and colleagues[48] found that language concordance was not required for patient satisfaction in cross-cultural interactions with pediatric patients; providers that used interpreters and were perceived as culturally competent had a positive impact with the parents' perception of how their care was delivered. The proper use of interpreters is a critical skill. Another significant cultural factor is an understanding of the impact of spirituality and religion. The cultural competency curriculum should provide an opportunity to examine religious practice, ethnic variations of the major faiths, and the cultural impact of spiritual observance on development.[49]

As also written about by Karnik and colleagues,[50] and Pumariega,[51] developmental formulations are an inescapable aspect of cultural child and adolescent psychiatry that may not be considered in other medical specialties. In creating a learning experience for trainees, the concept that normal behaviors and interactions are culturally determined must not be forgotten. Developmental milestones as varied as the age to start toilet training, the age when a child can stay at home alone, go out on a first date, or move out of the parents' home[4] may all have a good deal of cultural variability. With the ubiquitous presence of social networking and online information portals, providers ought to presume that the children of today are most likely being raised in a culture (quite) different from that of their parents'. Thus, attending to the therapeutic alliance not only with the patient, but also with the parent (and often, the teacher) becomes ever more important. Parents must feel that the provider conceptualizes the problem from their point of view, whereas the patient (especially true for teens) must feel that the psychiatrist is their ally, and not simply an agent of the parent. As such, skillful culturally attuned providers may have to play the roles of agent and ally to both parties.[45,52]

BARRIERS TO IMPLEMENTATION OF A CULTURAL COMPETENCY CURRICULUM

Barriers to cultural competency training may be institutional, logistical, or individual. An often-noted institutional barrier is that of available didactic time.[53] This is likely compounded by the perception that these topics are less important in clinical training.[54] An example of both institutional and logistical barriers is teaching about the use of interpreting services. The cost of interpreting services is a potential barrier to their use, which could be minimized by adequate third-party reimbursement.[55] Even when interpreting services are available, there must be consistent use by faculty and senior house-staff to effectively teach this skill to junior house-staff and students. Time constraints are a common explanation for failure to use existing services. Intuitively, one might expect that individual factors would be significant. This is borne out in the literature,[56] and measures are being developed to assess the ability to use interpreters effectively as part of medical practice.[57]

Another barrier is the appreciation that learning about cultural competence is the knowledge of what it is and what it is not. Cultural competence training is not the same as diversity training, which typically consists of much more general information that may not be provided in the framework of a particular social context.[45]

The sense of discomfort that may arise when the concept of bias is discussed between individuals with different cultural, racial, or ethnic backgrounds presents another roadblock to the implementation of such curricula. An example is the trepidation that may be experienced by the faculty member of color teaching a group of white residents about cultural competence.[58] Cultural competency is often a topic that some learners indicate they do not wish to learn about. As a result, these students may be particularly vocal in disputing the information provided, perhaps even "punishing" or "harassing" the instructor of the topic.[59] One might conceptualize that these learners are early in their personal development of cultural competency, and would do well to adopt Step 1 of the cultural sensibility approach (see the article by Karnik and Dogra elsewhere in this issue for further exploration of this topic), which consists of self-reflection of one's own experiences with cultures other than one's own, and potential biases. Some learners may even be most comfortable with ethnocentric monoculturalism, which is the predisposition of the majority (European American) culture to ignore or devalue other cultures.[58,60] It may be difficult to approach the concept of institutional, as well as individual racism. The topic of micro-insults (or micro-aggressions) is a necessary but difficult concept that involves "subtle verbal and non-verbal insults directed toward non-Whites, often done automatically and unconsciously. They are layered insults based on one's race, gender, class, sexuality, language, immigration status, phenotype, accent or surname....Micro-aggressions are also cumulative and cause unnecessary stress to people of color while privileging whites...."[61] Bias is a topic that may be difficult to approach because of the sensitivity of some learners. Care must be taken to help students overcome initial discomfort.

Dogra and colleagues[44] reviewed suggestions to overcome barriers in embedding diversity into the medical curriculum. While designed for the undergraduate medical curriculum, there are several principles (noted by **) that can easily be generalized to the training of child and adolescent psychiatrists:

1. Design a diversity and human rights education institutional policy
2. Create a safe learning environment**
3. Develop clear and achievable learning outcomes**
4. Develop content focused on the diversity of human experience (not simply race and ethnicity)**
5. Raise awareness of students' own biases and prejudices**
6. Integrate cultural diversity across the entire curriculum**
7. Make diversity patient-centered**
8. Teach outside the classroom and hospital setting**

9. Form multidisciplinary teams of educators**
10. Make training of faculty compulsory**
11. Develop clear and comprehensive assessment of policies, delivery, and learned outcomes of cultural diversity education.
12. Map what others are doing and challenge yourself as a role model.

It is useful to learn the institutional policy of the medical school and extrapolate that to the current didactic curriculum with specific learning objectives. For learners who are uncomfortable with the topic, couching this information in such a background can make it more palatable, and it may seem less personally directed. In addition, students and faculty must feel safe to discuss issues related to bias and discrimination to explore the impact of these on working with patients/families, and each other. In our experience, delving into such concepts in large or small group settings is potentially self-revealing with a risk for embarrassment or the potential for reprisal or rejection by others. Permission to speak frankly with colleagues in the spirit of mutual learning must be specifically sought and granted during the teaching process to help this work progress. Without this, reluctant learners may become more hostile or simply shut down and not participate.

It is helpful modeling if not just 1 or 2 faculty members are concerned about the effects of the variety of aspects of culture on patient presentation and care. As child and adolescent psychiatry training is often conducted in concert with psychology and social work training, the use of other disciplines in teaching cultural competency again models the need for all team members to consider these concerns in our work. If limited faculty are involved in this work, the topic may be marginalized and perceived by students as less important. The wider the range of faculty members that recognize, engage in, and express cultural aspects of work with their patients, the more likely it is that this behavior will become part of the academic culture.

Residents and students have been found to be more likely to have previous experience with multiculturalism during medical school and college than faculty members. They may have higher levels of comfort with, for example, sexual orientation issues and learning about non-Western approaches to the practice of medicine. As a result, one must consider that teaching about sociocultural aspects of diversity may not be purely a top-down experience. Learners may be able to provide new knowledge for faculty as well.[62]

CURRICULUM DEVELOPMENT

Dolhun and colleagues[63] note 8 specific content areas that can be covered in a cross-cultural education curriculum[(p616)] (**Box 1**).

In developing a cultural competency curriculum for subspecialists in psychiatry, such as child and adolescent psychiatrists, the development of specific objectives is key, particularly in light of the resistance that may come from trainees who are at earlier stages of cultural competency development, with less understanding both of the material and of the cultural attunement process. Clear objectives help concretize the need for the nuances of cultural competency that must be covered.

The August 2008 issue of *Academic Psychiatry* is a review of cultural competency in psychiatric education and is an excellent resource in developing a curriculum.[64] One example, the University of Toronto psychiatry cultural competence curriculum, is integrated throughout training beginning in the postgraduate year (PGY)-1 and ending in the PGY-5 year.[65] It is designed around the idea of competencies, each designated by the Canadian Medical Education Directions for Specialists (CanMEDS) paradigm. This

---

Box 1
Eight specific content areas that can be covered in a cross-cultural education curriculum

General concepts of culture (culture, individual culture, group culture)

Racism (racism and stereotyping)

Doctor-patient interactions (trust and relationship)

Language (meaning of words, nonverbal communication, use of interpreters, coping with language barriers)

Specific cultural content (epidemiology, patient expectations and preferences, traditions and beliefs, family role, spirituality and religion)

Access issues (transportation, insurance status, and immigration/migration)

Socioeconomic status (SES)

Gender roles and sexuality

Data from Dolhun EP, Muñoz C, Grumbach K. Cross-cultural education in US medical schools: development of an assessment tool. Acad Med 2003;78:615–22.

---

model delineates the roles of the physician specialist as a communicator, collaborator, manager, health advocate, scholar, and professional.[66] These are very similar to the Core Competencies of the ACGME: patient care, medical knowledge, practice-based learning and improvement, interpersonal and communication skills, professionalism, and systems-based practice.[67] Cultural Competency curricula span each of the categories in both models. Cultural Competency concepts span the 6 competencies and 7 roles of a physician and are delineated in **Table 1**.

In considering topics and specific content to be taught, as well as evaluated, the efficacy of the curriculum, an additional resource is the community. Bell and colleagues[58] note the importance of involving the community not only in research-related academic pursuits, but in practice-related matters, particularly in working with children and families that have a history of trauma. This can help prevent additional traumatization by health care providers through decreasing the number of micro-aggressions that are inadvertently committed by these providers.

The Committee on Culture and Diversity of the AACAP has developed a model curriculum for teaching cultural competency in child and adolescent psychiatry training programs, and the authors of this article have been involved in this project.[68] We have delineated 3 major goals to be covered by the end of child and adolescent psychiatry training.

Goal 1: Define the concept of cultural competence and describe its application in the practice of child and adolescent psychiatry with regard to knowledge, skills, and attitudes.

Goal 2: Differentiate normal development from pathology within the concept of cultural identity.

Goal 3: Describe the cultural competence model of service delivery and systems-based care. This includes the development of skills and the necessary attitudes and perspective to work in or consult to a system that provides care for children from culturally diverse populations and their families.

These goals can be integrated into currently existing topics and do not have to be separated into a separate course, although we have developed 3 model courses, with 6, 8, or 10 sessions throughout the training program. There are specific objectives

Table 1
Seven roles of a physician

ACGME Competencies	Definition	CanMEDS Roles	Definition
Patient care	Provide patient care that is compassionate, appropriate, and effective for the treatment of health problems and the promotion of health	Health advocate	Responsibly use their expertise and influence to advance the health and well-being of individual patients, communities, and populations
Medical knowledge	Demonstrate knowledge of established and evolving biomedical, clinical, epidemiologic and social-behavioral sciences as well as the application of this knowledge to patient care	Medical expert	Integrate all of the roles of CanMEDS, applying medical knowledge, clinical skills, and professional attitudes in their provision of patient-centered care
Practice-based learning and improvement	Demonstrate the ability to investigate and evaluate their care of patients, to appraise and assimilate scientific evidence and to continuously improve patient care based on constant self-evaluation and lifelong learning	Scholar	Demonstrate a lifelong commitment to reflective learning as well as the creation, dissemination, application and translation of medical knowledge
Interpersonal and communication skills	Demonstrate interpersonal and communication skills that result in the effective exchange of information and collaboration with patients, their families, and health professionals	Communicator	Effectively facilitate the doctor-patient relationship and the dynamic exchanges that occur before, during, and after the physician experience
Professionalism	Demonstrate a commitment to performing professional responsibilities and an adherence to ethical principles	Professional	Committed to the health and well-being of individuals and society through ethical practice, profession-led regulation, and high personal standards of behavior
Systems-based practice	Demonstrate an awareness of and responsiveness to the larger context and system of health care, as well as the ability to call effectively on other resources in the system to provide optimal health care	Collaborator and Manager	Effectively work within a health care team to achieve optimal patient care; and integrate participants in health care organizations, organizing sustainable practices, making decisions about allocating resources, and contributing to the effectiveness of the health care system.

Abbreviations: ACGME, Accreditation Council of Graduate Medical Education; CanMEDS, Canadian Medical Education Directions for Specialists.

within each goal that are identified as more or less complex by level of competency. Basic competency is the minimum level of cultural competency that a fellow should have on completion of child and adolescent psychiatry training. The next stage is intermediate, that level of cultural competency for a practitioner who is working in a community with a diverse patient population. Finally, advanced is the level of cultural proficiency to which a practitioner can aspire as a result of experience and scholarship.

We have identified several techniques for didactic sessions involving both passive and active learning techniques, including the use of several different movies and films. Because child and adolescent psychiatry fellows come from a diversity of training backgrounds and initial cultural competency work may have begun during medical school and/or general psychiatry training, a needs assessment is an appropriate way to ensure what topics most require coverage for each cohort of trainees. For each goal we have defined basic, intermediate, and advanced level competencies. These competencies can be cross-linked with the ACGME (and CanMEDS) competencies to help illustrate how cultural competency affects the functioning of a child and adolescent psychiatrist. Suggested methods for teaching each goal and a reference list are also provided. This curriculum will be available through the AACAP Web site (www.aacap.org).

EVALUATION

Although evaluation of a curriculum is typically regarded as important, there has been no consensus on how best to determine the impact of a cultural competency curriculum. The Tool for Assessing Cultural Competency Training has been developed to assess the presence of relevant topics in the medical school curriculum.[69] Using Miller's model (**Fig. 1**) to assess the learner's use of the information,[70] the pretest/posttest has been used to show the "knows" or "knows how." The Objective Structured Clinical Examination (OSCE) has been found to demonstrate that the learner can "show how" to use the knowledge. "Does" seems most effectively measured by the attending psychiatrist during observation of the resident with a patient. An evolved and useful adaptation of Miller[70] can be accessed at http://www.gp-training.net/training/educational_theory/adult_learning/miller.htm.[71]

One measure, the Intercultural Development Inventory, is a validated instrument found to be useful to assess the intercultural sensitivity of medical trainees before and after cultural training.[72] It has been found applicable to other professions as well, and its use simply requires (brief) formal training. Despite these measures, there remains a dearth of readily implementable evaluation tools to assess the efficacy of training and curricula.[73] Development of these measures is in progress,[53] and should include a variety of formative as well as summative components.[65]

FUTURE DIRECTIONS

The cultural sensitivity curriculum outlined in this article is based on the premise that teaching cultural psychiatry is a process of reflection on the ethological, social, and historical origins and contemporary meanings of culture in child psychiatry theory and practice. This involves questioning some of the assumptions of pediatric psychiatry that may be rooted in limited ethnocentric research that ignores cultural context. The hope is to inculcate in our trainees an open-mindedness to integrate the values and ideas of self and person that may be rooted outside of European American traditions. Clearing a space where one can begin to think about alternative ways of being

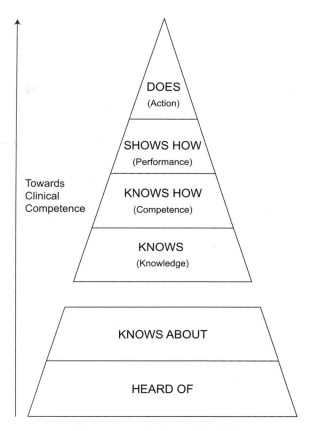

Pre assessment stages of familiarity

Fig. 1. Miller's prism of clinical competence (A.K.A. Miller's Pyramid). It is only the "does" triangle that the doctor truly performs. (*Based on* work by Miller GE. The assessment of clinical skills/competence/performance. Acad Med 1990;65(9):63–7 (with credit to adaptations by Drs R. Mehay and R. Burns, UK, January 2009); with permission.)

allows for more open dialog and negotiation with patients in clinical settings, as well as suggests fruitful topics for research and clinical innovation.[74]

REFERENCES

1. Betancourt JR, Green AR. Commentary: linking cultural competence training to improved health outcomes: perspectives from the field. Acad Med 2010;85(4): 583–5.
2. Kumagai AK, Lypson ML. Beyond cultural competence: critical consciousness, social justice, and multicultural education. Acad Med 2009;84(6):782–7.
3. Minde K. Transcultural child psychiatry: its history, present status and future challenges. Can Child Adolesc Psychiatr Rev 2005;14(3):81–4.
4. Ellis WG. The amok of the Malays. J Ment Sci 1893;39:325–38.
5. Littlewood R. The 'new cross-cultural psychiatry'. Br J Psychiatry 1990;157: 775–6.

6. Rutter M. Developmental psychiatry. Arlington (VA): American Psychiatric Press Inc; 1980.
7. Benedict R. Patterns of culture. New York: Houghton Mifflin; 1934.
8. Whiting JM, Child IL. Child training and personality. New Haven (CT): Yale University Press; 1953.
9. Betancourt JR, Green AR, Carrillo JE, et al. Defining cultural competence: a practical framework for addressing racial/ethnic disparities in health and health care. Public Health Rep 2003;118(4):293–302.
10. Nidorf JF, Morgan MC. Cross cultural issues in adolescent medicine. Prim Care 1987;14(1):69–82.
11. American Psychiatric Association Committee on Nomenclature and Statistics. Diagnostic and statistical manual of mental disorders. 4th edition [text revision]. Washington, DC: American Psychiatric Association; 2000.
12. Zayas LH, Lester RJ, Cabassa LJ, et al. Why do so many Latina teens attempt suicide? A conceptual model for research. Am J Orthopsychiatry 2005;75(2): 275–87.
13. Available at: http://www.umm.edu/gme/core_comp.htm. Accessed August 17, 2010.
14. Brotherton SE, Rockey PH, Etzel SI. US graduate medical education, 2003–2004. JAMA 2004;292(9):1032–7.
15. Kim WJ. A training guideline of cultural competence for child and adolescent psychiatric residencies. Child Psychiatry Hum Dev 1995;26(2):125–36.
16. Yager J. Specific components of bedside manner in the general hospital psychiatric consultation: 12 concrete suggestions. Psychosomatics 1989;30(2):209–12.
17. Sidelinger DE, Meyer D, Blaschke GS, et al. Communities as teachers: learning to deliver culturally effective care in pediatrics. Pediatrics 2005;115(Suppl 4): 1160–4.
18. Carrillo JE, Green AR, Betancourt JR. Cross-cultural primary care: a patient-based approach. Ann Intern Med 1999;130:829–34.
19. Thom DH, Tirado MD, Woon TL, et al. Development and evaluation of a cultural competency training curriculum. BMC Med Educ 2006;6:38.
20. US Census Bureau. Table 1a. Projected population of the United States, by race and Hispanic origin: 2000 to 2050. Washington, DC: US Census Bureau; 2004. Available at: http://www.census.gov/ipc/www/usinterimproj/natprojtab01a.pdf. Accessed August 17, 2010.
21. US Census Bureau. Table 1b Projected population change in the United States, by race and Hispanic origin: 2000 to 2050. Washington, DC: US Census Bureau; 2004. Available at: http://www.census.gov/ipc/www/usinterimproj/natprojtab01b.pdf. Accessed August 17, 2010.
22. Berger JT. Culture and ethnicity in clinical care. Arch Intern Med 1998;158: 2085–90.
23. Hill RF, Fortenberry JD, Stein HF. Culture in clinical medicine. South Med J 1990; 83:1071–80.
24. Flores G. Culture and the patient–physician relationship: achieving cultural competency in health care. J Pediatr 2000;136:14–23.
25. Betancourt JR. Cross-cultural medical education: conceptual approaches and frameworks for evaluation. Acad Med 2003;78:560–9.
26. Eisenberg JM. Sociologic influences on medical decision making by clinicians. Ann Intern Med 1979;90:957–64.
27. Stewart M, Brown JB, Boon H, et al. Evidence on patient–doctor communication. Cancer Prev Control 1999;3:25–30.

28. Robins LS, Fantone JC, Hermann J, et al. Improving cultural awareness and sensitivity training in medical school. Acad Med 1998;73(Suppl 10):S31–4.
29. Lu FG, Primm A. Mental health disparities, diversity, and cultural competence in medical student education: how psychiatry can play a role. Acad Psychiatry 2006;30:9–15.
30. US Department of Health and Human Services. Mental health: culture, race and ethnicity: a supplement to mental health: a report of the surgeon general. Rockville (MD): DHHS; 2001.
31. Institute of Medicine (US) Committee. Crossing the quality chasm: a new health system for the 21st century. Institute of MEdicine (IOM), 2001. Washington, DC: National Academies Press (US); 2001. Available at: http://www.nap.edu/openbook.php?isbn=0309072808. Accessed August 17, 2010.
32. Smedley BD, Stith AY, Nelson AR, editors. Unequal treatment: confronting racial and ethnic disparities in health care (Committee on Understanding and Eliminating Racial and Ethnic Disparities in Health Care, Board on Health Sciences Policy, Institute of Medicine). Washington, DC: National Academies Press; 2002.
33. Institute of Medicine of the National Academies. In the Nation's Compelling Interest: Ensuring Diversity in the Health Care Workforce. Available at: http://www.iom.edu/Reports/2004/In-the-Nations-Compelling-Interest-Ensuring-Diversity-in-the-Health-Care-Workforce.aspx. Accessed August 17, 2010.
34. Eaton D, Kann K, Kinchen S, et al. Youth risk behavior surveillance—United States, 2005. MMWR Morb Mortal Wkly Rep 2006;55:1Y108.
35. Garza-Trevino ES, Ruiz P, Venegas-Samuels K. A psychiatric curriculum directed to the care of the Hispanic patient. Acad Psychiatry 1997;21:1–10.
36. Harris HW, Felder D, Clark MO. A psychiatric residency curriculum on the care of African-American patients. Acad Psychiatry 2004;28:226–39.
37. Lu FG, Du N, Gaw A, et al. A psychiatric residency curriculum about Asian-American issues. Acad Psychiatry 2002;26:225–36.
38. Spielvogel AM, Dickstein LJ, Robinson GE. A psychiatric residency curriculum about gender and women's issues. Acad Psychiatry 1995;19:187–201.
39. Thompson JW. American Indians and Alaska Natives in psychiatry residency training. Acad Psychiatry 1996;20:5–14.
40. Weissman JS, Betancourt J, Campbell EG. Resident physicians' preparedness to provide cross-cultural care. JAMA 2005;294(9):1058–67. DOI: 10.1001/jama.294.9.1058.
41. Anandaraja N, Hahn S, Hennig N, et al. The design and implementation of a multidisciplinary global health residency track at the Mount Sinai School of Medicine. Acad Med 2008;83:924–8.
42. Pilcher ES, Charles LT, Lancaster CJ. Development and assessment of a cultural competency curriculum. J Dent Educ 2008;72(9):1020–8.
43. Poirier TI, Butler LM, Devraj R, et al. Instructional design and development: a cultural competency course for pharmacy students. Am J Pharm Educ 2009;73(5):1–7.
44. Dogra N, Reitmanova S, Carter-Pokras O. Twelve tips for teaching diversity and embedding it in the medical curriculum. Med Teach 2009;31:990–3.
45. Vaughn LM. Families and cultural competency—where are we? Fam Community Health 2009;32(3):247–56.
46. Britton CV. Ensuring culturally effective pediatric care: implications for education and health policy. Pediatrics 2004;114(6):1677–85.
47. Shin HB, Kominski RA. Language use in the United States: 2007. Washington, DC: U.S. Census Bureau; 2010. American Community Survey Reports, ACS-12.

Available at: http://www.census.gov/prod/2010pubs/acs-12.pdf. Accessed August 17, 2010.

48. Boudreau AD, Fluet CF, Reuland CP, et al. Associations of providers' language and cultural skills with Latino parents' perceptions of well-child care. Acad Pediatr 2010;10(3):172–8.

49. Mattis JS, Ahluwalia MK, Cowie SE, et al. Ethnicity, culture, and spiritual development. In: Roehlkepartain EC, King PE, Wagener L, et al, editors. The handbook of spiritual development in childhood and adolescence. Thousand Oaks (CA): Sage Publications; 2006. p. 283–96.

50. Karnik NS, Soller MV, Redlich A, et al. Prevalence differences of psychiatric disorders among youth after nine months or more of incarceration by race/ethnicity and age. J Health Care Poor Underserved 2010;21(1):237–50.

51. Pumariega A. Cultural competence in systems of care for children's mental health. In: Pumariega AJ, Winters NC, editors. The handbook of child and adolescent systems of care: the new community psychiatry. San Francisco (CA): Jossey-Bass; 2003. p. 82–104.

52. Joshi SV. Teamwork: the therapeutic alliance in pediatric pharmacotherapy. Child Adolesc Psychiatr Clin N Am 2006;15(1):239–62.

53. Chun MB, Takanishi DM. The need for a standardized evaluation method to assess efficacy of cultural competence initiatives in medical education and residency programs. Hawaii Med J 2009;68:2–6.

54. Samuel S, Lu F, Silberman E, et al. Residency training for ethnic minority psychotherapy: current practices and issues. American Association of Directors of Psychiatric Residency Training (AADPRT) Newsletter 1994;22(1):14.

55. Brotanek JM, Seeley CE, Flores G. The importance of cultural competency in general pediatrics. Curr Opin Pediatr 2008;20:711–8.

56. Diamond LC, Schenker Y, Curry L, et al. Getting by: underuse of interpreters by resident physicians. J Gen Intern Med 2009;24(2):256–62.

57. Lie D, Bereknyei S, Braddock CH, et al. Assessing medical students' skills in working with interpreters during patient encounters: a validation study of the interpreter scale. Acad Med 2009;84:643–50.

58. Bell CC, Wells SJ, Merritt LM. Integrating cultural competency and empirically-based practices in child welfare services: a model based on community psychiatry field principles of health. Child Youth Serv Rev 2009;31:1206–13.

59. Helms JE, Malone LT, Henze K, et al. First annual diversity challenge. How to survive teaching courses on race and culture. J Multicult Couns Devel 2003;31: 3–11.

60. Sue DW, Sue D. Counseling the culturally different: theory and practice. 3rd edition. New York: John Wiley & Sons, Inc; 1999.

61. Solorzano D, Allen WR, Carroll G. Keeping race in place: Racial microaggressions and campus racial climate at the University of California, Berkeley. Chicano-Latino Law Review 2002;23:15–112.

62. Tang RS, Bozynski ME, Mitchell JM, et al. Are residents more comfortable than faculty members when addressing socio-cultural diversity in medicine? Acad Med 2003;78:629–33.

63. Dolhun EP, Muñoz C, Grumbach K. Cross-cultural education in U.S. medical schools: development of an assessment tool. Acad Med 2003;78:615–22.

64. Lim RF, Lu FG. Culture and psychiatric education. Acad Psychiatry 2008;32(4): 269–71.

65. Fung K, Andermann L, Zaretsky A, et al. An integrative approach to cultural competence in the psychiatric curriculum. Acad Psychiatry 2008;32:272–82.

66. Frank JR, editor. The CanMEDS 2005 physician competency framework. Better standards. Better physicians. Better care. Office of Education. Ottowa, Ontario: The Royal College of Physicians and Surgeons of Canada. Available at: http://meds.queensu.ca/medicine/obgyn/pdf/CanMEDS2005.booklet.pdf.   Accessed May 31, 2010.
67. Accreditation Council of Graduate Medical Education. Common program requirements: general competencies. 2007. Available at: http://www.acgme.org/outcome/comp/GeneralCompetenciesStandards21307.pdf. Accessed May 31, 2010.
68. Al-Mateen C, Mian A, Cerda G, et al. AACAP (model curriculum). Approved by the AACAP Workgroup on Training and Education, in press.
69. Lie D, Boker J, Cleveland E. Using the tool for assessing cultural competence training (TACCT) to measure faculty and medical student perceptions of cultural competence instruction in the first three years of the curriculum. Acad Med 2006; 81(6):557–64.
70. Miller GE. The assessment of clinical skills/competence/performance. Acad Med 1990;65(9 Suppl):S63–7.
71. Mehay R, Burns R. Adaptation of Miller's Pyramid; free access. Available at: http://www.gp-training.net/training/educational_theory/adult_learning/miller.htm. Accessed August 17, 2010.
72. Altshuler L, Sussman NM, Kachur E. Assessing changes in intercultural sensitivity among physician trainees using the intercultural development inventory. Int J Intercult Relat 2008;27:387–401.
73. Price EG, Beach MC, Gary TL, et al. A systematic review of the methodological rigor of studies evaluating cultural competence training of health professionals. Acad Med 2005;80:578–86.
74. Kirmayer LJ, Rousseau C, Guzder J, et al. Training clinicians in cultural psychiatry: a Canadian perspective. Acad Psychiatry 2008;32:313–9.

International Medical Graduates in Child and Adolescent Psychiatry: Adaptation, Training, and Contributions

R. Rao Gogineni, MD[a,b,*], April E. Fallon, PhD[c,d],
Nyapati R. Rao, MD, MS[e,f]

KEYWORDS

- Diversity • Child/adolescent psychiatry
- International medical graduate • Acculturation

International medical graduates (IMGs) are a heterogeneous group who have immigrated to the United States from more than 140 countries and have diverse cultural, linguistic, and educational backgrounds. According to the American Psychiatric Association (APA) census of residents, currently, one-third of residency positions are filled by IMGs whereas according to the American Medical Association (AMA), nearly 30% of practicing psychiatrists in the United States are IMGs.[1] There is a growing literature on various aspects of IMGs, but it is mostly silent about IMGs as trainees in child psychiatry.

Child psychiatry is a shortage specialty, and considerable efforts are being made by its leaders to improve recruitment into the field. Historically, IMGs have played a critical role in filling positions in child psychiatry, but, of late, the IMGs selected for training in child psychiatry decreased from 250 in 2006 to 226 in 2009.

The authors have nothing to disclose.
[a] Department of Psychiatry, Robert Wood Johnson Medical School/UMDNJ, Piscataway, NJ, USA
[b] Division of Child and Adolescent Psychiatry, Cooper University Hospital, 401 Hadden Avenue, Camden, NJ 08103, USA
[c] School of Psychology, Fielding Graduate University, 2112 Santa Barbara Street, Santa Barbara, CA 93105-3538, USA
[d] Department of Psychiatry, Drexel University College of Medicine, Friends Hospital, Roosevelt Boulevard and Adams Avenue, Philadelphia, PA 19124, USA
[e] SUNY Downstate Medical Center, Brooklyn, NY, USA
[f] Department of Psychiatry and Behavioral Sciences, Nassau University Medical Center, 2201 Hampstead Turnpike, East Meadow, NY 11554, USA
* Corresponding author. 410 Baird Road, Merion Station, PA 19066.
E-mail address: rgoginenimd@yahoo.com

Child Adolesc Psychiatric Clin N Am 19 (2010) 833–853
doi:10.1016/j.chc.2010.07.009
1056-4993/10/$ – see front matter © 2010 Elsevier Inc. All rights reserved.

childpsych.theclinics.com

This article describes IMGs' history, demographics, training issues, and professional challenges as well as their strengths and weaknesses. The overarching theme is cultural for this discussion. Culture influences various aspects of the clinical endeavor, and IMG psychiatrists from various cultures bring their parental cultural expectations, judgments, and attitudes, albeit unconsciously, to their clinical work. An appreciation of such background facilitates the development of more focused training strategies that benefit IMGs and the patients that they serve. A review of history of IMGs in the United States is offered as a backdrop for the article.

HISTORY AND BACKGROUND

It is well known that physicians have always traveled to far-off lands in furtherance of their skills and knowledge. In the early twentieth century, it took the form of US physicians traveling to Europe for medical education, and in the middle to late twentieth century, the reverse was seen (ie, physicians from the world over sought training in the United States). The first among them arrived in the aftermath of World War II, seeking protection from persecution in Europe. Although the early migrants were welcomed with open arms, subsequent ones encountered increasing doubt about their competence and skills from the medical establishment in the United States. Consequently, rigorous testing of their readiness to practice medicine was introduced through the creation of the Educational Commission for Foreign Medical Graduates. In the past 10 years, the process has been considerably tightened. At the present time, IMGs are required to be certified in the same examinations that US medical graduates take. Alongside of this evolution in the testing rigor, there have been multiple changes in immigration laws according to the needs and priorities of society, and each one of them restricted the ease with which IMGs could enter graduate medical education in the United States. Due to the complexity of the US economy and the fast expansion of the US health care system, however, IMGs continued to be needed, and, consequently, in spite of these ups and downs, the presence of IMGs has continued unabated.[2,3]

The early generation of child psychiatrists was very much influenced by European child psychoanalysts. Consonant with the changes in immigration laws enacted in the 1960s that gave preference to technical skills over family ties, Asian nations, such as India, Pakistan, and the Philippines, became major sources of physicians and supplanted Europe and South America. Culturally, they came from non–Western European traditions that had significant differences in child rearing practices and relational paradigms, such as collectivism, versus individualism of the West. In addition, they lacked organized exposure to psychiatry in their home medical schools. Their commitment to psychiatry was suspect in the eyes of their teachers as were their clinical skills. Recently enacted health care reform and the expansion of American medical schools, without concomitant expansion of graduate medical education positions, have created an untenable situation for the IMGs—the former will result in increased demands for physicians whereas the latter can practically eliminate their presence of IMGs. In addition, recent difficulties in obtaining J1 and H1 visas have the potential to further reduce the number of candidates for child psychiatry. All in all, in 2010, the future does not look all that encouraging to IMGs in the United States.

What is the situation with child psychiatry's workforce? According to Thomas and Holzer,[4] the number and the distribution of child psychiatrists are in dire straits in the United States. The estimates of their supply vary from 10% to 45% of the number needed to meet the mental health needs of American youth, among whom it is estimated that 1 in 5 develop a mental disorder. According to the Department of Health and Human Services[4] the demand for child and adolescent psychiatric (CAP) services will double between 1995 and 2020, and there will be a need a for 12,624 child psychiatrists by 2020, whereas only 8312 will be available based on today's statistics. The number of IMGs who are child psychiatry residents has continued to diminish since 2004. The reasons for this decrease are not known, although the national security concerns that resulted in visa restrictions and the difficulties associated with IMGs taking the clinical skills assessment examination had much impact. Unless the Medicare cap is lifted and there is a broad expansion of residencies to accommodate the higher output of American medical schools and the IMG influx, the shortage of child psychiatrists may not improve.

COMPETENCE AND QUALITY OF IMGS

IMGs in CAP (IMG-CAP) face the same issues as their counterparts in general psychiatry. Weintraub[5] has written about the preponderance of myths about IMGs. These include that they are more passive, prefer organic and directive therapies, and have difficulty learning dynamic therapies and forming relationships with their patients than do American graduates.

It has been repeatedly reported in the literature that some IMGs have difficulty with the culture, the language, and the attitudes that are emphasized in the United States. Similarly, many investigators have identified the specific needs IMGs have in their education. Searight and Gaffert[6] looked at the behavioral science education of IMGs, and they observed that the IMG residents they interviewed reported limited education in psychiatry and behavioral science before starting residency. The specific deficits included medical interviewing, perceptions of family life in the United States, the doctor-patient relationship, and the mental health and psychosocial content of medicine. In a recent study, Dorgan and others[7] found two broad themes as barriers to effective communication between IMGs and their patients: educational and interpersonal. Each of these categories had secondary themes: in education-related barriers, there were science immersion and lack of communication training, whereas in interpersonal barriers, there were unfamiliar dialects, new power dynamics, and different rapport building expectations.

In summary, IMGs, the US medical education system, and the US hospital industry have an ambivalent and symbiotic relationship. Although this state of affairs served them well all these years, the significant changes in both medical education and health care industry require fresh thinking. Child psychiatry has to acknowledge its need for IMGs and offer creative models for using them to address its workforce issue and maldistribution challenges, including developing effective ways of selecting the best among them as trainees and providing them culturally sensitive training.

DEVELOPMENTAL CONSIDERATIONS

The transition from living in a native country to life as CAPs in the melting pot of the world is generally not without its vicissitudes. This section reviews the relevant issues of immigration and the problems related to training and socialization of IMGs into the field of CAP.

Migration, Immigration, and Acculturation

The process of leaving a homeland, settling into a new place and culture, and developing a comfort with this new arrangement is a process that few outsiders can truly comprehend. The majority of IMGs voluntarily emigrate for financial and professional reasons, so can return at will. Nothing in their backgrounds has readied them for this new life, however. The process of migration is a series of cumulative traumas, involving more than just leaving or arriving in a new country.[8] The term, *culture shock*, most aptly embraces the IMG experience of entering this country. Garza-Guerrero[9] has defined culture shock as "a reactive process stemming from the impact of a new culture upon those who attempt to merge with it as a newcomer".[(p410)] He views it as a violent encounter that confronts and threatens an immigrant's intrapsychic status quo. An immigrant initially faces an anxiety-provoking situation that "challenges the stability of his psychic organization".[9(p412)] When the crisis has been managed successfully, growth occurs. This evolution co-occurs with a process of mourning precipitated by the individual's "gigantic loss of a variety of love objects".[9(p410)] The coincidence of these two factors threatens an immigrant's identity.[10]

Grinberg and Grinberg[8] have delineated traced four stages in the psychobiologic adaptation to a new culture. Initially arising are feelings of intense sadness for all that is left or lost. A manic stage may follow in which the newcomer immigrant either minimizes the "transcendental significance of change in life or, on the contrary, magnifies and idealizes the change".[8(p37)] Later, nostalgia ensues and a sorrow for a paradise lost is experienced. At this point, immigrants have the opportunity to appreciate and work through previously unacknowledged emotions as they gradually assimilate the new culture. If this process is successful, aspects of the host culture are metabolized without rejecting previously embraced cultural values, "and as a result, the ego is enriched and the identity is consolidated".[10(p131)] Ticho[11] wrote that "Culture shock is the result of a sudden change from the average expectable environment to a strange and unpredictable one, and the experience of culture shock and the mastery of its disturbing effects seem to be preconditions for the integration of the new culture".[(p325)] Akhtar[12] refers this process of intrapsychic transformation as "the third individuation," which is akin to the second individuation precipitated by adolescence in the separation individuation process.[12] Learning psychiatry occurs against this tumultuous backdrop of immigration. In the initial phases, cultural adaptation takes priority over mastering psychiatry.[10] Rao writes, "the wounded self-esteem, stemming from slow and inadequate progress, or even the failure to learn psychiatry, will further add to an already overburdened self struggling with issues of loss and separation. This may manifest as a lack of enthusiasm for the field."[10(p132)]

If the IMG is not cognizant of the repercussions of culture shock, language, and communicational difficulties they blame themselves and the field of psychiatry rather than focusing on these other issues. Serious unresolved issues of culture shock may manifest as personality problems, academic underachievement, marital difficulties, clinical psychiatric problems, transfer to another specialty, and, finally, return to a native country in despair. Conversely, it may be displayed as excessive zeal for psychiatry, pseudo-Americanization, and rejecting behavior toward their native culture. Response from the host residency group may range from one extreme of unconditionally embracing IMGs and not requiring them to hold the same rigorous standards as their US compeers to scapegoating them for every system failure. Char[13] notes that IMG residents are "accepted into a training program as ambivalently valued objects. The foreign resident is valued because he is needed to fill the critical shortage of residents, and to satisfy our 'missionary' need to train foreigners, but he is rejected because of his handicaps."[(p237)]

Training Challenges for IMG-CAP

An in-depth examination of the choice of child psychiatry, difficulties with language and communication, and not growing up in America help explicate some of the training difficulties that IMG-CAP trainees experience.

The choice of child psychiatry

Many international graduates have little exposure to the field of psychiatry in their native country. For example, according to Das and colleagues[14] there are only 300 psychiatry training positions in India, which means that less than 0.6% of the graduating Indian medical students enter psychiatry training. Yet in the United States, 25% of IMGs become psychiatrists, with a disproportionate number of international graduates receiving further specialty training, including CAP. This suggests that IMGs make the choice of psychiatry, even if it is not the first choice. Thus, entrance into psychiatry is often akin to an arranged marriage (a culturally familiar process), a choice out of necessity and practicality, not initially out of passion or love. Most, at some point, however, fall in love with their profession and caring for patients and their families. How that process transpires is a question worthy of further study. It is known from social psychology research literature that mere exposure is likely to result in increased liking.[15,16] The phenomenon of cognitive dissonance (not wanting to view ourselves doing things that we do not agree with or believe in) may also play a role in increased interest in one's work.[17–19] It is likely also that interest and passion for patient care transcends the particular specialty. Regardless of how it happens, awareness of this dynamic is important to aid IMGs.

Little information is available as to why IMGs choose child psychiatry over general psychiatry or other specialties. Of all the specialties within psychiatry, the child and adolescent specialty remains a psychosocial field whose goals are consistent with protecting the next generation; it values the family, a goal consistent with Eastern cultural values. It is a field that encourages more introspection. The authors' informal survey of child psychiatry graduates reported that as child trainees, they thought they were more supported by their faculty than they were as adult trainees. On the one hand, they thought that they were given more autonomy and respect for their knowledge base. On the other hand, "regression in the service of training and learning" is more tolerated in CAP training programs. That is, child psychiatry residents are permitted to be professional yet still allowed to not know it all. Third, child and adolescent mental health programs and departments are filled with many caring, loving female staff, social workers, nurses, and teachers, who not only nurture patients and families but also nurture CAP trainees. This nurturing, in turn, can increase self-esteem and positive social mirroring. Lastly, the mere fact of providing care to adorable, undefended, and innocent children generally brings out the protective side in all of us, making us more humane and humble. All these factors can contribute to the psychological growth and development of IMG-CAP.

Difficulties with language and communication

For most IMGs, English is not their first language. Even though medical education is conducted in English in many parts of the world, the comprehension and expression of oral language may not be a well-learned skill. Communication is further made difficult by the use of idioms unique to the United States and dialects within subgroups.[20] Hein[21] articulated specific difficulties that IMGs have in communicating with their patients and other professionals, which included self-consciousness in new speaking situations or when speaking before groups; variations in the pronunciations, rhythm, and voice inflection; difficulty pronouncing certain English sounds; occasional feeling of being forced to use shorter answers to questions when longer responses are desirable; occasional embarrassment at being asked to repeat themselves; and continued concern for their accents. The authors frequently encourage residents to talk in the colloquial language familiar to children and their families. The residents, however, usually have only medical knowledge and formal English in their communication repertoire.

Greenson[22] suggested that the importance of the mother's speech represents both the means of maintaining and holding relations with the mother and also for withdrawing from her. If so, IMGs may be enacting some unconscious conflicts about separation by choosing the psychiatry specialty where language facility is crucial.[10] The guilt about leaving home may replay conflicts about using a new language. Connection to a mother tongue becomes heightened when beginning to live in a country with a different language.[8] There are two aspects to learning acquisition: learning the word and form (grammar and syntax), which is a cognitive task, and learning the accent and the intonation, which is an emotional task having to do with identification. Training programs must address the emotional aspects of learning a language, rather than treating this learning of a language as a purely cognitive issue. Process groups commonly used in residencies may help in this endeavor.

Not growing up in America

IMG-CAP do not have the same childhood experiences as their patients who have grown up in this country. They often do not have similar familial experiences of living between two households of divorced parents or attending day care or knowledge of the social scene and rules for dating and hooking up, beginning in middle school and intensifying during high school. They did not grow up with television as an auxiliary babysitter, with programs, such as *Barney*, *Sesame Street*, cartoons, doctor and cop shows, or the barrage of reality shows that the American child has exposure to from a young age. In short, they have not been exposed to the environment with which American children are making sense of their world. They do not have the familiarity with unstated norms and behavior that children incorporate into their psyche by mere exposure. Relating to adolescent patients is even more difficult because this lack of experience with American life—their dress norms and behavior, their music, and ways of relating through e-mail and Facebook—compounds the cultural divide. Even the educational system, a central aspect of work with children either directly or indirectly, is often different from an IMG-CAP resident's own experience. This makes it difficult to help parents with their behaviorally difficult children.

MAJOR CHALLENGES FACED BY IMG-CAP IN PRACTICE

Immigrant child psychiatrists face special issues arising from their sociocultural experiences. Understanding their impact on IMG-CAP is important in providing culturally sensitive treatments to children, adolescents, and their families. This article reviews issues most central to IMG-CAP. These include cultural differences; dealing with prejudice and discrimination; self-esteem and social mirroring; child rearing; and unique aspects of the treatment for IMG-CAP.

Appreciating Cultural Differences

Culture plays a significant role in the determination of perceptions and attitudes about the world. Appreciating the cultural differences between culture of origin and a host culture is important in understanding children and their families. The major areas that the authors view as essential and particularly applicable to IMG-CAP are differences in conceptualization of the self, relationships to others, social attitudes, health care and training systems, and boundaries.

Development of the self

Child psychiatrists and their patients (and families) bring to the treatment setting an unspoken perspective on how one defines the self. Roland[23] described the developmental differences between the Eastern, extended family as "we or familial self" and the Western individualistic "I self." In Western cultures, there are firm boundaries between the "you and I," a sharp differentiation between what is inside the self and what is part of others. Individualism supports having rights and obligations equal to each other. Decision making and responsibility are the individual's and not the group's.[24,25] All psychoanalytic theories of development reflect a "narrative of individualism".[23(p10)] In contrast, the Eastern "we self" incorporates more inner images of the extended family and community than the individualistic, more self-contained Western "I self."[23] Roland[23] describes the concept of a highly developed private self, which is the core of individuality. It is this private self that maintains an equilibrium between that and the semimerger experiences in ongoing extended family and community relationships in Eastern cultures, such as Pakistan, Japan, and India. A highly developed intuitive sensing of the group "other" is relied on. In contrast, verbal expression is used as part of proper social etiquette.

IMGs, often from an Eastern culture, come to a therapeutic relationship with a familial self-perspective. Without an appreciation for the difference in perspective, there may possibly be a misunderstanding of the nature of the psychopathology. That is, these differences in Eastern and Western philosophic, sociologic, and anthropological thought can influence the manner in which a child psychiatrist conceptualizes and then provides treatment for Western patients and their families, which can have a negative adverse influence treatment. Take, for example, a sophomore male college student from the mountains of New England who has ongoing daily contact with family to assure their agreement with his choices at school. Although it is possible that this behavior is well within the emerging helicopter parents phenomenon, New Englanders pride themselves on their view of individual responsibility and hardy self-reliance and, to some extent, represent the prototype of American individualism and self-directedness. Thus, an adolescent psychiatrist whose background is congruent with an Eastern perspective may underestimate the extent of maladaptive behavior that this student exhibits. CAPs who are able to recognize and hold their own perspective as potentially different from the adolescent being treated, are likely to be able to use that to their advantage in understanding a case, such as this one, within its cultural context.

Differences in relationship to others

In some cultures, relationships are more lineal, authoritarian, and hierarchical. The father or the eldest male in an extended family is seen as the absolute ruler.[24] This world view affects how the problem is seen, the advice given, and the therapeutic relationship. If a child psychiatrist brings this perspective to treatment with children and families who view relationships as more egalitarian, the treatment may be problematic on at least two levels. First, the CAP who carries a world view of being better than others' may view family dysfunction as due to lack of respect for this authoritarian hierarchical structure. Second, IMG-CAP may expect that families and children will follow their instructions or advice to the same degree and with the same reverence that a family from the native country might have. Not doing so, an IMG-CAP is likely to feel disrespected, disappointed, and angry with the family. The family, in turn, may view the psychiatrist as dictatorial and not understanding them. An IMG-CAP who comes to the treatment relationship with an understanding of differences in how different cultures might view relationships is more likely to take this difference into account when viewing and treating problems.

Differences in social attitudes

Many IMGs come from traditional extended families. They may have difficulty accepting evolving American cultural/social mores, such as living together without a marriage, youth sexuality, single parenthood, gay and lesbian relationships, and entitlement systems. Thus, IMG-CAP may find it challenging to develop a position of therapeutic neutrality vis-à-vis their patients and families and may miss or project aspects of psychopathology. Self-recognition of internalized prejudices, discriminations, and sensitivity training to accept these can be helpful for IMG-CAP. For example, a mother of 9 children presents to the clinic with her youngest child, the only one not placed in foster care. She requests that social security papers be completed for her 5-year-old boy, for whom she reports symptoms consistent with an attention-deficit/hyperactivity disorder diagnosis. In the session, the boy does not exhibit hyperactive behavior. Both American and IMG child residents may find it difficult to look beyond the manipulative elements in the mother's presentation and feel some disgust at this misrepresentation. IMGs may attribute this to a dysfunctional American system, whereas American graduates may attribute it to liberal mores. Such affects and blame may obscure other behavioral disorders that may be present in the child, the recognition of a need for educational parenting skills, and the mother's underlying motivations for such a request (eg, her own psychopathology, narcissism, or dependency that may be interfering with good parenting).

In another example, an upper middle class white family presented for treatment after the 16-year-old daughter ran away for 4 days. This running away was precipitated by the parents refusing to allow their daughter to attend the prom with an African American. Both attended the same private school. The parents stated that they would disown their only child, an adopted Asian girl, if she dated someone of color. As the mother stated, "I would sooner see these one hundred thousand dollar diamonds that I am wearing today go to Goodwill than give to a daughter who dated a Black boy." In this second example, race, gender, rules of dating, and issues of who has authority are significant aspects that are culturally determined. IMGs from a culture that respects authoritarian rule may be prone to side with parents' right to determine their own rules for their daughter. Yet it is culturally within the norm to permit adolescents to attend a prom with culturally diverse classmates. Educated parents from the dominant culture who do not adapt to these norms risk their child being ostracized. Not recognizing the importance of this aspect could lead therapists to underestimate the parents' need to control and the effect that their racial bias can have on encouraging their daughter's self-hatred of her color and culture of origin.

Discrepancies in systems of care and training

Pumariega and colleagues[26] outlined the importance of the congruence between the cultural competence of individual clinicians and that of the system of care they practice in. Some IMGs may experience culture shock between the health care and training systems of their native countries and the US model, particularly around understanding and accepting the complexity and multiplicity of the American systems. Most IMGs originally trained in a strictly medical model where doctors prescribe and those surrounding them are working to carry out the doctors' orders. But in the US system, there are complicated, overlapping, multiple systems with different lines of authority, such that it is difficult or impossible for IMG-CAP to be the solo authority. They may become frustrated easily, which accentuates feelings of immigrants' helplessness and can lead to giving up. Also, the multiple systems may have trouble accepting the legitimate and generally accepted leadership role of IMG-CAP because of their immigrant status. Members of a care team may also attribute culturally based stereotyped traits to an IMG-CAP and subtly put up multiple cultural roadblocks. IMG-CAP have to understand and perhaps empathize with the cultural variations of the system. Those who perceive these systemic issues are as personally intended end up feeling defeated, angry, and unable to work with school, welfare, primary care health, and governmental systems.

Boundary issues

On the APA Web site, a primer for residents discusses how gift taking, after-hours appointments, self-disclosure, and dual relationships are boundary crossings and leave residents vulnerable to being accused of boundary violations.[27] Although these may be somewhat intuitive for those reared in America, they are not so for IMGs. Myers[28] posits that differences in the collectivist (Eastern) versus the West European/American cultures contribute to differences in perspectives of appropriate relational boundaries (ie, group vs individualistic). Likewise, such differences in perspective also influence how privacy, confidentiality, and self-disclosure are conceptualized.

For instance it is common for IMG-CAP to have distant relatives and their friends calling or e-mailing them to discuss problems with their children. Such friends and relatives become confused and/or insulted if a child psychiatrist requested either to have the child come to the office or referred the child to a colleague. IMGs feel a loyalty conflict between what is appropriate back home and what is now appropriate with regard to good care and malpractice in America. If IMGs are burned enough times with this kind of interaction, they are likely to discontinue such practices easily enough. It is, however, the more subtle boundary crossings that are the cultural scotoma of immigrants.[28]

These guidelines apply not only to physician-patient relationships but also to physician-nurse, physician-therapist, and other professional relationships. In particular, male IMG-CAP should be aware of these cultural norm variations and individuation/self-concepts. In that respect, IMG-CAP may benefit from additional training in recognizing, preventing, and handling these delicate issues.

Facing Discrimination and Prejudice

Xenophobia can contribute to the marginalization of immigrant populations and can have adverse effects on ethnic identity formation.[29] IMGs face possible discrimination and prejudice from professionals and patients.

There is a perception among IMGs that there is some prejudice and discrimination against them by the medical establishment. In surveys of training programs, 80% of psychiatry and family practice and 70% of the surgery programs were perceived to show discrimination against international graduates.[30] Indeed, 80% of IMGs surveyed self-report considerable bias and prejudice,[31] although generalizations about group discriminations can be flawed particularly when applied to individuals.[32] An informal e-mail survey of recent IMG-CAP (Nyapati Rao, MD, MS and Rao Gogineni, MD. IMG–CAP: on training and cultural issues, unpublished data, 2010) found that graduates did not feel overt discrimination from their colleagues but thought they had to work harder to overcome xenophobic stereotypes and build their reputations. Many IMG-CAP that the authors have spoken to do not perceive much discrimination for entry-level jobs but perceive a made-in-America glass ceiling for higher-level positions. Surveys of practice reveal that IMGs occupy less-attractive positions and care for the most indigent, difficult, and chronic children and adolescents in the country.[33,34] They are more likely to work in the public sector, administering direct care, and less likely to occupy administrative and medical school positions.[34] These differences remain significant even after age, gender, race, and board certification are controlled for.

IMG-CAP report that they need to work harder not only to work through the cultural and psychological barriers of systems but also with patients and their families. Surveys of patients in a general medical population showed discrimination against diverse groups of physicians based on emotional reasons rather than medical concerns.[35] A few examples illustrate the different problems.

Over the course of professional lives, racial and ethnic slurs have been mounted against IMG-CAP, who have been called various derogatory names, most often by oppositional, uninhibited, and conduct-disordered youth. It is important to ascertain the meaning of name calling within the therapeutic context because it could be a clinical issue. To do so requires a certain ability to stand apart from the perceived or intended narcissistic insult. If a CAP is reactive, then a clinical opportunity is lost. In cases where such an act seems primarily related to resistance, careful processing with patients can address it and help develop a stronger working alliance. For example, such name calling by a child with an oppositional defiant disorder and an excessive need for autonomy could be seen as an effort to push away the psychiatrist, consistent with behavior in the rest of this child's life. In other cases, where it seems primarily to push the boundaries of acceptable etiquette, some limit setting must be considered.

What is more common among children and adolescents is a less overt and dramatic display of prejudice. For example, an 8-year-old boy with a history of oppositionality underlying narcissistically vulnerability and impulsive aggression presented for treatment. Input from other residential staff revealed that the parents were racist. In the therapy sessions, the boy was withdrawn and had no eye contact and it was a struggle to develop a connection with him. It was suspected that some of the parents' prejudice was internalized by the boy and he felt reluctant to trust the child psychiatrist. The psychiatrist continued working with the boy but worked with the parents through intermediaries (teachers and support staff) to see the doctor as a caring expert professional who could help their child. This case required careful working through of these projected negative feelings with the parents and child. The parents never gave up their racist attitudes but began to contain their racism and develop trust in the psychiatrist to treat their son. This case was particularly difficult because the negative projections toward minorities always remained in the periphery of treatment and were a constant reminder to the psychiatrist of his foreign and unacceptable status. The psychiatrist was watchful of the potential for induced countertransference rage and helplessness that could invade their work together.

Another common demonstration of prejudice and discrimination is the preference for certain families to see a white pediatrician and/or a white master's-level clinician rather than a board certified IMG-CAP who has experience in providing both medication and therapy. At times they might reluctantly tolerate an IMG-CAP to prescribe medications but not therapy. Unfortunately, some agencies covertly or overtly promote this kind of prejudicial and discriminatory practice. The question becomes, What should an IMG-CAP do? This is a political issue that requires attention at the national level. At the local level, consultation and discussion with a trusted colleague or mentor often are helpful.

Self-esteem and Social Mirroring in IMG-CAP

Two common problems immigrants struggle with are immigration-induced or precipitated low esteem and problems with social mirroring. Superficially, both may seem to look like low self-esteem. They can be and should be distinguished from each other, however, for the understanding and remediating of each. Self-esteem is an intrapsychic notion based on self-respect and self-worth.[36,37] Although self-esteem is considered an enduring personality trait, immigrant guilt (leaving families behind, betrayal of culture, and loyalty conflicts), grief reactions to losses, and anxiety and depressive reactions contribute to lowering self-esteem.

Social mirroring originated with Winnicott's notion of mirroring wherein a child's sense of self is profoundly shaped by the reflections mirrored back to him or her by significant others.[38] This mirroring is essential for healthy development.[39] This concept was broadened and applied to minority and immigrant experiences.[40–42] IMGs do not necessarily think they are less but think that others do not value or undervalue them. An IMG looks into the eyes of the dominant culture and sees back a reflection of the dominant culture's view on him or her; that is, the IMG does not see the sparkle of approval from teachers and others but rather disapproval and disappointment. Often what IMGs experience in this social mirroring is that they are now minority physicians with inferior status, no longer considered trained and respected professionals but foreigners who must again prove their skills.

With immigration-induced low self-esteem and/or negative social mirroring, IMGs may feel vulnerable and less worthy. Feeling less wanted, they may compensate by working more than their peers or they may withdraw, which potentiates further projections onto IMGs. They may also become defensive and angry and these emotions may adversely affect treatment.

A story from a colleague illustrates issues with social mirroring. While attending his third meeting in a professional group whose membership is by invitation only, this colleague thought, "Nobody is talking to me, everyone is ignoring me. They don't like me. I am not at their level. They are real American professors and I am just an immigrant." When he noticed that he was feeling this way he decided to challenge his negative cognitions. He then realized that there was little reality to his thinking. It was the leaders who were not fraternizing with him and they were only talking among themselves and not to the newer members. It seemed, however, that it had not affected his overall self-esteem. It was more of a social mirroring problem rather than a self-esteem issue because he saw himself as accomplished but thought that the larger group did not recognize his contributions. With his understanding of the difference between self-esteem and social mirroring, the feelings dissolved quickly.

Recognition of immigration-induced self-esteem problems and the impact of social mirroring can help trainees put in perspective issues of worth and helps preceptors to mentor them. This same awareness is also helpful for immigrant and minority patients and families.

For example, a 13-year-old Latino boy presented with symptoms of depression and irritability, saying that nobody liked him or wanted to be his friend. Neither he nor the family could provide information on any major new stresses. Further examination revealed that he always felt inferior to whites and never felt he was equal in the school or on the playground. With the onset of adolescence and increase in cognitive capacities, he now "realized" more about his "lesser" status. Further explorations clarified this cognition as more of a projection of immigrant minority status and thus a social mirroring problem. When the therapist gave the social mirroring explanation to the family, the boy was visibly relieved and reported feeling much better in ensuing weeks.

Child Rearing Practices

Many investigators, such as Canino and Spurlock,[43] have described the influence of culture on child rearing practices. Healthy parenting practices differ across cultural groups.[44] Child rearing practices and parent-child relationships play a significant role in socialization, personality, and symptom expression of illness. Some of the areas of cultural difference are in the promotion of the self, promotion of individuation, promotion of social skills, sleeping arrangements, sex roles and expectations, discipline, adaptive social behaviors, family values, role of extended family, and handling of habits and fears. For example, with sleeping arrangements in Western culture, infants are moved to their own crib and room early in life. This is in contrast to cultures where sleeping with parents until school age is not uncommon. Likewise, cultures manage promotion of individuation differently. In Western cultures, there is a tendency to positively reinforce being separate and pursuing one's own interests early whereas the Eastern family discourages by fear or shame early individuation and separateness of the child.

Ethnic identity and ethnic pride often are embedded in child rearing practices. We credit our children's accomplishments to our "correct" upbringing and in turn blame others' child rearing practices for their children's failures. In the mental health field, until recently there has been a great deal of blame placed on parents for their children's difficulties. Proud IMG-CAP unwittingly blame Western child rearing for substance abusing, oppositional, impulsive, conduct disordered, and promiscuous American teen patients. This can result in negative therapeutic reactions. Conversely, they sometimes perceive that Western child rearing practices are attributed to the advancement of the West, further contributing to low self-worth on the part of IMG-CAP. The latter is likely to result in an under treatment of Western patients.

UNIQUE TREATMENT ASPECTS

For IMG-CAP (and child psychiatrists of immigrant origins in general), there are several unique aspects of treatment worthy of discussion. This article discusses therapeutic alliance, resistance, transference, and countertransference. Assessment, understanding, and making necessary interventions to address these four areas are vital for good outcomes. In the treatment of children and adolescents by IMG-CAP, there at least three different elements. First, the children we treat experience their own treatment alliance and manifest resistances and transferences. Second, parents and caregivers are actively involved experiencing and manifesting these same phenomena, which may be different from their children's. The child psychiatrist's countertransference is often entirely different to children than to their parents. Third, cross-cultural/immigrant status of the physician further complicates these elements.

Treatment Alliance

The establishment of a trusting, confiding, and collaborative therapeutic relationship[45] has been empirically shown to affect treatment outcomes.[46] It accounts up to for 30% of the variance in outcomes even when pharmacotherapy is the primary intervention.[47] In treating children, the clinician needs to establish a treatment alliance with the patients and with parents/care-givers and other systems involved in a child's life (eg, school or probation officer). Having originated from another culture can have an impact on the early connection with the child and family. Although speaking the same language, other than English, can enhance the therapeutic alliance, a recognizable accent or differences in communication style can interfere with it. Often the upfront acknowledgment of this difference and its possible impact help bridge the connection because families are appreciative of an IMG-CAP's ability to recognize their perspective and reluctance. For example, a psychotic inpatient boy insisted he had met his new doctor before. "I know, I've seen you before." The new doctor, recognizing the youth's lack of discernment, said, "No you haven't, but we Indians all look alike." This addressed the unspoken anxiety and allowed the youth to move on. Maintaining cultural neutrality and judicious accommodation to the cultural differences are also crucial for establishing a workable therapeutic alliance.[48] The authors find the concept of multidirectional partiality as advocated by Boszormenyi-Nagy and Krasner[49] particularly useful. This is the ability of a therapist to give all family members, both those who are present in the session and those who are absent, a sense of being understood, accepted, and important.

Resistance

Resistance, the compromise between the striving for recovery and maintaining the status quo, manifests in many ways.[47,50] Many resistances by children are even normative and culturally based, such as the striving of Western youth for autonomy and the distractions from many culturally sanctioned activities, such as socialization via cell phones and text messaging. Understanding and managing the resistance of patients and families are crucial to adherence to continued treatment. Instead of understanding and realizing the ubiquitous nature of these resistances as part of treatment, an IMG-CAP may take them personally, blame the patient for character flaws, or attribute these resistances to a decadent and unhealthy aspect of Western society. In doing so, IMG-CAP allow their patients and families to do the same, instead of helping them understand the integral part of understanding resistance in successful treatment. Such attributions can result in premature termination, premature dismissal, low self-esteem on the part of the therapist, or intense feelings of narcissistic injury, anger, guilt, and/or shame on the part of the patient as well as the clinician.

Transference

Comas-Diaz and Jacobsen,[51] in writing about ethnocultural transferences in the therapeutic dyad, suggested that there are intraethnic and interethnic transferences. Interethnic transferences can be manifested in overcompliance and friendliness, denial of ethnicity and culture, mistrust, suspicion, ambivalence, and hostility. In intraethnic transference, the omniscient-omnipotent therapist, the traitor, the autoracist, and ambivalent reactions emerge. In short, the reactions emerge from "like me" and "not like me" projections.

Interethnic transferences can be negative or positive. Being asked by an adolescent boy if you are related to Osama bin Laden is not likely to be missed. The seemingly more positive transferences, however, are often not examined. In resident clinics where children and adolescents are transferred every 6 months to a year, many parents request their children be transferred to someone ethnically similar to their previous doctor. This sometimes carries with it an assumption that the painful aspects of the loss will be minimized. Or, projecting their values onto the treating psychiatrist, they hope that this next doctor will have the same understanding as the previous one because he or she is Hispanic or Indian.

The following is an example of a positive interethnic transference that proved difficult to work through with the adolescent and her family. A male Filipino CAP was seeing a 16-year-old Korean girl in therapy for oppositionality and defiance with intense battles with her parents over autonomy and individuation. The therapist thought that they had developed a good relationship. The adolescent seemed to make progress working on her contributions in her interaction with her parents. The therapist also reported that she expressed curiosity about his interests. After approximately 6 months of therapy, she reported that she had begun dating a Filipino boy. She gleefully reported that her parents would "kill her" if they found out that she was dating anyone but especially a non-Korean. How much of her acting out was due to the projection of the idealized positive transference toward the therapist or to her need to be separated from her ethnocentric Korean parents? How much of it was her internalization of American multiculturalism? After careful working through, it became clear it was projection of the idealized transference and she was able to move on to the presenting issues.

Intraethnic transferences are less common. Many professionals assume that immigrant patients prefer to see someone from their native country. This is not always the case for many reasons. An example illustrates this problem. A white therapist was referred a Nigerian family. On the telephone, the therapist had some difficulty understanding the father's English and suggested the name of an excellent Nigerian child psychiatrist. It was evident that the father was reluctant to take the referral, so the therapist agreed to see the family. Later he learned how insulted the father had been. The father, a successful businessman, had wanted to see "the best." Referring to another Nigerian implied to him that he was being sent to someone who had as inferior status as he had, betraying a certain degree of ethnic self-hate often seen in minorities and immigrant groups. What the therapist also later learned was that this family was from a different part of Nigeria from the child psychiatrist and they would have had to communicate in English because they did not have the same mother tongues.

Patients or families may choose an immigrant therapist for unconscious reasons. Such a choice may lead to idealization or devaluation of an IMG psychiatrist. In the example previous example, the father devalued the psychiatrist's sameness. Patients can also project jealousy and racism onto the treating psychiatrist. In some instances, patients might be initially positive about seeing an IMG only later to express anger and dissatisfaction as they project their own self-hatred onto the psychiatrist.

IMG status of the clinician also can lead to triangulations. A 9-year-old boy was struggling with difficult-to-treat Asperger syndrome and mood disorders. His father, an immigrant Muslim, chose a Pakistani Muslim CAP outside of his health network with the hope that the psychiatrist would collude with his denial, prejudice against mental illness, and his harsh disciplinary tactics toward the boy. The Pakistani psychiatrist worked delicately with the child and the family to help them accept the illness and provide appropriate parenting. The family eventually accepted a transfer to a psychiatrist in their health network.

Language may play a significant role in treatment and the transference.[52,53] If therapist and patient speak the same language, affective communication is made easier and may contribute to the idealization of the therapist by parents and child. Parentification of a child patient can often minimized as the parents communicate directly with the psychiatrist without using their child as a translator. (This happens because the child is often more fluent in English than the parents). Conversely, a language barrier can contribute to fear of being misunderstood and can cause initial mistrust, particularly when the psychiatrist's accent is significant.[52]

Countertransference

Although traditionally taught in the context of psychotherapy supervision, the importance of countertransference extends beyond the psychotherapeutic relationship. The recognition and the ability to manage countertransference is a skill that is considered second only to the ability to perform a comprehensive diagnostic interview.[54–56]

Comas-Diaz and Jacobsen[51] divide the topic into interethnic and intraethnic countertransferences. They discuss how interethnic countertransference can result in denial of ethnocultural differences, the clinical anthropologist syndrome (excessive curiosity about the cultural background of the patient/family), guilt, pity, aggression, and ambivalence.[51] Intraethnic countertransference can contribute to an IMG distancing, cultural myopia, anger, survivor guilt, hope, and despair. These counter-transference reactions can lead to emergence of conflicts underlying therapeutic issues as trust, ambivalence, and anger.

With patients of the same cultural background, there is often an assumption that they are "like us." For example, a 21-year-old upper-caste intelligent Indian student was referred for anxiety, depression, and panic to an Indian psychiatrist. The CAP felt honored to get this referral of a smart and cultured girl. He started treating her as if she were an anxious, depressed young woman. Within a few weeks she developed an extremely ambivalent, demanding/blaming relationship with the therapist concomitant with agitation, pan anxiety, and deep depression. The psychiatrist quickly recognized that his cultural myopia and immigrant guilt had blinded him from examining her history of chronicity, past brief psychotic-like episodes, and severe past trauma that resulted in an underestimation of the intensity of transference reactions by patients with borderline characteristics. This newfound recognition enabled the clinician to change the treatment approach and address more a serious nature of illness. There might have been some degree of stereotypic idealized coun-tertransference reaction by the psychiatrist—"people from my ethnic groups never get messy personality disorders."

Interethnic countertransference can surface with significant world events. After 9/11, many South Asians and Arabs, even if they were not from the same country or same religion, suffered from guilt and shame because their patients made direct or indirect accusations about their relationship to the perpetrators. It is easy to become defensive and angry because patients inaccurately assume that there is some connection to the 9/11 aggressions. A sense of humor, understanding of transference, the role of negative cognitions, and the ability to carefully monitor countertransfer-ences is important. IMG-CAP, in turn, can also have their own prejudices, elevating their own cultural heritage and undervaluing Western mores. The next example illus-trates the interplay of interethnic transference and countertransference. A 42-year-old mother sought help parenting her two excessively attention-demanding children. The mother was a high school graduate, living in a blue-collar small town. The mother seemed depressed and was a survivor of sexual abuse. As they worked on parenting issues, transferences of ambivalence and projection of the aggressor role onto the therapist were apparent. She viewed the CAP as a dominant Muslim man who controlled women and demanded submissiveness. The psychiatrist saw her as a blue-collar, undercivilized, needy, dependent woman, these feelings partly induced by the patient. The therapist's recognition of the transference and of his countertrans-ference prejudices helped the mother to become more assertive and parent more effectively her overanxious children.

Immigrant guilt at having achieved success can also have an impact on CAPs' ability to provide the best treatment. When overidentifying with a sufferer, whether or not an immigrant or an impoverished minority, they often experience guilt and shame. This can at times manifest itself as rescue fantasies, overidentification, and even boundary crossings as they want to "give" more than is therapeutic. It can set up re-enactments, poor outcomes, narcissistic injury, and anger.

Although cultural similarities in a therapeutic dyad can enhance treatment by facil-itating understanding regarding cultural traditions and language, a therapist can unconsciously identify with something that has been stirred up in a patient and a parallel process for therapist and patient can occur.[57] For example, a parallel process between CAPs' acculturation, that of their children and family, and the accul-turation/identity formation of minority children they treat can potentially contribute to positive and negative outcomes both personally and in their therapeutic work (Andres Pumariega, MD, personal communication, July 2010). When IMG-CAP listen to a parent's helplessness and anger, their reaction may be reflective of their own struggles with children who have rebelled against the traditional and embraced a new culture.

Immigrant clinicians, because of their own experiences, share a special empathy for those who have had similar experiences. In a parallel process, IMG-CAP have an unconscious identification process that occurs between themselves and patients. IMG-CAP could examine these parallels and their impact in the context of supervision or within another psychological safe setting.[58] For example, an intelligent African American male was admitted to a magnet high school. Within 2 months he was withdrawn, depressed, and anxious, requesting to return to the local high school. The boy spoke to the CAP of having difficulties learning the formal and informal rules. The psychiatrist remembered his first months in the United States—his loneliness and difficulties transitioning from being a respected attending to a lowly postgraduate year 1 resident in the new hierarchical structure. In discussing this case with the guidance team, a group he trusted and respected, the CAP was irritated with what he thought was a rigid protocol for the boy's return to his former school and suggested special consideration for the boy. Reflecting back on his unusual demanding behavior, he recognized a parallel process between his interaction with staff and what the boy was experiencing but not directly expressing. As he thought about the boy and his complaints, he realized that in his empathic stance, he had not paid sufficient attention to the difficulty the boy was having in no longer being "a star." The boy expected that he be given special treatment and felt narcissistically injured when he was not. The CAP had not been aware of it because he too had difficulties dealing with his own anger when he too went from being a respected professional in his own country to being a resident in his new country. With his newfound understanding, he was able to help the boy with his disappointment and anger that he was not at the top of his class and that he had to accept his ordinary treatment and status in this school of exceptional children.

RECOMMENDATIONS FOR TRAINING AND SUPPORT

With a large portion of CAPs coming from other parts of the world, it behooves training programs and national organizations to consider the special needs of this group for training and ongoing support. Their experience with immigration and as a member of a minority group gives them a special empathy toward children and adolescents of diverse backgrounds. This section focuses on specific areas to augment their education and training, enhance their treatment skills, further their personal growth, and provide advocacy for minorities and the disadvantaged.

Some of the strategies recommended by various investigators to improve education and training include evaluating language skills and offering remediation opportunities, accenting reduction strategies, providing cultural education the first year of training, and the use of senior faculty to teach courses.[59] Faculty involved with IMG training should be conversant with the core cross cultural differences present in their residents.[10] On university campuses, English and speech therapy departments can be enlisted to aid in language and accent improvement.

One such program that has attempted to address these issues is one sponsored by the APA under the directorship of Rao and Hales.[60] In this day-long course, lectures and small groups are used help IMG trainees identify areas of need and adapt to the fundamentals of psychiatric practice. There have been efforts to train the teachers of IMGs on issues most relevant to this group.[61] In this 6-module training curriculum, Steinart and Walsh[61] elaborate on the possible differences in previous education based on hierarchical structures and propose various didactic and evaluative skill-training strategies. Clinical skills verification, if administered as residents enter a CAP residency program, can then be used to tackle problem areas not previously addressed in the adult training program. This same process could be used to focus on insufficiencies in psychosocial interventions, psychological theory, and psychotherapy theory and practice. Structured supervision can reinforce the biopsychosocial model over the linear medical model. Mentoring should be used to enhance treatment skills, not just case management and psychopharmacologic interventions. Learning how relationships affect physicians, therapists, patients, families, schools, and other social service agencies is particularly important for CAPs. This is often an unspoken dynamic that American graduates learn by growing up in the culture. IMGs often recognize their own lack of familiarity, but no one has helped articulate how these dynamics are in play in the treatment setting. Related to this is the application of cultural specific psychotherapeutic interventions.

It is also recommended that IMG-CAP develop greater familiarity with American culture—such as child rearing practices, history, literature, and religious and secular holidays. In addition to reading textbooks, familiarization can be aided by reading newspapers, watching TV, attending ethnic movies, watching cartoons, traveling within the new country, attending American cultural functions, and attending variety of religious activities. Help can be sought from training directors to find appropriate events. Teaching cross-cultural seminars using IMG and American graduates teaching each other can help address stereotypes, xenophobia, and the reality of diverse cultures. With this dyad, not only do IMGs learn about US culture but also US graduates learn about cultural diversity through the cultures and values from which IMGs originate (Andres Pumariega, MD, personal communication, July 18, 2010). Both IMG and American medical graduates need to recognize the lack of cultural uniformity and also learn that different subgroups and geographic regions may have variations in language and culture.

Often IMGs do not come from a culture that nurtures academic and research interests. The AMA has been a major advocate of using additional resources and training to enhance academic and research skills of IMGs. CME activities can be helpful in this regard. Participation in professional organizations and advocacy groups for children, adolescents, and their families are also professional and societal obligations. In particular, advocacy by IMG-CAP on behalf of minorities and other patients from disadvantaged and discriminated groups can be a special area of focus. IMG-CAP, in collaboration with many of these groups, can promote culturally sensitive, educational programs, lectures, and workshops in various communities. Some organizations covertly or overtly promote anti-IMG practices (discussed in the discrimination and prejudice section of the article). These should be addressed organizationally as well as politically.

An often-neglected area is personal growth and personal care. For IMG-CAP, the stress of acculturation, excessive guilt, and loyalty conflicts can hinder promoting themselves, promoting their own growth, and placement of the "I self" before "we self." Personal psychotherapy and the development of a family genogram can be invaluable processes through which IMG-CAP can explore and address such conflicts. As many self-help gurus and resiliency enhancing strategists advocate, it is necessary to focus on personal growth to master a profession. The art of thinking positively, expressing oneself more openly, and the importance of making reasonable compromises also aid in adjustment to a new culture and improve personal and professional functioning. As IMG-CAP are completing training, the focus often needs to be on assistance in securing a position, career planning, settling down, and even estate planning.

FUTURE CONSIDERATIONS AND SUMMARY

With globalization of medicine, the AMA and various national and international organizations are advocating a global focus on the learning and practice of medicine. As Mezzrich[62] has suggested, the IMGs add a cultural richness to their environment. Due to their dualistic cultural identity and an array of professionally relevant, comparative experiences, they have the unique potential to contribute to the advancement of psychiatric concepts and deliver sensitive and effective patient care. They also provide an important liaison between the United States and the rest of the world, functioning as cultural ambassadors between American psychiatry and international psychiatry.

The United States has been welcoming of immigrants for the past 400 years. It also has opened doors to CAPs born and trained abroad to enhance mental health care for its children, adolescents, and their families. It behooves us to ensure their success in accomplishing this mission. Addressing the important adaptational issues, reviewed in this article, through the needed enhancements in training and supports, IMG-CAP can provide effective and culturally sensitive treatments for the most underserved population of children and enhance their own professional lives.

REFERENCES

1. American Medical Association. Physician Characteristics and Distribution in the U.S. Chicago (IL): American Medical Association; 2008.
2. Rao N, editor. IMGs in American medicine: contemporary challenges and opportunities. Chicago: American Medical Association; 2009. Available at: http://www.ama/assn.org/ama1/pub/upload/mm/18/img-workforce-paper.pdf. Accessed July 18, 2010.
3. Schowalter JE. A history of child and adult psychiatry in the United States. Psychiatric Times 2003;20:9.
4. Thomas CR, Holzer CE. The continuing shortage of child and adolescent psychiatrists. J Am Acad Child Adolesc Psychiatry 2006;45(9):1023–31.
5. Weintraub W. International medical graduates as psychiatric residents: one training director's experience. In: Husain SA, Munoz RA, Balon R, editors. International medical graduates in the United States: challenges and opportunities. Arlington (VA): American Psychiatric Press; 1997. p. 53–64.
6. Searight HR, Gaffert J. Behavioral science education and the international medical graduate. Acad Med 2006;81:164–70.
7. Dorgan KA, Lang F, Floyd M, et al. International medical graduate-patient communication: a qualitative analysis of perceived barriers. Acad Med 2009;84:1567–75.
8. Grinberg L, Grinberg R. Psychoanalytic study of migration: its normal and pathological aspects. J Am Psychoanal Assoc 1984;32:13–38.
9. Garza-Guerrero AC. Culture shock: its mourning and vicissitudes of identity. J Am Psychoanal Assoc 1974;22:408–29.
10. Rao NR. The influence of culture on learning in psychiatry; the case of Asian-American International Medical graduates. Int J Appl Psychoanal Stud 2006;4:128–43.

11. Ticho G. Cultural aspects of transference and countertransference. Bull Menninger Clin 1971;35:313–4.
12. Akhtar S. A third individuation: immigration identity and the psychoanalytic process. J Am Psychoanal Assoc 1995;43:1051–84.
13. Char WF. Psychiatric training for foreign medical graduates II the foreign resident: an ambivalently valued object. Psychiatry 1971;34(3):234–8.
14. Das M, Gupta N, Dutta K. Psychiatric training in India. Psychiatr 2002;26:70–2.
15. Bornstein RF. Exposure and affect: overview and meta-analysis of research, 1968–1987. Psychol Bull 1989;106:265–89.
16. Zajonc RB. Feeling and thinking: preferences need no inferences. Am Psychol 1980;35:151–75.
17. Baron RA, Byrne D. Social psychology. 10th edition. Boston: Pearson Education, Inc; 2004.
18. Chen MK, Risen JL. How choice affects and reflects preferences: revisiting the free-choice paradigm. J Pers Soc Psychol 2010. [Epub ahead of print].
19. Petty RE, Briñol P, DeMarree KG. The Meta-Cognitive Model (MCM) of attitudes: implications for attitude measurement, change, and strength. Social Cognition 2007;25(5):657–86.
20. Bates J, Andrew R. Untangling the roots of some IMG's poor academic performance. Acad Med 2001;76:43–6.
21. Hein JM. International graduates and communication. In: Husain SA, Munoz RA, Balon R, editors. International medical graduates in the United States: challenges and opportunities. Arlington (VA): American Psychiatric Press; 1997. p. 31–44.
22. Greenson RR. The mother tongue and the mother. Int J Psychoanal 1950;31: 18–23.
23. Roland A. Cultural pluralism and psychoanalysis: the Asian and North American experience. New York: Routledge; 1996.
24. Sue DW, Sue D. Counseling the culturally different. 3rd edition. New York: Wiley; 1999.
25. Mahler M, Pine F, Bergman A. The psychological birth of the human iinfant: symbiosis and individuation. New York: Basic Books; 1973.
26. Pumariega A, Rothe E, Rogers K. Cultural competence in child psychiatric practice. J Am Acad Child Adolesc Psychiatry 2009;48:362–6.
27. Watrous S. Boundary issues in psychiatry. Residents guide to surviving psychiatric training. 2nd edition; 2007. p. 112–5. Available at: www.psych.org. Accessed July 18, 2010.
28. Myers GE. Addressing the effects of culture on the boundary-keeping practices of psychiatry residents educated outside of the United States. Academic Psychiatry 2004;28(1):47–55.
29. Pumariega A, Rothe, E. Leaving no children or families behind: the challenges of immigration. Am J Orthopsych, in press.
30. Desbiens NA, Vidaillet HJ Jr. Discrimination against international medical graduates in the United States residency program selection process. BMC Med Educ 2010;10:5.
31. Woods S, Harju A, Rao S, et al. Perceived biases and prejudices experienced by international medical graduates in the post-graduate medical education system. 2006. Available at: www.medonline.org. Accessed August 15, 2010.
32. Varki V. Of pride, prejudice, and discrimination, why generalizations can be unfair to the individual. Ann Intern Med 1992;116(9):762–4.
33. Balon R, Mufti R, Williams W, et al. Possible discrimination in recruitment of psychiatry residents? Am J Psychiatry 1997;154(11):1608–9.

34. Blanco C, Carvalho C, Olfson M. Practice patterns of international and U.S. medical graduate psychiatrists. Am J Psychiatry 1999;156:445–50.
35. Druzin P, Shier I, Yacowar M, et al. Discrimination against gay, lesbian and bisexual family physicians by patients. Can Med Assoc J 1998;158(5):593–7.
36. Maslow AH. Motivation and personality. 3rd edition. New York: Harper & Row; 1987.
37. Greenberg J. Understanding the vital human quest for self-esteem. Perspect Psychol Sci 2008;3:48–55.
38. Winnicott DW. Mirror-role of the mother and family in child development. In: Lomas P, editor. The predicament of the family: a psycho-analytical symposium. London: Hogarth; 1967. p. 26–33.
39. Kohut H. Analysis of the self: approach to treatment of narcissistic personality disorders. New York: International Universities Press; 2000.
40. Gogineni RR. Identity formation in children of immigrants. American Psychiatric Association Annual Meetings, Washington DC, 2008.
41. Gogineni RR. Children of immigrants: identity formation. American Academy of Child and Adolescent Psychiatry Annual Meetings. Boston, October 25, 2007.
42. Suarez-Orozco C, Suarez-Orozco M. Children of immigrants. Cambridge (MA): Harvard; 2001.
43. Canino IA, Spurlock J. Culturally diverse children and adolescents: assessment, diagnosis and treatment. New York: Guilford Press; 1994.
44. Lubell KM, Lofton T, Singer HH. Promoting health parenting practices across cultural groups: a CDC research brief. Atlanta (GE): Centers for Disease Control and Prevention, National Center for Injury Prevention and Control; 2008.
45. Good GE, Beitman BD. Counselling and psychotherapy essentials. New York: Norton; 2006.
46. Luborsky L. Therapeutic alliances as predictors of psychotherapy outcomes: Factors explaining the predictive success. In: Horvath AO, Greenberg LS, editors. The working alliance: theory, research, and practice. Oxford (UK), England: John Wiley & Sons; 1994. p. 38–50.
47. Schowalter JE. Psychodynamics and medication. J Am Acad Child Adolesc Psychiatry 1989;28(5):681–4.
48. Ahktar S. Immigration and identity: turmoil, treatment, and transformation. New Jersey: Jason Aronson; 1999.
49. Boszormenyi-Nagy I, Krasner B. Between give and take: a clinical guide to contextual therapy. New York: Bruner-Mazel, Inc; 1986.
50. Gabbard GO. Long-term psychodynamic psychotherapy. Washington D.C: American Psychiatric Press Inc; 2004.
51. Conas-Diaz L, Jacobsen FM. Ethnocultural transference and countertransference in the therapeutic dyad. Am J Orthop 1991;61(3):392–402.
52. Lijtmaer RM. Language shift and bilinguals: transference and countertransference implications. J Am Acad Psychoanal 1999;27:611–24.
53. Kernberg O. Countertransference. J Am Psychoanal Assoc 1965;13:38–56.
54. Langsley D, Yager J. The definition of a psychiatrist: eight years later. Am J Psychiatry 1988;145:469–75.
55. Rao NR, Meinzer AE, Berman SS. Countertransference: its continued importance in psychiatric education. J Psychother Pract Res 1997;6:1–11.
56. Langs R. The technique of psychoanalytic psychotherapy, vol. 2. New York: Jason Aronson; 1974.
57. Rodriguez C, Cabaniss D, Arbuckle M, et al. The role of culture in psychodynamic psychotherapy: parallel process resulting from cultural similarities between patient and therapist. Am J Psychiatry 2008;165(11):1402–6.

58. Alonso A. The quiet profession: supervisors of psychotherapy. New York: Macmillan Publishing Co; 1993.
59. Brody EB, Modarressi TM, Penna M, et al. Intellectual and emotional problems of foreign residents learning psychiatric theory and practice. Psychiatry 1971;34: 238–47.
60. Rao N, Hales D. Course helps IMGs adapt to psychiatric practice in the U.S. Psychiatr News 2009;44(4):4.
61. Steinert Y, Walsh A. Faculty development program for teacher of international medical graduates. Association of Faculties of Medicine of Canada; 2006. Available at: http://www.afmc.ca/img/modules_en.htm. Accessed August 15, 2010.
62. Mezzich J. International medical graduates and world psychiatry. In: Husain SA, Munoz RA, Balon R, editors. International medical graduates in the United States: challenges and opportunities. Arlington (VA): American Psychiatric Press; 1997. p. 1–7.

Psychopathology, Families, and Culture: Autism

Raphael Bernier, PhD[a],*, Alice Mao, MD[b], Jennifer Yen, MD[c]

KEYWORDS

- Autism spectrum disorders • Culture • Families
- Developmental disabilities

BACKGROUND AND OVERVIEW

Autism spectrum disorders (ASDs) are now considered to be the most common of the developmental disorders. However, the effect of cultural influences on the diagnosis and treatment of ASDs has received limited attention. The lengthy diagnostic processes, complicated treatment planning, and associated medical symptoms pose challenges to clinicians in considering the cultural influences on the disorder. Furthermore, cultural factors affecting diagnostic processes, adaptation of the family to having a child with autism, and treatment differences may have received less attention because neurodevelopmental changes seem to be much more significant in contributing to the abnormal social interaction, behaviors, and communication problems. Although symptoms of biologic disorders may be similar across cultures, symptom description, interpretation, and acceptance can vary tremendously. Despite the limited research data available at present, evidence suggests that culture does play a role.

This article reviews the available literature on cultural differences in diagnosis, acceptance, and treatment of ASD. It is important to focus on both macrolevel cultural factors—factors at the dominant culture level that affect the people in that society and microlevel factors—factors at the family level that affect response to diagnosis or treatment choice. Both can play a role in the course and outcome of an individual with ASD. Macrolevel factors, such as the availability of services, societal acceptance of the disorder, and existence of national- and/or state-funded treatment options,

The authors have nothing to disclose.

[a] Department of Psychiatry and Behavioral Sciences, University of Washington, Box 357920, Seattle, WA 98195, USA

[b] Depelchin Children's Center, Baylor College of Medicine, 4950 Memorial Drive, Houston, TX 77007, USA

[c] Depelchin Children's Center, Baylor College of Medicine, 6655 Travis, Suite 700, Houston, TX 77030, USA

* Corresponding author.

E-mail address: rab2@u.washington.edu

Child Adolesc Psychiatric Clin N Am 19 (2010) 855–867
doi:10.1016/j.chc.2010.07.005
1056-4993/10/$ – see front matter © 2010 Elsevier Inc. All rights reserved.

childpsych.theclinics.com

significantly affect the quality of diagnostic and intervention services provided, which directly influences the outcome for an individual with autism. In addition, cultural factors at the microlevel within families, such as individual response and acceptance of the diagnosis, vary considerably and can affect outcome. Although parenting behavior and parenting style are clearly not related to the development of ASD, parental perspectives of ASD and parental responses to receiving a diagnosis influence educational and treatment choices. As outlined later, research into macrolevel cultural factors and family-specific factors indicate that both the factors significantly affect the understanding of ASD, the diagnosis and treatment of the disorder, and the course of the disability.

PREVALENCE OF ASD ACROSS CULTURES

Median prevalence rates of ASD across international surveys are estimated to be 13 per 10,000 for autistic disorder, 21 per 10,000 for pervasive developmental disorders not otherwise specified, and 2.6 per 10,000 for Asperger disorder.[1] These estimates range from 91 per 10,000 in the United States[2] to 22 per 10,000 in the United Kingdom,[3] 7.2 per 10,000 in Denmark,[4] and 13.2 per 10,000 in Iceland.[5] In a review of epidemiologic studies of ASD, Fombonne[1] found that the prevalence rates were related to sample size and reported a large sample variability both within and between countries because of different methodologies. The diagnostic process and the ability to accurately diagnose ASD within the spectrum also vary within and across countries. Obtaining accurate prevalence estimates in some countries may be hampered by increased childhood mortality, poverty, and health issues. Furthermore, some cultures may not recognize ASD as a disorder or may group individuals with ASD under another diagnostic category. Inconsistent medical record keeping in some countries makes estimating ASD prevalence impossible. In addition, cultural beliefs and practices can affect identification and integration of individuals with ASD into a society. As a result, some individuals with ASD may be missed in epidemiologic studies, with true estimates significantly affected.[6] Fombonne[1] concluded that the unique design features of epidemiologic studies account for the between-study variability, suggesting that the true prevalence rates are likely to be comparable across countries.

Kogan and colleagues[7] found differential prevalence rates as a function of racial or ethnic background in the United States. Through a nationwide phone survey, they found that the odds of having an ASD were 57% lower for non-Hispanic African American children than for non-Hispanic White children. The odds of having an ASD diagnosis was 42% lower for non-Hispanic multiracial and non-Hispanic other single race (not African American or White) children when compared with non-Hispanic White children.[7] The investigators attribute the difference in rates to parental reporting of current diagnosis and suggest that the differential age of diagnosis and availability of services for ethnic/racial minorities and low socioeconomic status may account for the observed disparity. Similar findings were noted by the Autism and Developmental Disabilities Monitoring Network; the investigators concluded that ascertainment issues, environmental risk factors, and genetic susceptibility may influence the observed racial/ethnic differences.[2] However, a study of birth cohorts in California over a 7-year period failed to find any differences in prevalence rates between racial and ethnic groups.[8] The conflicting findings indicate that further exploration of effects resulting from differential access to treatment and diagnostic services is warranted.

Kanner[9] noted that some parents of children with autism had substantial educational backgrounds and were employed as physicians, lawyers, and professors.

Subsequent reports[10,11] indicated elevated rates of ASD in families of higher socio-economic status. However, the reports are likely a result of bias, because individuals of high socioeconomic status have greater access to service or time to participate in research.[12] More recent reports failed to find an association between socioeconomic status and ASD.[8]

Long-term cohort studies, such as the Taiwan Birth Cohort Study,[13,14] are currently underway in Hong Kong and Taiwan to study ASD in native populations. A review of cases of children diagnosed with autism in different areas of Taiwan found that children living in urban areas were more likely to undergo a shorter diagnostic process and receive the autism diagnosis at a younger age compared with suburban and rural peers.[15] Much of the disparity occurred from a lack of specialty and coordinated services in the suburban and rural areas because most of the specialty providers were concentrated in urban regions in the Northern areas of Taiwan, with no significant differences in socioeconomic status.

CULTURAL PERSPECTIVES ON ASD SYMPTOMS, DIAGNOSIS, AND CHARACTERIZATION

The birth of a child is universally accepted as a life-changing event. Most adults anticipate the birth of their child with a combination of joy and trepidation. Inevitably, expectations of the child's appearance, temperament, and developmental path arise based on wishes and past experiences. When a child is noted to have delays in speech development, abnormal repetitive behaviors, and problems with reciprocal social interaction, a decision to seek evaluation may be prompted. Because diagnostic instruments and standards may be different in different cultures, there may be significant differences in time from detection to diagnosis.

One of the core problems of ASD is in reciprocal social interaction. As a result, differences in cultural beliefs about appropriate social behavior can affect the accurate diagnosis of ASD. For instance, in Asian culture, direct eye contact with authorities is considered to be a sign of disrespect.[16,17] However, reduced eye contact is considered to be a part of the impaired nonverbal behavior criteria for diagnosis of ASD. By extension, children raised in Asian culture may avoid eye contact not because of ASD but because of the social norms of their culture.

In a review of the Indian literature on ASD, Daley[18] considered that the greater emphasis on conformity to social norms and the value placed on social relatedness in Indians could result in Indian parents recognizing social symptoms earlier and seeking treatment. However, despite social difficulties being observed by Indian parents earlier, the median age range of recognition is 25.7 months versus the 14.9 to 19.1 months in the West. In many cases, the parents delayed seeking helps as long as 2 years and 8 months after initial symptom presentation, because of the cultural beliefs of the parents and family. Examples of misinterpretation of symptoms leading to delayed diagnosis include the following cases[18]:

1. A parent with a 3-year-old girl who did not relate socially with peers her age considered her a mature child because she responded well to adults.
2. A mother was not alarmed that her son was still not speaking at age 4 years because Indian boys talk later.
3. A child who keeps quiet and to oneself was perceived as a good child because he or she is trouble free.

Macrolevel cultural factors that can contribute to delayed diagnosis also include requirements of the society for continuing medical education and recertification. The lack of requirements for recertification and requirements to keep up-to-date on new medical information may contribute to delayed diagnosis.[19] The older and well-respected Indian doctors were speculated to have possibly had an outdated view of autism, resulting in the late or misdiagnosed cases in the review.[18]

CULTURAL INFLUENCES IN DIAGNOSIS AND ASSESSMENT OF ASD

The gold standard assessment tools for diagnosing ASD are the Autism Diagnostic Observation Schedule (ADOS)[20] and Autism Diagnostic Interview.[21] These instruments have drastically improved the standardization of assessment and characterization of ASD; however, they were not designed to consider cultural variables or influences. Although the behavior-based ADOS has been translated into 12 languages, the effect of potential cultural confounds on the validity and reliability of the instrument has not been thoroughly assessed.

There is limited research examining the diagnosis and characterization of ASD in non-Western countries. This may be, in part, because in many cultures there is not a single word or label for ASD. For example, in Native Hawaiian and Native American languages, ASD is defined by longer descriptions of behaviors than by a single term.[22] In addition, some Asian languages do not have a word for ASD,[23] whereas others use a term that does not accurately reflect what is known about the disorder at present.

A recent report describing referral patterns in a sample of 50 consecutive clinic cases of ASD in a hospital in Saudi Arabia found that the presenting complaint for most of the cases was communication problems and that girls were diagnosed at a later age than boys, although in the similar 3:1 ratio as previously reported.[24] The investigators suggest that the delay in diagnosis in girls may result from societal expectations that boys be more outgoing, therefore, those girls with social deficits may be considered simply shy or lacking opportunities to interact.

In many parts of India, there are few professionals experienced in ASD and religious healers are often first consulted to help children with ASD. When medical provision is sought, medication or vitamin prescriptions are often the first method of intervention rather than referral for behavioral interventions that have been shown to be effective, although this pattern is changing.[25] In the United States, parents and professionals are more likely to detect general developmental delays or regression in language skills.[26] Language delays are not considered to be a core feature of ASD by some Indian parents and professionals because of the belief that boys acquire speech later than girls.[27] Daley[27] hypothesizes that these differences in what behaviors are first observed and considered as core to ASD are due to increased importance of social conformity in Indian culture when compared with the dominant US culture, which is more focused on language development.

There is limited research on ASD in Africa; however, a recent study examined health care workers' knowledge of ASD in Nigeria and highlighted gaps in understanding social impairments and repetitive and restricted interests. Further, more than half of the 134 interviewed health care professionals held the belief that facilities providing services and laws covering children with ASD were lacking.[28] Grinker[25] reported that Africans are less likely to use psychiatric treatment and more likely to pursue traditional healers because of cultural beliefs embedded in historical experiences. It was also reported that a common belief held by Europeans who colonized Africa was that Africans were assumed to be too primitive to suffer from mental illnesses because of their lack of exposure to stresses associated with life in industrialized societies. As a result, when Africans did show signs of mental illness, they were incarcerated rather than treated at hospitals.[25]

In the United States, research examining the effects of race and ethnicity on diagnosis indicates that the age at which children are diagnosed with ASD varies as a function of ethnic background. A study of Medicaid-eligible children with ASD in Philadelphia County found that on average, White children receive a diagnosis about 1.5 years earlier than African American children and 2.5 years earlier than Latino children.[29] Further, African American children spend more time in treatment before receiving the diagnosis of ASD. In a follow-up study, Mandell and colleagues[30] found that the African American children ultimately diagnosed with ASD were nearly 3 times more likely than White children to first receive another diagnosis, such as conduct or adjustment disorder. The investigators concluded that African American parents might be more likely to emphasize on disruptive behavior during the assessment rather than social oddities in their children. Other possible explanations are that general prejudices held by the clinician, specific stereotypes about health-related behaviors, and statistical discrimination in which the clinician has different expectations on the probability of ASD occurring in children of different ethnicities result in the observed differences in diagnostic outcomes.[31]

CULTURAL INFLUENCES IN PARENTAL ADJUSTMENT TO AN ASD DIAGNOSIS

One of the most difficult tasks that a parent faces is the response to the diagnosis of ASD. The most important adjustment for a parent raising a child with ASD is to successfully modify the original expectations of raising a typically developing child and to accept the child and the child's unique developmental trajectory and behavioral differences. Therein lie the unique challenges for the parent of the child with autism. For the family caring for a child with autism, the hardship is tangible and creates more substantive changes to the family system because of the permanence of the condition. Cultural factors affect the family's ability to accept the child and provide the resources necessary to promote the child's adaptation and development.

After the diagnosis of autism, many parents experience shock, trauma, and grieving for the loss of the normally developing child that they had planned for. Feelings such as denial about the diagnosis, anger about the unfairness of having to raise a child with developmental delays, and fear for the future of the child are all common reactions to the diagnosis. In some cases, the imperfect child, who is perceived as a reflection of the parent's own competence, may represent a narcissistic injury. The stark contrast between the imagined parenting experience and the reality of caring for a child with autism and intellectual disability may lead to intense disappointment and self-blame. Unlike other illnesses or events that may be time limited, having a child with autism creates a lifetime of multidimensional issues and demands for the family. Families may develop a new sense of self-organization as they are coping but may still feel marked by a distinct sense of tragedy.[32]

Variations in coping styles of parents have tremendous effect on their ability to accept and care for their child with ASD. When compared with White parents, Asian parents use reframing techniques[33] and redirect their energy toward positive actions such as the main coping strategies.[34] A recent study of Southeast Asian parents revealed 9 distinct set of coping style patterns when dealing with a child with autism, including denial or passive coping, empowerment, redirecting energy, shifting of focus, rearranging life and relationships, changed expectations, social withdrawal, spiritual coping, and acceptance.[35] Traditionally, Southeast Asian families lived in clans and depended on each other for all the family's needs. In addition, the researchers found that parents relied heavily on their extended family, when available, and that mothers resented the lack of adequate support from spouses and had an overall frustration about their weakness in English-speaking skills, which they thought impeded their abilities to maximize help for their children.[35] As a result, consideration of the immigrating families' experience in being physically detached from most of their extended family members is essential.

Stigma exists about mental illness in Chinese culture, and many families feel ashamed about having a child with a disability, thinking that mental illness is the punishment for a parent's behavior, particularly, the mother's behavior.[36] In addition, societal pressures for conformity in Chinese culture allow little room for the acceptance of individual differences, such as a child's disabilities. In China, 43 caregivers of children with ASD were interviewed about the experiences of raising a child with ASD.[37] Despite societal disapproval of ASD, parents reported wanting only what was best for their children. Most of the families in the study devoted considerable financial resources and time to their child. All the interviewed caregivers conveyed fear that their child's disability would result in discrimination and that the family would be judged in accordance with the traditional Chinese belief that a child's behavior and success directly reflects on the parents. Caregivers also reported concerns that their children would not receive proper care and services, citing that the stigma can discourage families from seeking out an evaluation and reporting a diagnosis to the school.

The reported reluctance to seek services or treatment for a disability because of the stigma is found in other cultures. South Asian families reported a reluctance to refer their child for services because of the stigma associated with the diagnosis and highlighted fears of a possible negative effect on arranged marriages, particularly for girls.[38]

CULTURAL INFLUENCES ON ASD TREATMENT

In addition to diagnostic differences in ASD, usage rates of special education and treatment services differ as a function of race and ethnic background. Dyches and colleagues,[39] in a review of the US Department of Education's 2001 Individuals with Disabilities Education Act report, found that students identified as African American or Asian or Pacific Islander received educational services under the category of ASD at twice the rate of American Indian/Alaskan or Hispanic students. The investigators concluded that the reluctance of families within some cultures to use the ASD label could account for the discrepant usage rates.

Disparities in access to and use of services of racial and ethnic minorities have been noted in children both with and without ASD.[40,41] Decreased access to treatment for Latino, African American, and socioeconomically deprived children with ASD have been noted.[42] Racial and ethnic minority families are also less likely to use the services of professionals such as case managers, psychologists, and developmental pediatricians.[43] It has been proposed that the disparity may be explained by the poor outreach and cultural competency of providers,[44] general mistrust of the system as a function of institutionalized discrimination,[45] and greater reliance on extended family members and friends than professionals.[46]

Perceptions of treatments are influenced by cultural values. In mental health, the choice of treatment is based on the family's belief about the cause of the diagnosis, but understanding of the cause varies across cultures. African American, Asian American, and Latino families may be less likely to view a child's symptoms as related to a health condition and therefore be less likely to seek out traditional medical treatments. Instead, these families may explore alternative therapies such as diet changes and supplemental vitamins.[47,48] For example, one study found that Latino children diagnosed with ASD were 6 times more likely to be treated using nontraditional strategies than children of other ethnicities.[49]

A 2006 study examining mothers' experiences of raising a child with ASD in an ultraorthodox Jewish community in Israel suggested that in this culture, ASD is believed to be associated with mystical forces.[50] Facilitated communication, repeatedly found by controlled studies to be an ineffective intervention,[51] involves the use of an adult's support to a child's hand while a child types on a keyboard to communicate. This technique continues to be used in the ultraorthodox Jewish community in Israel because it is considered as a way for children with autism to "impart hidden knowledge from heaven."[50(p20)]

Treatment goals are also influenced by cultural perspectives. For example, a high value is placed on individualism in Anglo-American culture, whereas some other cultures have a more collectivist orientation, prioritizing the group over the individual. As a result, some families may focus on treatment of behaviors that facilitate family and community activities rather than individual competence and autonomy. This approach could clash with behavioral treatments often aimed at fostering independence and self-help skills.[6] Differences in child-rearing practices and cultural values between and among racial and ethnic groups have implications that providers must consider when designing and implementing a treatment plan. For example, child-rearing practices of Mexican American mothers tend to focus more on teaching politeness and obeying authority figures, whereas Anglo-American mothers more often value self-directed learning and independent thinking.[52] Cultural differences have also been noted with regard to families' treatment decisions when dealing with a child with autism. Complementary and alternative medicine (CAM) use and Asian cultures are frequently associated with each other in the literature; however, recent research indicates that CAM use depends on the type of CAM.[53] In a cross-sectional survey of children's CAM use in Hong Kong, Wong[53] found that Western families used biologic therapies such as dietary management, whereas the 3 most common CAM types used by families in Hong Kong were acupuncture, sensory integration, and Chinese medicine. In addition, 76.9% of the families held expectations that it would augment the conventional treatments. The use of CAM in Hong Kong (40.8%) was less than that in Canada (52%) or the United States (74%). The father's job and the mother's religion were the 2 factors that were most significantly related to CAM use.[53] A study in Hong Kong reviewed the application of the Treatment and Education of Autistic and related Communication-handicapped CHildren (TEACCH) program in Chinese preschool children with autism. When compared with the control group, which received the typical in-school services through Individualized Education Plan and private therapy, the children in the TEACCH program showed significantly more improvement in perception and fine motor and gross motor tasks at 6 months and had gradual and significant improvement in all developmental domains at 12 months.[54]

Many ASD interventions include goals focusing on recognition and expression of emotion. However, some cultures value private over public displays of emotion and discourage outward emotional displays.[55] A treatment attempting to elicit outward emotional expression may contradict the values of these cultures. In addition, in many ASD interventions parents are encouraged to be an active member of the treatment team and implement interventions at home and in other settings for their child. However, expectations about the role of parent, teacher, and provider vary across cultures. In some cultures, parents do not expect to have a role and may expect therapists and educators to be the primary providers. These differences in focus can affect treatment goals in a service plan. To effectively collaborate with families in developing treatment goals and plans, cultural influences must be considered.

DEVELOPMENTAL CONSIDERATIONS

For a family with a child with ASD, early childhood is characterized by the family's recognition of the child's impaired social interaction, speech delay, and unusual behaviors. After diagnosis, there is a gradual appreciation and acceptance of an atypical developmental trajectory. Often, stress on the parents is increased by the extended family members' responses to the diagnosis, which although well-meaning, may include suggestions for intervention that may be unrealistic or impractical. Many parents stop working to coordinate their children's treatment and are thus faced with increasing financial burden.[56] Furthermore, parents may experience stress related to their children's inappropriate and disruptive social behaviors. The stereotyped, unpredictable, and repetitive behaviors of autistic children limit the family's opportunities for social activities and disrupt the family's daily routine, thereby compounding stress.

Typical problems that parents confront during this period include the child's irregular sleep patterns, hyperactive or disruptive behavior, lack of communication skills, restricted eating habits, and inability to achieve independent elimination habits. Concerns about keeping the child safe and an inability to obtain appropriate daycare or respite further increase stress. Unpredictable, disruptive, and unusual behaviors frequently lead parents to avoid public situations because they fear others' responses; however, this can lead to feelings of isolation and frustration. Normally developing siblings may resent missing activities because they are not tolerated by the child with autism. Parents may have to divide time so that one parent may accompany the sibling to a cherished activity.

Significant tasks for the family during this stage involve accepting the diagnosis, obtaining community services, and integrating complex treatment interventions. Clinicians must consider the macrolevel and microlevel cultural influences on the acceptance of the diagnosis and consideration of treatment options. The behaviors that are considered to be significant and first noted by parents may vary as a function of cultural background. For example, White families may be keenly aware of language delays and are concerned with communication problems, whereas families from other cultures with a focus on social conformity, such as Indian culture, may focus more on the socially disrupted behaviors. In some cultures, the stigma that is attached to having a child with a disability can affect the family's experience of receiving a diagnosis and so clinicians must rely on culturally specific coping strategies to make the diagnostic process successful. For example, many Asian families rely on reframing and directing their energy toward positive actions such as coping techniques. Clinicians could build on this approach by exploring options for positive outlets to direct family actions, such as directing energy toward treatment or participating in research to enhance understanding about the disorder. Ultimately, in the early phase after the diagnostic evaluation, clinicians can help the families by providing education about the disorder, discussing the variations in the developmental trajectory for children with ASD, and, most importantly, providing information about local resources for family support, educational programs, speech therapy, behavioral interventions, and physicians who are comfortable with working with children who have ASD.

Middle childhood may become challenging as parents search for appropriate educational settings for their children. Options vary by depending to a large degree on the intellectual level of the child. Children with ASD who have moderate intellectual disability may be able to participate in special education public school settings with ASD educational programs. Often families who are not able to afford a private program relocate to obtain services from a public school district that has appropriate programs for children with ASD. If the child has a significant intellectual disability and is not toilet trained, the search for appropriate school settings is much more difficult. Few private schools for children with ASD accept children who are not toilet trained because of the significant staff time required to provide individualized intensive interventions. Often parents have to develop a unique program for their child based on a combination of public and private resources encompassing behavioral interventions, such as applied behavioral analysis (ABA) or Floor Time therapy, speech and occupational therapy, and social skills training. The stress of implementing intensive ABA programs has been noted to contribute to maternal stress and depression.[57] The focus of the programs, in addition to traditional education, may be on the development of adaptive behaviors in the areas of self-care, domestic chores, and social behaviors. Clinicians must consider the cultural influences on treatment goal choice and treatment choice in general during this time. Although White families tend to emphasize independence and language development, which are the traditional goals for behavior-based interventions, these treatment goals may not be appropriate for children across all cultures. Clinicians must explore treatment goals with the family to ensure that the goals synthesize with the culturally relevant goals of the family. Further, during middle childhood, intense sadness can often arise in situations in which parents are confronted by the contrast between their child's developmental delays and those of a typically developing child. Clinicians can aid parents by predicting that these feelings of grief will occur and are common among parents raising a child with autism. Given the important role of extended family members in many cultures, such as Asian and Latino families, helping parents to find activities that they can share with their child allows them to be among other parents and family members and can be invaluable.

Adolescence and young adulthood are marked by transitions that are influenced by a family's cultural background. For example, some cultures value interconnected family networks closely, whereas others value independence. The treatment goals of this developmental period could vary as widely as skills for independence to foundational social skills to increase family interaction. Clinicians must be sensitive to the family culture to ensure that these treatment goals mesh with the cultural expectations.

CONSIDERATIONS FOR PRACTICE

Clinicians must be aware that the diagnostic process, developmental progression, and treatment selection in autism are influenced by culture at the macro- and micro-levels. Diagnosticians and treatment providers must have the basic knowledge about how family members of differing cultures may perceive autism and must be aware that differing levels of cultural identity and personal experience can affect a family member's adherence to or acceptance of those cultural norms. Clinicians must also have the skills to consider and incorporate these family and cultural norms into the diagnostic and treatment processes for individuals with autism.

It is essential for clinicians to consider the stigma that is associated with autism in many cultures and how it influences both their work with families with autism and the family's perception of the child with autism. To consider stigma at the societal and cultural levels, clinicians must be aware of their own cultural biases on how autism is characterized and treated.

Clinicians must be aware of the cultural influences on a family's perception of what autism is and what the diagnostic process means. Families in many cultures underuse mental health services for the evaluation and treatment of autism. By conducting the diagnostic evaluation and communicating about the process in a manner that is consistent with the cultural perceptions of autism, it may be possible to keep families engaged and potentially improve outcomes.

Clinicians must consider that the goals of treatment may vary as a function of culture and modify those treatment goals accordingly. CAM usage also varies by cultural groups, and given the widespread use of treatments that have not been empirically evaluated, clinicians must provide a framework for families to evaluate the applicability and utility of these treatments for their children.

SUMMARY

Regardless of the developmental stage or progression, a clinician's understanding of the parents' experience of their child's diagnosis and the cultural influences on the family's perception of diagnosis and treatment is paramount to providing services that are beneficial to the family.

There is limited research on the cultural influences in the diagnosis, treatment, and course of ASD, and much work is needed in this area. Existing studies examining prevalence rates suggest differential diagnostic rates as a result of differential usage rates of treatment services, age differences in diagnosis, and ethnic or racial group membership algorithms; however, environmental exposure or genetic factors cannot be ruled out. An important next step in ASD research is identifying the true prevalence rates and exploring each of these potential factors. Research needs to be conducted to identify and eliminate the barriers to service use for both diagnosis and treatment to increase usage rates and decrease the age of diagnosis for minority children. Other important steps for future research include validity testing of the existing gold standard diagnostic instruments in other languages and cultures and the examination of the efficacy of existing interventions (eg, ABA-based therapies) in differing cultures. ASDs are the most prevalent developmental disorders and affect families from all ethnic and racial backgrounds. Identifying the cultural factors at the macro- and microlevel that influence early detection, the diagnostic process, and treatment is the important next step to advance the understanding of ASD in a way that is helpful and influential for people of all backgrounds.

REFERENCES

1. Fombonne E. Epidemiology of autistic disorder and other pervasive developmental disorders. J Clin Psychiatry 2005;66(Suppl 10):3.
2. ADDM. Prevalence of autism spectrum disorders—autism and developmental disabilities monitoring network, United States, 2006. MMWR Surveill Summ 2009;58:1–20.
3. Chakrabarti S, Fombonne E. Pervasive developmental disorders in preschool children: confirmation of high prevalence. Am J Psychiatry 2005;162:1133.
4. Madsen KM, Hviid A, Vestergaard M, et al. A population-based study of measles, mumps, and rubella vaccination and autism. N Engl J Med 2002;347:1477.
5. Magnusson P, Saemundsen E. Prevalence of autism in Iceland. J Autism Dev Disord 2001;31:153.
6. Bernier R, Gerdts J. Autism spectrum disorders: a reference handbook. Santa Barbara (CA): ABC-CLIO; 2010.
7. Kogan MD, Blumberg SJ, Schieve LA, et al. Prevalence of parent-reported diagnosis of autism spectrum disorder among children in the US, 2007. Pediatrics 2009;124:1395.
8. Croen L, Grether JK, Selvin S. Descriptive epidemiology of autism in a California population: who is at risk? J Autism Dev Disord 2002;32:217.
9. Kanner L. Autistic disturbances of affective contact. Nerv Child 1943;2:217.

10. Lotter V. Epidemiology of autistic conditions in young children: I. Prevalence. Soc Psychiatry 1966;1:124.
11. Treffert DA. Epidemiology of infantile autism. Arch Gen Psychiatry 1970;22:431.
12. Fombonne E. Epidemiological surveys of pervasive developmental disorders. In: Volkmar FR, editor. Autism and pervasive developmental disorders. 2nd edition. New York: Cambridge University Press; 2007. p. 33–68.
13. Lung FW, Shu BC, Chiang TL, et al. Efficient developmental screening instrument for 6- and 18-month-old children in the Taiwan Birth Cohort Pilot Study. Acta Paediatr 2008;97:1093.
14. Lung FW, Shu BC, Chiang TL, et al. Parental mental health, education, age at childbirth and child development from six to 18 months. Acta Paediatr 2009; 98:834.
15. Chen CY, Liu CY, Su WC, et al. Factors associated with the diagnosis of neurodevelopmental disorders: a population-based longitudinal study. Pediatrics 2007; 119:e435.
16. Lian M-GJ. Teaching Asian American children. England. In: Duran E, editor. Teaching students with moderate/severe disabilities, including autism: strategies for second language learners in inclusive settings. 2nd edition. Springfield (IL): Charles C Thomas, Publisher; 1996. p. 239.
17. Sue DW, Sue D. Counseling the culturally diverse: theory and practice. 5th edition. Hoboken (NJ): John Wiley & Sons Inc; 2008.
18. Daley TC. From symptom recognition to diagnosis: children with autism in urban India. Soc Sci Med 2004;58:1323.
19. Joshi M. India. In: Sexton V, Hogan J, editors. International psychology: views from around the world. Lincoln (NE): University of Nebraska Press; 1992. p. 206.
20. Lord C, Rutter M, DiLavore P, et al. Autism diagnostic observation schedule - WPS (ADOS-WPS). Los Angeles (CA): Western Psychological Services; 1999.
21. Lord C, Rutter M, Le Couteur A. Autism diagnostic interview—revised: a revised version of a diagnostic interview for caregivers of individuals with possible pervasive developmental disorders. J Autism Dev Disord 1994;24:659.
22. Connors JL, Donnellan AM. Walk in beauty: Western perspectives on disability and Navajo family/cultural resilience. In: McCubbin HI, Thompson EA, Thompson AI, et al, editors. Resiliency in Native American and immigrant families. Thousand Oaks (CA): Sage Publications, Inc; 1998. p. 159.
23. Dobson S, Upadhyaya S, McNeil J, et al. Developing an information pack for the Asian carers of people with autism spectrum disorders. Int J Lang Commun Disord 2001;36:216.
24. Al-Salehi SM, Al-Hifthy EH, Ghaziuddin M. Autism in Saudi Arabia: presentation, clinical correlates and comorbidity. Transcult Psychiatry 2009;46:340.
25. Grinker R, editor. Unstrange minds: remapping the world of autism. New York: Basic Books; 2007.
26. Coonrod EE, Stone WL. Early concerns of parents of children with autistic and nonautistic disorders. Infants Young Child 2004;17:258.
27. Daley TC, Sigman MD. Diagnostic conceptualization of autism among Indian psychiatrists, psychologists, and pediatricians. J Autism Dev Disord 2002; 32:13.
28. Bakare MO, Ebigbo PO, Agomoh AO, et al. Knowledge about childhood autism and opinion among healthcare workers on availability of facilities and law caring for the needs and rights of children with childhood autism and other developmental disorders in Nigeria. BMC Pediatr 2009;9:12.

29. Mandell DS, Listerud J, Levy SE, et al. Race differences in the age at diagnosis among Medicaid-eligible children with autism. J Am Acad Child Adolesc Psychiatry 2002;41:1447.

30. Mandell DS, Ittenbach RF, Levy SE, et al. Disparities in diagnoses received prior to a diagnosis of autism spectrum disorder. J Autism Dev Disord 2007;37:1795.

31. Balsa AI, McGuire TG, Meredith LS. Testing for statistical discrimination in health care. Health Serv Res 2005;40:227.

32. Gombosi PG. Parents of autistic children. Some thoughts about trauma, dislocation, and tragedy. Psychoanal Study Child 1998;53:254.

33. Twoy R, Connolly PM, Novak JM. Coping strategies used by parents of children with autism. J Am Acad Nurse Pract 2007;19:251.

34. Ma J, Lai K, Pun S. Parenting distress and parental investment of Hong Kong Chinese parents with a child having an emotional or behavioural problem: a qualitative study. Child Fam Soc Work 2002;7:99.

35. Luong J, Yoder MK, Canham D. Southeast Asian parents raising a child with autism: a qualitative investigation of coping styles. J Sch Nurs 2009;25:222.

36. Tsang HWH, Tam PKC, Chan F, et al. Stigmatizing attitudes towards individuals with mental illness in Hong Kong: implications for their recovery. J Community Psychol 2003;31:383.

37. McCabe H. Parent advocacy in the face of adversity: autism and families in the People's Republic of China. Focus Autism Other Dev Disabl 2007;22:39.

38. Raghavan C, Weisner TS, Patel D. The adaptive project of parenting: South Asian families with children with developmental delays. Educ Train Ment Retard Dev Disabil 1999;34:281.

39. Dyches T, Wilder L, Obiakor F. Autism: multicultural perspectives. In: Wahlberg T, Obiakor F, Burkhardt S, et al, editors. Autistic spectrum disorders: educational and clinical interventions. Oxford (England): Elsevier Science, Ltd; 2001.

40. Newacheck PW, Hung Y-Y, Wright KK. Racial and ethnic disparities in access to care for children with special health care needs. Ambul Pediatr 2002;2:247.

41. Stevens GD, Shi L. Racial and ethnic disparities in the primary care experiences of children: a review of the literature. Med Care Res Rev 2003;60:3.

42. Liptak GS, Benzoni LB, Mruzek DW, et al. Disparities in diagnosis and access to health services for children with autism: data from the National Survey of Children's Health. J Dev Behav Pediatr 2008;29:152.

43. Thomas KC, Ellis AR, McLaurin C, et al. Access to care for autism-related services. J Autism Dev Disord 2007;37:1902.

44. Lau AS, Garland AF, Yeh M, et al. Race/ethnicity and inter-informant agreement in assessing adolescent psychopathology. J Emot Behav Disord 2004;12:145.

45. Schnittker J. Misgivings of medicine?: African Americans' skepticism of psychiatric medication. J Health Soc Behav 2003;44:506.

46. Terhune PS. African-American developmental disability discourses: implications for policy development. J Pol Pract Intellec Disabil 2005;2:18.

47. Bussing R, Schoenberg NE, Perwien AR. Knowledge and information about ADHD: evidence of cultural differences among African-American and White parents. Soc Sci Med 1998;46:919.

48. Yeh M, Hough RL, McCabe K, et al. Parental beliefs about the causes of child problems: exploring racial/ethnic patterns. J Am Acad Child Adolesc Psychiatry 2004;43:605.

49. Levy SE, Mandell DS, Merhar S, et al. Use of complementary and alternative medicine among children recently diagnosed with autistic spectrum disorder. J Dev Behav Pediatr 2003;24:418.

50. Shaked M, Bilu Y. Grappling with affliction: autism in the Jewish ultraorthodox community in Israel. Cult Med Psychiatry 2006;30:1.
51. Schreibman L. The science and fiction of autism. Cambridge (MA): Harvard University Press; 2005.
52. Rodriguez BL, Olswang LB. Mexican-American and Anglo-American mothers' beliefs and values about child rearing, education, and language impairment. Am J Speech Lang Pathol 2003;12:452.
53. Wong VC. Use of complementary and alternative medicine (CAM) in autism spectrum disorder (ASD): comparison of Chinese and Western culture (Part A). J Autism Dev Disord 2009;39:454.
54. Tsang SK, Shek DT, Lam LL, et al. Brief report: application of the TEACCH program on Chinese pre-school children with autism—does culture make a difference? J Autism Dev Disord 2007;37:390.
55. Sue DW, Sue D. Counseling the culturally diverse: theory and practice. 4th edition. New York: John Wiley & Sons, Inc; 2003.
56. Luther EH, Canham DL, Young Cureton V. Coping and social support for parents of children with autism. J Sch Nurs 2005;21:40.
57. Schwichtenberg A, Poehlmann J. Applied behaviour analysis: does intervention intensity relate to family stressors and maternal well-being? J Intellect Disabil Res 2007;51:598.

Trauma and Diverse Child Populations

Toi Blakley Harris, MD[a],*, L. Lee Carlisle, MD[b], John Sargent, MD[c],
Annelle B. Primm, MD, MPH[d,e]

KEYWORDS

• Culture • Childhood • Adolescence • Trauma

The importance of cultural diversity in the study of childhood trauma has long been appreciated intuitively. Acquiring the empiric evidence to guide assessment and treatment, however, has been a slow and arduous process, which is not difficult to understand given that culture is a fluid entity relevant to infinite subpopulations. Despite the difficulties, research in the area of childhood trauma has increasingly endeavored to examine and understand issues of culture and diversity.

TYPES OF TRAUMA

Estimates of lifetime prevalence rates of trauma exposure have been challenging because of difficulties with attempts to quantify the nature of trauma, duration, diagnostic criteria used, cultural factors related to the meaning of the traumatic event, and the available support during and after the trauma.[1] There are varying reports of the prevalence rates of childhood trauma in the literature. In 2008, Cohen and colleagues[2] reviewed data and reported that up to 68% of youth in a primary care setting had been exposed to potentially life-threatening events (PTE) and greater than half of these individuals have encountered multiple PTEs. A prospective study involving controls and childhood maltreatment survivors found 98.9% of the 882 participants reported at least 1 traumatic event by the 40 years of age. In this study, the rates of multiple interpersonal traumas were more pronounced in child maltreatment survivors, but the rate of other types of traumatic exposures (ie, natural disasters, combat experience,

The authors have nothing to disclose.
[a] Menninger Department of Psychiatry and Behavioral Sciences, Baylor College of Medicine, 1 Baylor Plaza BCM 350, Houston, TX 77030, USA
[b] Department of Psychiatry and Behavioral Sciences, University of Washington, Box 356560, Seattle, WA 98195-6560, USA
[c] Department of Psychiatry, Tufts Medical Center, 800 Washington Street, Boston, MA 02111, USA
[d] Department of Psychiatry, Johns Hopkins School of Medicine, Baltimore, MD, USA
[e] Minority and National Affairs, American Psychiatric Association, 1000 Boulevard, Suite 1825, Arlington, VA 22209-3901, USA
* Corresponding author.
E-mail address: toih@bcm.edu

Child Adolesc Psychiatric Clin N Am 19 (2010) 869–887
doi:10.1016/j.chc.2010.07.007
1056-4993/10/$ – see front matter © 2010 Elsevier Inc. All rights reserved.

human made disaster, and so forth) were similar to controls. These results, in keeping with previous studies, pointed to greater revictimization rates among individuals with childhood trauma histories.

LITERATURE REVIEW

In this section, the authors summarize key findings of a review of the current literature (**Figs. 1** and **2**) as it pertains to the influence of culture on: (1) incidence of trauma, (2) mental health impact of trauma, (3) resilience, and (4) cultural approaches to care and healing.

Incidence and Prevalence

A comprehensive literature search of trauma and diverse child populations for the years 2000 to 2010 is presented in **Fig. 1**. The pie chart is a visual representation of the most likely types of sources of trauma found in the backgrounds and histories of these children and corresponds to the following percentages: sexual abuse 24%, physical abuse 9%, psychological maltreatment 0%, neglect 21%, terrorism 9%, natural disasters 1%, refugee trauma or war zone trauma 1%, domestic violence 11%, complex trauma 0%, traumatic grief 0%, community violence 1%, school violence 2%, medical trauma or medical child abuse 0%, and other trauma 43%.

Another search using identical parameters and databases as in **Fig. 1**, but expanding them to include the years 1990 to 2010 is represented in **Fig. 2**. The bar graph demonstrates a dramatic increase in the volume of research relating to trauma and diverse childhood populations from 1990 to the present.

The development of trauma-related maladaptive symptoms has been shown to vary dependent upon trauma type and cumulative rates of exposure because of cultural and ethnic variables. In 2009, Kar delineated youths' risk for subsequent posttraumatic stress disorder (PTSD) associated with trauma type noting natural disasters

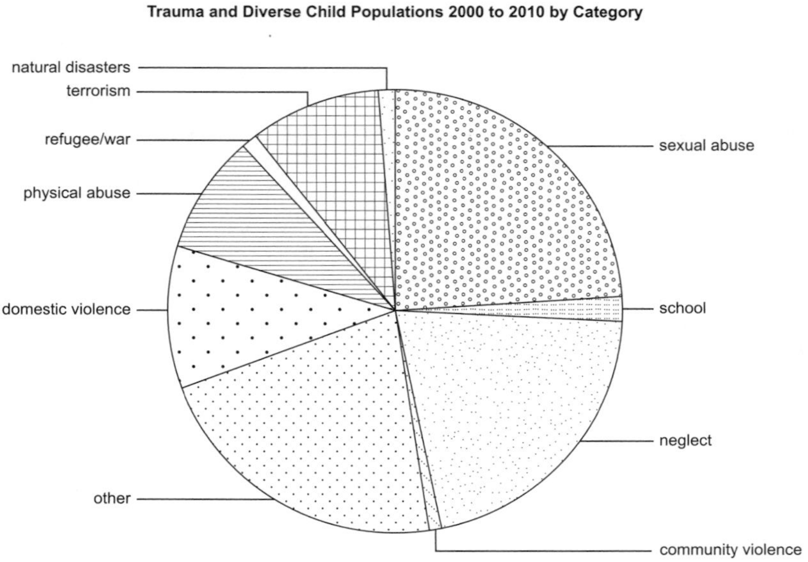

Fig. 1. Trauma and diverse child populations 2000 to 2010 by category. (*Courtesy of* Lee Carlisle, MD, Seattle, WA.)

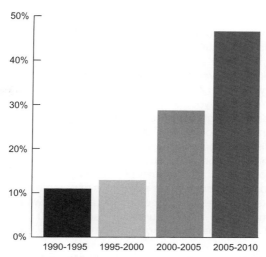

Fig. 2. Trauma and diverse child populations. (*Courtesy of* Lee Carlisle, MD, Seattle, WA.)

(earthquakes, hurricanes, floods, tsunami, cyclone, and so forth) in the range of 5% to 43% or greater, and man-made disaster survivors (community violence, war, terrorism, and so forth) with higher rates of PTSD (30% to 100%).[1] In 2009, Courtois and Ford outlined Terr's (1991) differentiation of trauma types and prevalence rates.[3,4] Trauma types were delineated based upon frequency, type I traumas were described as the result of single, unexpected occurrences; whereas, type II (complex traumas) were described as repetitive or chronic in nature. The prevalence rates varied between types. According to research, type II trauma is more prevalent and is associated with a greater risk for developing PTSD versus type I trauma (33%–75% vs 10%–20%).[3]

Research concerning effects of cultural diversity on child sexual abuse (CSA) accounted for the greatest number of studies and more empiric data than any of the other childhood traumas. It also generated the greatest amount of questions, confusion, and conflicting evidence. For example, studies of cross-cultural differences in CSA have generated widely varying results. In 1984, Kercher and McShane[5] found that more Latino women reported child sexual abuse than African Americans or non-Latino whites. In 1986, Lindholm and Wiley[6] found African American children reported higher rates than Latino or non-Latino whites, who both had similar rates. In yet another study from 1994, Urquiza and Goodin-Jones[7] found lower levels of CSA among Latino college students.

Similar inconsistencies have been present in studies addressing willingness to disclose, severity of abuse, and emotional response to CSA. Comparisons across studies were difficult because of varying research methods, nonuniform definitions of CSA, and the presence of study subjects from multiple cultures within broad ethnic groups researched.

Among Asian Americans, Zhai and Gao[8] found lower rates and lower recurrence of child maltreatment as compared with other cultural populations. In regard to the type of abuse, Asian Americans had lower rates of neglect and sexual abuse and higher rates of physical abuse when compared with other cultural groups. The investigators proposed that beliefs in physical punishment and the value of parental authority were risk factors for physical abuse in this population.

In a unique study, Freisthler, Bruce, and Needell[9] applied spatial regression procedures to 940 census tracts in California to explore the impact of neighborhood processes on child maltreatment. For African American children, they found higher rates of maltreatment were associated with higher rates of poverty. In addition to this expected finding, however, they also found a higher density of off-premise alcohol outlets correlated with higher rates of maltreatment. Decreased rates of child maltreatment for African American youths were associated with an increase in population since the 1990 census, neighborhoods consisting of a higher percentage of African Americans, and neighborhoods with an influx of more new residents. Similarly, percentages of Hispanic youth in neighborhoods also correlated with decreases in reports of child maltreatment. The investigators hypothesized that neighborhoods were less likely to report child maltreatment as they became more segregated or that these neighborhoods became less suspicious of parenting choices of their neighbors as caseworkers and residents became more familiar with the parenting styles. Child-care burden, defined by the number of adults (>20 years of age), children (<13 years of age), and the percentage of elderly residents, was also assessed. Higher rates of child maltreatment were correlated with increased child-care burden only in non-Hispanic white children, contrary to the hypothesis that neighborhood disorganization results in higher maltreatment reports. What may be representative of disorganization in one culture may be strength in another culture.

Mental Health Impact of Trauma

Roberts and colleagues[10] looked at race/ethnic differences related to PTSD trauma type and help seeking. African Americans and Hispanics had higher risk of child maltreatment; whereas, Asian Americans, African American men, and Hispanic women had higher risk of war-related events than non-Hispanic whites. Among those exposed to trauma, PTSD risk was slightly higher among African Americans and lower among Asian Americans compared with non-Hispanic whites.

A prospective study of 574 children aged 5 to 21 years, by Lansford and colleagues,[11] explored early physical abuse and its association with adolescent sequelae in work, romantic relationships, parenthood mental health, and violent delinquency. With a particular focus on race and gender, they found significantly greater effects of early physical abuse on later violence in African American youth as compared with non-Hispanic whites and girls versus boys. Researchers speculated poorer outcomes for African Americans were caused by minority status associated with increased rates of residential instability, residing in violent neighborhoods, experiences with racism, fewer opportunities for mental health care, or inadequate mental health care.

Studies have documented the risk for revictimization is greatest among CSA survivors. Other investigators delineated adverse childhood experiences, such as emotional withdrawal by a caretaker, physical neglect by a caretaker, a caretaker's failure to provide protection, sexual abuse by a non-caretaker, and any type of sexual abuse, were found to be predictive of future victimization.[12,13]

Traumatic experiences have been documented to occur within the context of immigration. Literature findings delineating the adverse mental health sequelae that were outside of the scope of this literature review have been summarized by these authors. Trauma exposure for immigrant children, in addition to encompassing the same, full spectrum of risk as other youth, is aggravated by the unique process of immigration, a process that, by itself, is inherently traumatic. Immigration trauma can be broken down into 3 phases: preimmigration, migration/journey, and resettlement.

Preimmigration trauma occurs in the child's homeland and often includes exposure to violence and persecution. Bolea and colleagues[14] explored the experiences of Sudanese immigrants in the Midwest for whom murders of parents and siblings were common in this phase. Children have also witnessed torture and rape of family and community members; whereas, others have been coerced into committing these acts as child soldiers. The investigators propose that the grieving process associated with these traumas is often overlooked because, despite the fact the traumas occurred there, these children still experience the loss of their homeland. Finding the support from family or immigrating community may be difficult because parents and other adults are suffering from the same traumas.[15]

Migration traumas include dangerous, often long, journeys, separation from parents or other family members, and those associated with detention facilities and refugee camps. In their flight to safety, Sudanese immigrants experienced starvation, attacks by lions, and near drowning in rivers inhabited by crocodiles. The camps were also dangerous, with scarcity of water, food, and medicine. The foster parents of one child substantiated the reports of the lack of safety in the camps as exemplified by their foster child hiding his clothes and shoes each night because they had been stolen as he slept in camps.[14] Children who are separated from family members experience higher rates of trauma and associated depression, anxiety, and PTSD symptoms as compared with accompanied minors.[16] Growing up with the uncertainty associated with these camps and facilities causes many children to lose hope of ever getting a new home.[15]

Resettlement traumas are about adapting to a new culture. Immigrant children, in addition to dealing with racism and stigmatization in both the neighborhood and school, have been described as cultural brokers because of their tendency to acquire language faster, which often leads to intergenerational tensions at home.[16]

Ngo and Le[17] investigated serious violence in immigrant youth of Chinese and Southeast Asian origins. The Cambodian and Laotian youth were exposed to the highest levels of stressors. Physical abuse in all groups except Chinese youth was a predictor of violence. The individual's level of perceived support buffered against most stressors. This finding was in contradistinction to acculturation, intergenerational conflict, and individualism, which predicted more violence.

Additional data obtained outside of the literature review in **Fig. 1** revealed factors associated with the negative impact of natural disasters on childhood mental health. In 2006, Thienkrua and colleagues[18] reported on data collected at 2 and 9 months after the tsunami. These researchers utilized a modified version of the PsySTART Rapid Triage System, the University of California at Los Angeles PTSD Reaction Index, and the Birleson Depression Self-Rating Scale and noted that the presence of PTSD and depression was highest among children who were displaced and resided in camps. A total of 75% of the children in displacement camps had direct contact with tsunami exposure. PTSD symptoms were seen in 13% of children in the camps in comparison to those from unaffected villages (6%). PTSD symptoms persisted in the children residing in camps at 9 months (10%). The prevalence of depressive symptoms remained the same in children residing in camps: 11% at 2 months and 12% at 9 months. Risk factors for PTSD symptoms included delayed evacuation times, displacement, increased exposure to disaster, perceived life danger of either self or loved ones, experiencing fear or anxiety during traumatic exposure, and sustaining a physical injury. Risk factors for depressive symptoms included perception of life or family endangerment and older age.

When youth have been exposed to natural disasters, war, and family violence, the risk for subsequent psychiatric sequelae are increased. In 2008, Catani and colleagues[19] examined this relationship with childhood tsunami survivors and found higher rates of PTSD (30.4%) and major depression (19.6%) and previous and current periods of suicidality (22.6% and 17.2% respectively) in children with prior war exposure, family violence, and father's history of alcohol intake.

In a prior review of Hurricane Katrina's impact on childhood mental health, Drury and colleagues[20] cited disrupted mental health services, and inadequate, poorly coordinated governmental responses as infrastructure deficits that contributed to initial challenges with supporting the mental health of Katrina survivors. These investigators reported data from the Kaiser Foundation (2007) that noted worsening of mental health status of adults (15%) and their children (4%) and lack of access to mental health services for children in the 6 months before this study (9%).[21] One study reviewed in this manuscript identified PTSD symptoms in a multiethnic school-age population to be 50% (62.5% who remained in New Orleans vs 43.5% who evacuated before the hurricane).[22] Of the children who screened positive for PTSD, 88.% were found to have a comorbid psychiatric disorder with separation anxiety disorder and oppositional defiant disorders most common. Two favorable intervention studies were cited; group formats utilizing relaxation and exposure therapy, and cognitive behavioral therapy and narrative therapy in either group or individual formats were all found to reduce anxiety symptoms in hurricane survivors.

Recent cross-sectional data from Peters and colleagues[23] identified the risk of increased alcohol and drug use among 170 African American and Hispanic-American males after Hurricane Ike. These researchers identified statistically significant use of substances was increased in boys (aged 9–19 years) who attempted to suppress thoughts related to the hurricane: alcohol ($P<.5$), marijuana ($P<.1$), codeine cough syrup ($P<.00$), antienergy drinks ($P<.00$), crystal methamphetamine ($P<.00$), and sildenafil citrate (Viagra; [$P<.00$]). Similar to other studies that identified increase substance use in adults following disasters, Peters and colleagues found increased rates of substance use in a child and adolescent population.

Resilience: Protective and Risk Factors

Given high rates of lifetime trauma exposure, attention to protective and risk factors will aide in the understanding of which youth are most likely to suffer adverse and long-standing sequelae of trauma. Both biologic and psychosocial factors have been associated with psychological resilience. More recent attention has been focused on exploration of the role of environment and genetic influences on the stress response during development. Heritability has been shown to contribute to 30% to 40% of the risk to develop mood and anxiety disorders including PTSD.[24]

Gillespie and colleagues[24] summarized data reported on this topic. Stressful life events experienced during development have been shown to alter the hypothalamic-pituitary-adrenal (HPA) axis, which can result in subsequent anxiety or mood disorders. Predisposing genetic variables lend either toward the development of vulnerabilities or resilience in youth exposed to traumatic events. Scientists have identified FKBP5 and CRHRI as 2 genes involved in the regulation of the HPA axis following exposure to traumatic events. Additional data reviewed by Gillespie and colleagues suggested that a critical period exists during which brain exposure to corticosterone affects fear learning that is modulated by the quality of maternal care. Therefore, when trauma is experienced within a supportive environment, an amygdala-dependent emotional circuit is developed that can distinguish between nonthreatening and threatening environmental cues.

Resilience has emerged as an independent research issue involving a plethora of interesting social and cultural considerations. DuMont and colleagues[25] prospectively followed a cohort of CSA, physical abuse, and neglect cases matched with nonabused children of similar age and ethnicity over 22 years. Eight domains of resilience were measured: education, psychiatric disorder, substance abuse, official reports of arrest, self-reports of violent behavior, employment, homelessness, and social activity. Overall, 48% of abused children compared with 61% of controls were resilient in adolescence, and in young adulthood, 30.2% compared with 46%, respectively. Nonwhites were statistically more likely to be resilient in adolescence. Individuals who were shown to be consistently resilient throughout adolescence and young adulthood had the following characteristics: female and either lived with both parents, had a long first placement, or had a highly supportive relationship. Nonresilience was associated with being male, white, and either having a brief first placement, less likely to live with both parents, or less likely to have a supportive relationship. This study contributed to the field's understanding of resilience identifying that female, African Americans who were maltreated in childhood appeared to be more resilient in this sample.

Children exposed to trauma demonstrate higher rates of delinquency. Several studies have now demonstrated that a strong ethnic identity can be a mitigating factor in delinquency following childhood trauma. Bruce and Waelde[26] studied 307 adolescents in the California Bay Area and found higher levels of ethnic identity correlated with less delinquency in the presence of increasing trauma symptoms. This protective effect of ethnic identity is much stronger for minorities than for non-Hispanic whites.

Zhai and Gao[8] found lower rates of neglect and CSA among Asian Americans. Protective factors were thought to arise from the focus on family harmony, reputation, and high degree of indulgence of preschool children. However, when CSA did occur in a study involving South Asian immigrant women, Singh and colleagues[27] used semistructured interviews and found the following protective factors: sense of hope, South Asian social support system, social advocacy, and intentional self-care.

Castro and colleagues[28] identified resilience in Latino adolescents whose fathers were illicit drug users. Family traditionalism, specifically the conservative cultural values of respect for elders and family traditions, and sense of social responsibility toward the cultural community were all found to be protective. Austin[29] studied connections between use of alcohol, tobacco, and other drug use and violence among rural native Hawaiians and suggested ethnic pride to be protective against violent behavior. Siqueira and Crandall[30] looked at differences in risk and protective factors for binge drinking among adolescents from 6 Hispanic subgroups in Florida. Their conclusion was that prevention programs focused on Hispanic subgroups ethnically rather than addressing all Hispanics as one culture.

Moscardino and colleagues[31] used semistructured interviews with caregivers of child survivors of the terrorist school siege in Beslan, Russia in 2004 and suggested return to normality, reinforcement of the positive, good social supports, and culturally shared values toward the common threat of possible future terrorist attacks as protective factors. Spilsbury and colleagues[32] found, as have others, nonwhite ethnicity to be a protective factor for behavioral problems in children exposed to domestic violence.

The escalating HIV/AIDS epidemic in Tanzania and Kenya raised concern by Lalor[33] of increased CSA related to a practice in which infected individuals use sex with a child to cleanse themselves. Plummer and Njuguna[34] collected data from 36 professionals from a variety of tribal groups across Kenya and found their concerns to be similar. Protective factors were based on traditions and religion, criminal punishment, rigid gender roles, and the high value placed on a female child's virginity. Risk factors, which included strict patriarchy, inflexible gender roles, and low emphasis on children's rights, were likewise deeply rooted in culture, the same culture in which the protective factors were present. The consensus of this study was that sexual abuse is clearly intertwined with culture and therefore any prevention and treatment approach would, by necessity, need to be culturally relevant.

Psychological resilience after trauma has been documented in diverse child and adolescent populations. Individual, family, community, and cultural variables have been identified that can support posttraumatic growth and development in children exposed to trauma. Further study is warranted to develop clinical application.

Cultural Approaches to Care and Healing

When experiencing psychological distress, racial and ethnic minorities are less likely to follow up with traditional mental health providers while experiencing psychological distress and more likely to seek help through family, faith leaders, or through folk medicine.[35] All minority groups (African Americans, Asian Americans, Hispanic Americans) were less likely to seek treatment for PTSD than non-Hispanic whites and fewer than half of minorities with PTSD sought treatment in the study conducted by Roberts and colleagues.[10] These authors reviewed the following factors contributing to decreased help seeking: (1) stigma related to mental health disorders and treatment, (2) lack of desire to pursue and receive psychological support outside of the family unless under extreme conditions, (3) perceived ethnic or racial bias in mental health or health care providers, and (4) decreased access to health and mental health care in lower socioeconomic communities. The findings from Roberts and colleagues indicated that PTSD and other psychiatric sequelae of childhood trauma among US race and ethnic minorities have been largely undiagnosed and untreated, indicating a need for investment in accessible, culturally sensitive treatment options.

CLINICAL ASSESSMENT/DIAGNOSTIC CHALLENGES

A myriad of adverse health and mental health sequelae of childhood trauma have previously been described in the literature. When conducting a mental health evaluation of a youth following a traumatic event, there are many broad areas or domains to be assessed. In addition to information gathered through clinical interviews and collateral reports, psychometric instruments have been useful to assist with the assessment process of children and adolescents who have experienced trauma; low agreements between caregiver and youth reports of internalized symptoms warrant multiple informants and psychometrics. **Box 1** contains a review of psychometric tools used in diverse youth populations.[36–38]

The authors of this article used Kendall-Tackett's outline of 4 potential pathways following childhood maltreatment as a framework for child trauma assessment.[12] In addition to the 4 areas identified by Kendall-Tackett (behavioral, social, cognitive

---

Box 1
Trauma and diverse child populations

Semistructured and self-report measures have been summarized in the literature by Spates and colleagues,[36] Lemos-Miller and Kearney,[37] and Hawkins and Radcliffe[38]:

1. Semi-structured: Child and Adolescent Psychiatric Assessment: Life Events Section and PTSD Module, Children's PTSD inventory

2. Self-report: Children's PTSD Inventory, Trauma Symptom Checklist for Children, Child PTSD Symptom Scale, Screen for Child Anxiety Related Emotional Disorders, Children's Depression Inventory, Posttraumatic Cognitions Inventory, Adolescent Dissociative Experiences Scale

and emotional), the authors included a fifth pathway to address cultural factors to be considered in the clinical evaluation of a youth.

Behavioral

Among all of the pathways, the behavioral outcomes of trauma are the best described, including harmful activities, such as the misuse and abuse of substances (tobacco, alcohol, and illicit substances); disordered eating; self-injurious behavior; suicide attempts and ideation; high-risk sexual behavior; and poor sleep hygiene. These harmful behaviors often result in subsequent medical and psychiatric sequelae. During initial and subsequent evaluations, traumatized youth warrant screening for individual (suicidality; self-injurious behavior; substance intoxication/withdrawal; high-risk sexual practices; and aggression toward others, property, and so forth), family (domestic violence, physical, sexual, or psychological abuse by current caretakers), and community (community violence) safety concerns. Vital signs; urine toxicology screens; and laboratory data to assess the nutritional and metabolic status, the presence or absence of sexually transmitted diseases, and general health of the youth have been recommended based upon clinical history. In addition to the monitoring of safety concerns, the encouragement of consistent feeding and sleeping schedules and the return to normal routines have been shown to improve clinical outcomes of trauma survivors.

Social

Social pathways of childhood trauma survivors lead to adverse outcomes in adulthood. These adverse outcomes are related to interpersonal styles, victimization rates, and rates of homelessness. Kendall-Tackett reviewed the data of Becker-Lausen and Mallon-Kraft (1997) that described the maladaptive interpersonal styles of childhood maltreatment survivors.[39] Becker-Lausen and Mallon-Kraft characterized individuals as either manifesting avoidant or intrusive patterns of interacting with others based upon varying degrees of interdependency, self-disclosure, and warmth. When comparing the interaction styles, individuals who demonstrated an avoidant style were described as having low self-disclosure, low interdependency, and low warmth, and individuals who demonstrated intrusive styles were described as having high interdependency, high self-disclosure, and an excessive need for closeness. Both of these patterns of interpersonal styles led to impaired social interactions and limited social support. Prior studies have highlighted the association between adequate social support and good health behaviors, particularly in individuals of lower socioeconomic status. Obtaining historical information from the youth and collateral reports will assist in identifying potential maladaptive interpersonal styles to be addressed during treatment planning.

As previously discussed, there is a high risk of revictimization among CSA survivors. With revictimization, the trauma survivor has an increased risk of acquiring a sexually transmitted disease and for chronic stress negatively impacting health and psychological wellbeing. Given the risk of revictimization, ongoing surveillance for safety concerns is indicated in conjunction with treatment plans, including a formal mechanism to improve safety awareness.

Homelessness has been identified as another potential social consequence of childhood trauma. Sexual and physical abuse in studies involving women have shown that abused women with similar socioeconomic status were more likely to be homeless in comparison to their counterparts who were domiciled. The association between family violence, separations caused by foster care placements, and homelessness place children with histories of family violence at risk for subsequent traumas and fragmented social networks. In addition, a disproportionate number of minority children from underrepresented backgrounds have been placed in the foster care system, which carries added risk for potential homelessness.[40] Homelessness has caused and exacerbated harmful health effects related to malnutrition, lack of medical care, inclement weather exposure, increased risk of physical injury, and lack of routine hygiene.

Cognitive

Beliefs and attitudes have been shown to impact health. The internal working model has been studied as a framework individuals have used to interpret the motives or actions of others and stressful or negative life events. Childhood trauma survivors have been described to distort reality in multiple domains, negatively interpreting life events, underestimating their own capacity to deal with real and perceived danger, and overestimating adversity and danger. Cognitive distortions such as these have increased psychological distress in trauma survivors and increased the likelihood of depression. Interpersonal trust and optimism have both been linked to longevity; however, childhood trauma survivors have less potential for both of these cognitive patterns based on prior adversities. Other investigators have also described the relationship between traumatized youth's cognitions and psychological symptoms. Cognitions related to traumatic experiences have been shown to be key factors for the onset of PTSD and emotional dysregulation. Obsessive thoughts; negative self-appraisals; and avoidant coping strategies, such as thought suppression, have been found in maltreated youth.[37] Within the context of a mental health assessment, eliciting information regarding the youth's cognitions and related emotions associated with traumatic events has been an essential component of case formulation and the identification of appropriate treatment recommendations.

Along with having a propensity to develop cognitive distortions, the literature has described a frequent misperception of perceived danger in childhood trauma survivors. These misperceptions have resulted in increased levels of cortisol or stress hormone levels leading to immune system suppression, neurotoxicity, increased rates of chronic diseases, and slower wound healing. Mulvihill further reviewed adverse health outcomes of childhood trauma and noted the increased rates of chronic diseases, including ischemic heart disease, liver disease, cancer, chronic lung disease, and skeletal fractures.[41] As previously discussed, the mental health evaluation and treatment of childhood survivors has health implications that call for collaboration with primary care physicians to assure optimum physical health over the lifespan of this patient population.

Emotional

Over the past 3 decades, researchers have identified the significance of negative emotions related to childhood trauma. Researchers have described unique challenges that clinicians may face who attempt to conduct culturally sensitive evaluations during or after a traumatic event for youth and families.[1] In conjunction with being attuned to the cultural nuances of clinical presentations, health and mental health care providers who work with the pediatric population are also called to take into consideration the developmental phase and cognitive capacity of the individual. The limited verbal abilities and level of cognitive development have been identified as barriers clinicians encounter during the assessment and treatment process. Recognizing the impact of development on clinical symptoms, the *Diagnostic and Statistical Manual of Mental Disorders* (DSM) has added specific descriptors for children and adolescents to aide in the diagnosis of psychiatric disorders. Symptoms following traumatic exposure may overlap with the symptoms of several diagnostic categories, including anxiety, mood, disruptive, and substance abuse disorders. Following exposure to traumatic events, if symptomatic, the majority of youth will experience either anxiety, or mood symptoms following a traumatic event.[38] This next section will focus specifically on pediatric and adolescent posttraumatic stress disorder and associated impairments and conditions following traumatic exposures.

Since the introduction of PTSDs, many investigators have proposed alternate criteria to delineate the full range of symptoms extending beyond PTSDs classic triad of intrusion, avoidance, and hyperarousal seen in youth with complex trauma histories. In 2009, Courtois and Ford reviewed the scientific literature's call for attention to post-traumatic adaptation and a broader examination of the complete range of symptoms following childhood complex trauma.[3] They cited the work of van der Kolk[42] and the National Child Traumatic Stress Network, which has supported the incorporation of Developmental Trauma Disorder (DTD) in the upcoming addition of DSM V (Fifth Edition).

Similar to disorders of extreme stress not otherwise specified described by Herman and van der Kolk in adults,[3,43] DTD would include developmentally adverse interpersonal trauma as an objective Cluster A1 criteria. DTD would also provide criteria to denote 3 additional features outside of classic PTSD that highlight behavioral and relational challenges more pronounced in traumatized youth: (1) dysregulation triggered by trauma related stressors negatively impacting emotions, cognitions, physical/somatic, behavior, self attributions, and behavior; (2) beliefs altered by recurrent betrayals and occurrences of abandonment that have negatively impacted personality structure development, creating a lack of trust in others and future expectations of revictimization and self-blame; and (3) impairments in major domains of functioning (interpersonal relationships [family or peer], school, employment, and legal issues). The range of dysfunction caused by complex trauma spans all 5 axes, including (1) Axis I: frequent comorbidity with mood disorders, somatoform disorders, eating disorders, substance abuse disorders, and other anxiety disorders; (2) Axis II: personality disorders; (3) Axis III: acute and chronic health conditions described previously; (4) social, educational, vocational, and legal challenges; and (5) overall impaired functioning.

Cultural

As previously described, exposure to traumatic events in childhood has occurred globally in varying degrees among all ethnic groups. Culture has been shown to influence and modify behavioral and emotional responses to trauma, the cognitive beliefs regarding the trauma itself, and impact of the societal roles of the family, and the community's individual and collective response to trauma. Since the establishment of cultural psychiatry in 1969, this field has highlighted the importance of factoring in cultural influences when evaluating behaviors, help-seeking patterns, and response to psychiatric treatment. Cultural perspectives are needed to differentiate between normative and maladaptive behaviors. Models for conducting culturally sensitive assessments for children, adolescents, and families have been described.[44] Hays's model, which incorporates various aspects of an individual's identity and group affiliations, has been described in the literature.[45,46] Brown describes Hays's acronym ADDRESSING to delineate the following social locations: A: age-related factors (chronologic age and cohort); DD: disability (acquired and developmental ability, visible, and invisible); R: religion and spirituality; E: ethnic origins, culture, race/phenotype; S: social class, current, and former; S: sexual orientation (lesbian, gay, bisexual, heterosexual, questioning); I: indigenous heritage/colonization (history of colonizer); N: national origin (immigration status, personal or family; refugee); G: gender and biologic sex (male, female, intersex); and gender identity (masculine, feminine, or transgender).

The challenges associated with the evaluation of children and adolescents within an appropriate sociocultural context have been well documented. Lack of knowledge about a particular culture and personal clinician bias negatively impact clinical encounters.[44] Likewise, an individual or family's negative bias against mental health care and the mental health provider's cultural background also threaten or interfere with the successful establishment of a therapeutic alliance.

Within the DSM, there are 2 sections of content that have been helpful to identify cultural considerations for mental health clinicians. The DSM-IV-TR (Text Revision) outline for cultural formulation (2000) has been used as a tool to improve the skill of the clinician to address these cultural concerns in a systematic manner; this issue of the DSM also included a glossary of culture-bound syndromes.[47] In 2001 Gaw reviewed culture-bound syndromes and idioms of distress related to acute stress disorder, such as falling out in African American and Caribbean cultural groups, and proposed utilizing DSM IV diagnostic categories for clinical application.[48] For additional information regarding conducting culturally relevant child and adolescent mental health assessments, refer to article by Pumariega and colleagues elsewhere in this issue.

Treatment

Because of the multiple domains that childhood trauma affects, a multidisciplinary team that addresses the biologic, psychological, and sociocultural sequelae has been proven most effective. Using the behavioral-social-cultural-cognitive-emotional framework proposed in the assessment section, the authors recommend a similar approach for treatment. Safety concerns of the youth or family identified in the evaluation are addressed throughout the assessment and treatment phases. Using this clinical vignette, the authors explore a step-wise assessment and treatment process of a traumatized youth based upon clinical guidelines and research evidence.

CASE PRESENTATION
Preflight

Astrid is a fictitious name used to protect the identity of a 12-year-old Haitian girl. Before January 12, 2010 she lived in Port-au-Prince, Haiti in a small concrete house with her mother and 2 younger sisters. Before her father left the household, he would frequently physically abuse Astrid's mother. His departure led to a worsened financial state for her family.

Flight

When the earthquake occurred that afternoon, Astrid was playing outside with her 8-year-old sister. As the quake shook her house, Astrid and her sister were terrified. While they watched, their house collapsed, killing Astrid's mother and her 5-year-old sister. Astrid was terrified during the earthquake and then horrified as she ran to the house, lying in rubble. She looked for her mother and sister and did not find them. An adult neighbor found Astrid and her sister and got food for them amid the chaos. Astrid and her sister had not been physically injured but were frightened and crying. Over the next 2 weeks, Astrid stayed with her neighbor's family and obtained food periodically. They slept outdoors. Astrid was withdrawn and generally noncommunicative. In an effort to cope with the recent tragedy, Astrid and her sister drank teas to heal the soul from mourning daily and attended prayer vigils with their neighbors held across the city; however, no formal mental support was accessed.

Resettlement

Astrid's maternal aunt, Ruby, lives in the Haitian community in Boston. She had immigrated to Boston 15 years previously to attend college and remained as a teacher in a public high school. Ruby is married to a fellow Haitian and has 2 children (5 years old and 2 years old). She learned of her sister's death in the earthquake, which left Astrid and her sister orphaned. In the 2 weeks immediately following the earthquake, Ruby made arrangements to bring Astrid and her sister to Boston. They were able to come to Boston to stay with her aunt in early February. Astrid spoke Creole, which her aunt's family also spoke. She shared a room in the family's apartment with her sister and was registered to attend the neighborhood middle school in Boston.

Shortly after arriving in Boston, Astrid began waking up each night crying with nightmares. She also began complaining of chest pain, abdominal pain, and dizziness followed by syncopal-like episodes at school, regularly visiting the school nurse. She also began complaining before school. Her aunt became alarmed and took Astrid to visit the local health center. Astrid would not speak with her doctor but her physical examination, chest radiograph, and cardiogram were all normal. The physician asked how Astrid was doing emotionally and Ruby assured the doctor that she was "OK."

Astrid's teacher, Mrs Lewis, contacted Ruby about Astrid's behavior and performance in school and recommended that she take Astrid for a mental health evaluation. Ruby became very defensive and did not want to discuss Astrid's difficulties with her teacher. Ruby felt that Astrid was behaving appropriately at home, and knew that she was having significant difficulty concentrating in school and was not attempting schoolwork. She was aware that Astrid's emotions fluctuated between crying; withdrawal; and complaining of pain, dizziness, and periods of blacking out. Ruby felt more comfortable sharing Astrid's struggles with her parish's priest, who recommended prayer sessions with church leaders to heal Astrid's soul.

After a month of taking Astrid to meet with the priest and participate in prayer sessions, a fellow congregant mentioned that her cousin had received help from the Boston Haitian Mental Health Network for similar problems following the earthquake. Ruby was encouraged to take Astrid to a local neighborhood mental health center that had an affiliation with the Haitian Mental Health Network. Ruby relayed to the counselor the difficulties that Astrid had been having at school. Ruby stated that Astrid did play with her sister and would interact with her younger cousins but that at times she would isolate in her room.

The counselor contacted a member of the Haitian Mental Health Alliance who met with Astrid and her aunt. This therapist spoke with Astrid in Creole and helped Astrid explain her pain and discomfort. The Haitian American clinician also helped Astrid begin to talk about what happened during the earthquake. Astrid spoke of her terror when the ground shook and of her guilt about her mother's death and her sadness at missing her mother. She fluctuated between being in pain, being tearful, and acting stoic and dazed. The Haitian American therapist agreed to continue to meet with Astrid. Astrid did seem relieved after talking with the Haitian American counselor.

Five months after the earthquake Astrid was continuing to have nightmares, but was attending school. Astrid was able to play with her sister and was learning English. She was continuing in weekly therapy with the Haitian American therapist.

Astrid's problem list included displacement from her homeland and subsequent language barrier and cultural dissonance between Astrid and her school environment, death of caregiver, and prior and acute trauma exposure from domestic violence and the recent disaster. Using the framework discussed previously, based upon

Kendall-Tackett's and Hay's models, the authors identified the following factors in her assessment. In the *behavioral* pathway, Astrid had not demonstrated any safety concerns or harmful behaviors based upon clinical examination and collateral reports from her aunt and teachers; however, she did receive continued screening for such behaviors throughout treatment.

Historical details from Astrid's case highlighted deficits in her *social* functioning. Following the earthquake, Astrid and her sister experienced an abrupt change in their home life with the traumatic loss of their mother, homelessness, and the temporary lack of basic needs. Case management is beneficial in such instances in assisting with the immediate and ongoing needs of children and families impacted by trauma. Case managers can help families navigate the complexities of interfacing with governmental, social, educational, and mental health agencies and organizations.

During the initial phases of her resettlement with her maternal relatives in the United States, Astrid did manifest a maladaptive interpersonal style seen commonly in childhood survivors as indicated by her avoidant interaction patterns with peers and family. Psychoeducation provided to Astrid, her family, and school personnel assisted with a greater understanding of her trauma sequelae and supported the need for treatment. School-based group cognitive behavioral therapy programs promoting adaptive interpersonal skills have proven effective for trauma survivors (cognitive behavioral interventions for trauma in schools) and could prove beneficial to Astrid.[2] Group interpersonal psychotherapy to target mood, anxiety, and conduct symptoms in refugee children with war-related traumas successfully reduced depressive symptoms in female, but not male, children who participated in Verdeli's 2008 study.[49] In 2008, Rousseau and Guzder reviewed alternate school-based prevention programs aimed at supporting successful postmigration and found them to have longitudinal outcomes that encourage their use to promote protective factors in refugee youth.[50] Astrid and her sister could benefit from participation in school-based intervention to address existing difficulties and prevent subsequent psychiatric sequelae related to trauma, loss, and migration.

With the aid of the DSM cultural-bound syndromes, a consideration for falling out will be made based upon Astrid's symptoms of dizziness that proceed collapse, which may correspond to either a conversion disorder or dissociative disorder. Falling out, or blacking out, as a culture-bound syndrome has been described in the DSM as a culturally recognized idiom of distress in Caribbean populations and seen in the southern United States.[47]

Relocation with her maternal relatives provided Astrid and her sister with a family unit that has previous history with cultural differences between their native country and host country. Her aunt could potentially identify with Astrid's acculturation issues. Ruby initially sought help in her community of faith, but pursued the congregant's suggestion of a formal mental health assessment. In other refugee families, this might not be the case where the practice of voodoo, sometimes seen in this cultural group, and the use of indigenous healers would be the preferred sources of psychological support.

Astrid's initial tendency to use avoidant coping strategies enhanced her likelihood to develop psychiatric sequelae following trauma. Along with these maladaptive strategies, Astrid's *cognitive* distortions were recognized during the clinical interview previously discussed. Within the context of individual psychotherapy, data supports that these cognitive distortions could be addressed using cognitive and behavioral therapy or trauma-focused cognitive behavioral therapy.

In reviewing the *emotional and cultural* pathways of Astrid's case, her diagnoses consisted of acute stress reaction with the potential for posttraumatic stress disorder and possibly the culture-bound syndrome of falling out. During the initial aftermath of traumatic events after the disaster, emotional first aid strategies and their benefits toward fostering social support and emotional regulation following traumatic events have been well delineated in the literature.[1] A myriad of psychotherapy and pharmacotherapy options could be used in treatment of her symptoms of acute stress. Along with cognitive behavioral therapy modalities, additional recommendations for evidence-based psychotherapy include the use of brief psychoanalytic psychotherapy to explore the traumatic events. This practice has been shown to assist the childhood survivor with anxiety reduction, prevent progression of depression, and process grief.[1]

For refugee children traumatized by war-related violence, narrative exposure therapy (KidNet) demonstrated reduction in PTSD symptoms in this patient population, which was sustained for up to 1 year.[51] This treatment option may have a role in all forms of trauma to assist with the habituation of the trauma response while constructing a narrative of the youth's life events, including past traumas. For Astrid's younger 5-year-old sibling, play therapy and parent-child psychotherapy would be appropriate interventions given her developmental level and cognitive abilities.

Astrid's psychiatric symptoms (anxiety, mood, somatic, and sleep) have improved with mental health services and community support. Therefore, a pharmacologic intervention was not indicated at this point. The role of pharmacotherapy in the context of treating traumatized youth has limited evidence; however, use of psychotropic agents to treat comorbid psychosis, agitation, mood dysregulation, anxiety, and impaired sleep has been recommended clinically. In 2010, Harris and Sargent outlined the current recommendations for adult and pediatric populations, which include (1) antidepressants (selective serotonin reuptake inhibitors, selective serotonin-norepinephrine reuptake inhibitors), (2) adrenergic agents (clonidine, prazosin), (3) atypical antipsychotics, (4) anticonvulsants, and (5) benzodiazepines.[52]

When prescribing for diverse patient populations, observation for the potential impact of cultural and ethnic differences on medication response and or adverse effects is warranted. For more than 30 years, varying responses to psychotropic medications have been described in the literature.[53] In addition to ethnic specific mutations that can impact the metabolism of drugs, there are nonbiologic factors, including diet (herbs, caffeine, and so forth), smoking, gender, and age, that justify consideration.[54] For a more comprehensive discussion of specific ethnic differences in metabolism of psychotropic agents, please refer to Ruiz and colleagues (2000),[55] Ng and colleagues (2008),[56] and article by Lawson and colleagues elsewhere in this issue.

FUTURE DIRECTIONS/SUMMARY

Although some responses to trauma are universal, culture counts in the impact of trauma in children and youth from ethnically and racially diverse groups. Risk and incidence of trauma, manifestations of idioms of distress, psychopathology, and maladaptive responses to traumatic experiences are all culturally modified. Culture plays an important role in what, if any, help is sought for posttraumatic mental health need, whether it be from a mental health professional or someone in the sociocultural realm of the child. This help may be from a family member, a religious leader, or a traditional healer. Culture is an important factor in determining resilience. Both perceived social support and strong ethnic identity have been found to foster resilience in children and youth from US ethnic and racial minority groups.

The statement that risk factors are not predictive factors because of protective factors is highly applicable to diverse children and youth exposed to trauma. Given the high exposure of minority youth to negative social determinants of health, such as poverty and adverse living environments, it is imperative that we invest in preventive approaches and as much as possible shore up protective factors to buffer against inevitable stress and trauma in distressed, diverse communities. We must also anticipate posttraumatic mental health needs by providing early intervention to eliminate, or at least mitigate, the impact on development and adult outcomes. Future research should explore culturally tailored approaches to intervention and determine promising practices to maximize posttrauma resilience.

Psychiatrists and other mental health professionals must develop relationships across systems and sectors. These outreach efforts include establishing liaison relationships with educational systems, pediatric and adolescent medicine, and faith-based groups to reduce the stigma of mental health help seeking, provide psychological education about the impact of trauma and useful models of treatment (ie, emotional first aid), and maximize our reach for case finding as early as possible so that we may address, in a timely fashion, posttraumatic mental health needs in children and youth to achieve optimal outcomes.

ACKNOWLEDGMENTS

The authors wish to express their sincere gratitude to Thomas Kimpel, MD, Jean Raphael, MD, MPH, Carl C. Bell, MD, and the All Healers Mental Health Alliance for their assistance with this manuscript.

REFERENCES

1. Kar N. Psychological impact of disasters on children: review of assessment and interventions. World J Pediatr 2009;5(1):5–11.
2. Cohen JA, Kelleher KJ, Mannarino AP. Identifying, treating and referring traumatized children: the role of pediatric providers. Arch Pediatr Adolesc Med 2008; 162:447–52.
3. Courtois CA, Ford JD. Treating complex traumatic stress disorders: an evidence-based guide. New York: The Guilford Press; 2009. p. 16–18, 23.
4. Terr L. Childhood traumas. Am J Psychiatry 1991;148:10–20.
5. Kercher GA, McShane M. The prevalence of child sexual abuse victimization in an adult sample of Texas residents. Child Abuse Negl 1984;8(4):495–501.
6. Lindholm K, Wiley R. Ethnic differences in child abuse and neglect. J Hispanic Behav Sci 1986;8:111–25.
7. Urquiza AJ, Goodin-Jones BL. Child sexual abuse and adult revictimization with women of color. Violence Vict 1994;9:223–32.
8. Zhai F, Gao Q. Child maltreatment among Asian Americans: characteristics and explanatory framework. Child Maltreat 2008;20:1–17.
9. Freisthler B, Bruce E, Needell B. Understanding the geospatial relationship of neighborhood characteristics and rates of maltreatment for black, Hispanic and white children. Soc Work 2007;52(1):7–16.
10. Roberts AL, Gilman SE, Breslau J, et al. Race/ethnic differences in exposure to traumatic events, development of post-traumatic stress disorder, and treatment-seeking for post-traumatic stress disorder in the United States. Psychol Med 2010;29:1–13.
11. Lansford JE, Miller-Johnson S, Berlin LJ, et al. Early physical abuse and later violent delinquency: a prospective longitudinal study. Child Maltreat 2007;12:233–45.
12. Kendall-Tackett K. The health effects of childhood abuse: four pathways by which abuse can influence health. Child Abuse Negl 2002;26:715–29.

13. Zanarini MC, Frankenburg FR, Bradford R, et al. Violence in the lives of adult borderline patients. J Nerv Ment Dis 1999;187:65–71.
14. Bolea PS, Grant G, Burgess M, et al. Trauma of the Sudan: a constructivist exploration. Child Welfare 2003;82(2):219–33.
15. Fantino AM, Colak A. Refugee children in Canada: searching for identity. Child Welfare 2001;80(5):587–96.
16. Brymer MJ, Steinberg AM, Sornborger J, et al. Acute interventions for refugee children and families. Child Adolesc Psychiatr Clin N Am 2008;17:625–40.
17. Ngo HM, Le TN. Stressful life events, culture and violence. J Immigr Minor Health 2007;9(2):75–84.
18. Thienkura W, Cardozo BL, Chakkraband S, et al. Symptoms of posttraumatic stress disorder and depression among children in tsunami-affected areas in Tsunami-Affected Areas in Southern Thailand. JAMA 2006;296(5):537–48.
19. Catani C, Jacob N, Schauer E, et al. Family violence, war, and natural disasters: a study of the effect of extreme stress on children's mental health in Sri Lanka. BMC Psychiatry 2008;8:33.
20. Drury SS, Scheeringa MS, Zeanah CH. The traumatic impact of hurricane Katrina on children in New Orleans. Child Adolesc Psychiatr Clin N Am 2008;17:685–702.
21. Abramson D, Garfield R. The recovery divide: poverty and the widening gap among Mississippi children and families affected by hurricane Katrina. New York: Mississippi Child & Family Health Study, National Center for Disaster Preparedness, The Children's Health Fund; 2007.
22. Scheeringa M, Zeanah C. Reconsideration of harm's way: onsets and comorbidity patterns in preschool children and their caregivers following hurricane Katrina. J Clin Child Adolesc Psycholo 2008;37(3):508–18.
23. Peters RJ, Meshack A, Amos C, et al. The association of drug use and post-traumatic stress reactions due to hurricane Ike among fifth ward Houstonian youth. J Ethn Subst Abuse 2010;9(2):143–51.
24. Gillespie CF, Phifer J, Bradley B, et al. Risk and resilience: genetic and environmental influences on development of the stress response. Depress Anxiety 2009;26:984–92.
25. DuMont KA, Widom CS, Czaja SJ. Predictors of resilience in abused and neglected children grown-up: the role of individual and neighborhood characteristics. Child Abuse Negl 2007;31:255–74.
26. Bruce E, Waelde LC. Relationships of ethnicity, ethnic identity and trauma symptoms to delinquency. J Loss Trauma 2008;13:395–405.
27. Singh AA, Hays DG, Chung Y, et al. South Asian immigrant women who have survived child sexual abuse: resilience and healing. Violence Against Women 2010;16(4):444–58. Available at: http://www.library.nhs.uk/booksandjournals/details.aspx?t=Healing&stfo=True&sc=bnj.ovi.amed,bnj.ovi.bnia,bnj.ebs.cinahl,bnj.ovi.emez,bnj.ebs.heh,bnj.ovi.hmic,bnj.pub.MED,bnj.ovi.psyh&p=11&sf=srt.publicationdate&sfld=fld.title&sr=bnj.ebs&did=2010612464&pc=3273&id=188. Accessed July 26, 2010.
28. Castro FG, Garfinkle J, Naranjo D, et al. Cultural traditions as "Protective Factors" among Latino children of illicit drug users. Subst Use Misuse 2007;42(4):621–42.
29. Austin AA. Alcohol, tobacco, other drug use, and violent behavior among native Hawaiians: ethnic pride and resilience. Subst Use Misuse 2004;39(5):721–46.
30. Siqueira LM, Crandall LA. Risk and protective factors for binge drinking among Hispanic subgroups in Florida. J Ethn Subst Abuse 2008;7(1):81–92.

31. Moscardino U, Axia G, Scrimin S, et al. Narratives from caregivers of children surviving the terrorist attack in Beslan: issues of health, culture and resilience. Soc Sci Med 2007;64(8):1176–87.
32. Spilsbury J, Belliston L, Drotar D, et al. Clinically significant trauma symptoms and behavioral problems in a community-based sample of children exposed to domestic violence. J Fam Violence 2007;22(6):487–99.
33. Lalor K. Child sexual abuse in Tanzania and Kenya. Child Abuse Negl 2004;28(8):833–44.
34. Plummer CA, Njuguna W. Cultural protective and risk factors: professional perspectives about child sexual abuse in Kenya. Child Abuse Negl 2009;33(8):524–32.
35. Lim R. Clinical manual of cultural psychiatry. Arlington (VA): American Psychiatric Publishing, Inc; 2006.
36. Spates RC, Waller S, Samaraweera N, et al. Behavioral aspects of trauma in children and youth. Pediatr Clin North Am 2003;50:901–18.
37. Lemos-Miller A, Kearney CA. Depression and ethnicity as intermediary variables among dissociation, trauma-related cognitions, and PTSD. J Nerv Ment Dis 2006;194(8):584–90.
38. Hawkins SS, Radcliffe J. Current measures of PTSD for children and adolescents. J Pediatr Psychol 2006;31(4):420–30.
39. Becker-Lausen E, Mallon-Kraft S. Pandemic outcomes: the intimacy variable. In: Kantor GK, Jasinski JS, editors. Out of darkness: current perspectives on family violence. Newbury Park (CA): Sage; 1997. p. 49–57.
40. Ko S. Culture and trauma briefs: promoting culturally competent trauma informed practices. In: National Center for Child Traumatic Stress, Vol 1, No. 1, 2005. Available at: http://www.nctsnet.org/nctsn_assets/pdfs/culture_and_trauma_brief.pdf. Accessed May 15, 2010.
41. Mulvihill D. The health impact of childhood trauma: an interdisciplinary review, 1997–2003. Issues Compr Pediatr Nurs 2005;28:115–36.
42. Van der Kolk BA. Developmental trauma disorder. Psychiatr Ann 2005;35:401–8.
43. van der Kolk BA, Roth S, Pelcovitz D, et al. Disorders of extreme stress: the empirical foundation of a complex adaptation to trauma. J Trauma Stress 2005;18:389–99.
44. Ecklund K, Johnson WB. Toward cultural competence in child intake assessments. Professional psychology. Res Pract 2007;38(4):356–62.
45. Hays PA. Addressing cultural complexities in practice: a framework for clinicians and counselors. Washington, DC: American Psychological Association; 2001.
46. Brown LS. Cultural competence. In: Courtois CA, Ford JD, editors. Treating complex traumatic stress disorders: an evidence based guide. New York: The Guilford Press; 2009. p. 166–82.
47. American Psychiatric Association. Diagnostic and statistical manual of mental disorders. Text revision. 4th edition. Washington, DC: American Psychiatric Association; 2000. p. 897–903.
48. Gaw AC. Cross-cultural psychiatry. Washington, DC: American Psychiatric Publishing, Inc; 2001. p. 73–98.
49. Verdeli H, Clougherty K, Onyango G, et al. Group interpersonal psychotherapy for depressed youth in IDP Camps in Northern Uganda: adaptation and training. Child Adolesc Psychiatr Clin N Am 2008;17:605–24.
50. Rousseau C, Guzder J. School-based prevention programs for refugee children. Child Adolesc Psychiatr Clin N Am 2008;17:533–49.
51. Neuner F, Catani C, Ruf M, et al. Narrative exposure therapy for the treatment of traumatized children and adolescents (KidNET): from neurocognitive

theory to field intervention. Child Adolesc Psychiatr Clin N Am 2008;17: 641–64.

52. Harris T, Sargent J. Trauma and associated disorders. In: Cheng K, Myers KM, editors. Child and adolescent psychiatry, the essentials. 2nd edition. Philadelphia: Lippincott, Williams, and Wilkins; 2011. p. 122–39.

53. Kalow W, editor. Pharmacogenetics of drug metabolism. New York: Pergamon; 1992.

54. Smith MW. Ethnopsychopharmacology. In: Lim R, editor. Clinical manual of cultural psychiatry. Arlington (VA): American Psychiatric Publishing, Inc; 2006. p. 207–36.

55. Ruiz P, editor. Ethnicity and psychopharmacology [Review of Psychiatry Series, Vol. 19, No. 4, Oldham JO and Riba MB, series editors.]. Washington, DC: American Psychiatric Press; 2000. p. 1–130.

56. Ng CH, editor. Ethnopsychopharmacology advances in current practice. Cambridge (UK): Cambridge University Press; 2008. p. 1–176.

Index

Note: Page numbers of article titles are in **boldface** type.

Child Adolesc Psychiatric Clin N Am 19 (2010) 889–895
doi:10.1016/S1056-4993(10)00089-1
1056-4993/10/$ – see front matter © 2010 Elsevier Inc. All rights reserved.

childpsych.theclinics.com